KAISER PERMANENTE

HEALTHWISE®

H A N D B O O K

A Self-Care Guide For You And Your Family

- *Over 180 Health Care Problems*
- *Prevention*
- *Home Treatment*
- *When To Call Your Doctor*

DONALD W. KEMPER

THE HEALTHWISE STAFF

THE KAISER PERMANENTE PHYSICIANS
AND STAFF OF COLORADO

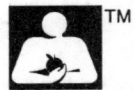

A Healthwise® Publication
Healthwise, Incorporated, Boise, Idaho
(A not-for-profit organization)

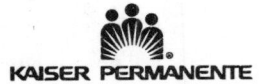

KAISER PERMANENTE®

First Edition, 1976
Second Edition, 1978
Third Edition, 1979
Fourth Edition, 1983
Fifth Edition, 1985
Sixth Edition, 1986
Seventh Edition, 1987
Eighth Edition, 1989
Ninth Edition, 1990
Tenth Edition, 1991
Eleventh Edition, 1994
Kaiser Permanente Colorado Edition (First Printing), 1997
K-col-1st-2-97

ISBN:1-877930-17-2

Library of Congress Catalog Card Number: 89-84789

Printed in the United States of America

Table of Contents

Part II. Health Problems

Part IV: Self-Care Resources

To Our Readers

No book can replace the need for doctors — and no doctor can replace the need for people to care for themselves. The purpose of this book is to help you and your doctors work together to manage your health problems.

The *Healthwise Handbook* includes basic guidelines on how to recognize and cope with over 180 of the most common health problems. These guidelines are based on sound medical information from leading medical and consumer publications, with review and input from doctors, nurses, pharmacists, physical therapists, and other health professionals. We have worked to present the information in a straightforward way that is free from medical jargon. We hope you find it easy to read and easy to use.

While this book does not eliminate the need for professional medical help, it does provide a better basis for you to work with your doctors to prevent and jointly care for health problems. Should you receive professional advice in conflict with this book, look first to your health professional. Because your doctor is able to take your specific history and needs into consideration, his or her recommendations may prove to be the best. Likewise, should any self-care recommendations fail to provide positive results within a reasonable period, you should consult a health professional.

This book is as good as we can make it, but we cannot guarantee that it will work for you in every case. Nor will the authors or publishers accept responsibility for any problems that may develop from following its guidelines. This book is only a guide; your common sense and good judgement are also needed.

We are continually adding to and improving this book. If you have a suggestion that will make this book better, please send it to Healthwise Handbook Suggestions, c/o Healthwise, P.O. Box 1989, Boise, ID 83701.

We wish you the best of health.

About Healthwise

Healthwise is a nonprofit organization working to help people do a better job of staying healthy and taking care of their health problems. Since its founding in 1975, Healthwise has won awards of excellence and recognition from the Centers for Disease Control, The U.S. Department of Health and Human Services, the American Society on Aging, and the World Health Organization.

Healthwise works with organizations wishing to enhance the individual's role in health care. Our clients range from volunteer organizations and church groups to Fortune 500 companies, major unions, state governments, hospitals, insurers, and health maintenance organizations.

Healthwise has published seven books, all with workshops and training to support them:

The *Healthwise Handbook* and the Healthwise Workshop.
The use of informed medical self-care to improve the quality of care given at home and to help reduce health care costs.

Healthwise for Life: Medical Self-Care for Healthy Aging and the Healthwise for Life video.
Medical self-care for people aged 50 and better, including fitness, nutrition, caregiving, and medication management.

Pathways: A Success Guide for a Healthy Life and the Pathways to Health Workshop.
A guilt-free approach to health changes in 10 areas, including stress, nutrition, fitness, smoking, alcohol and other drugs, and relationships. The book and workshops are designed to help people make the healthy changes they most want to make.

The Growing Younger Handbook and the Growing Younger Workshops.
Fitness, relaxation, nutrition, and self-care for adults aged 60 and better.

Growing Wiser: The Older Person's Guide to Mental Wellness and the Growing Wiser Workshops.
Memory improvement, mental vitality, coping with loss and life change, maintaining independence, and self-esteem for older adults.

It's About Time: Better Health Care in a Minute (or two).
A medical consumerism booklet, with quick, easy-to-use action steps that promote good doctor-patient relationships.

La salud en casa: Guía Práctica de Healthwise.
A Spanish translation of the Healthwise Handbook.

In addition to these books and workshops, Healthwise has produced videotapes and other instructional aids to support health promotion efforts. For more information, contact Healthwise at P.O. Box 1989, Boise, ID 83701, (208) 345-1161.

Acknowledgements

This 11th Edition of the *Healthwise Handbook* combines the best of old and new. The original 1976 1st Edition was written and edited with major contributions from Kathy McIntosh and Toni Roberts. Since then, scores of people have helped to improve and update the book. Their combined work resulted in the book's winning of the American Health Book Award.

Starting with the 10th Edition, we conducted exhaustive research on every topic, carefully reviewed and evaluated reader suggestions, and reorganized and updated it. Over 20 new topics have been added and many sections are completely rewritten. We hope you like it.

Special thanks go to Diana Stilwell, MPH, who coordinated the research and medical reviews, wrote many of the updates, and edited the entire book. Molly Mettler was also a major contributor to the writing and editing and shares with Diana responsibility for the quality of the book. The design, layout, and production work of Andrea Blum and Terrie Britton, and the layout work of Carrie Wiss and Sue Armstrong, as well as the editorial and proofreading assistance of Jean Miller and Jane Woychick, are greatly appreciated. Many thanks also go to Cindy Hovland, who provided invaluable assistance.

This book would not have been possible without the extensive help and guidance from health professionals. Steve Schneider, MD, was the principal medical reviewer for this edition. The following other health professionals were also particularly helpful.

Physicians

Janet Aguilar, MD	Edwin Matthes, DDS
Richard Aptaker, DO	James T. Pozniakas, MD
Bruce Davis, MD	Cajsa Schumacher, MD
Gail Eberharter, MD	Warren Scott, MD
Michael Felder, MD	Stanford Shoor, MD
Andrew Fox, MD	David Sobel, MD, MPH
Steven Freedman, MD	Gary Stein, MD
William Fuchs, MD	William Teubl, MD
Marty Gabica, MD	Marti W. Nelson, MD
Matthew Handley, MD	Michael Weiss, MD, MPH
Elisabeth Kelley, MD	

Nurses

	Sherri Rickman, RN
Marian Broida, RN	Margo Sturgis, RN, GNP
Gene Drabinski, RN	Susan Van Houten, RN, BSN
Judy Dundas, RN	Susie Whittinghill, RN
Jayne Hanich, RN	The staff of Employee Managed
Randi Holland, RN	Care Corporation

Physical Therapist
Lynn Johnson, PT, ATR

Health Educators
Bob Gorsky, PhD
Joan Greathouse, MED
Jim Giuffré, MPH

Nutritionist
Ruth Schneider, RD, MPH

We also wish to thank those health professionals and consumers whose review, suggestions, and input on previous editions were the foundation for the current book.

Most of all, we would like to thank the hundreds of thousands of medical consumers who use the *Healthwise Handbook*. It is your actions that reward us the most and inspire us to constantly look for ways to improve this handbook.

Funding for the original development of the *Healthwise Handbook* was provided by the W.K. Kellogg Foundation of Battle Creek, Michigan.

Donald W. Kemper
February, 1997

Kaiser Permanente Colorado Acknowledgements

We wish to thank and acknowledge Kaiser Permanente colleagues in Northern California who successfully piloted use of the *Healthwise Handbook* in 1993, providing the groundwork for many Kaiser Permanente divisions to implement self-care programs. We extend special thanks to Steven Freedman, MD, Pamela Larson, MPH and David Sobel, MD, MPH. This book has benefited from careful review by many people within Kaiser Permanente, both in California and Colorado. Within Colorado, we thank the Best Practices Team, Primary Care Redesign Team, Public Affairs, Health Plan Executive Team and the Department of Community Medicine for their time and energy devoted to this edition of the *Healthwise Handbook*. In particular, we appreciate the contributions of:

Michael Alexander
Sue Broadbooks, PA-C
Sally Butler, LCSW
Tim Clarkson, MD
Toby Cole, MD
Shelley Cooper
Sue Jane Fox, RN, MN
Eric France, MD
Steven Gardner, MD
Maureen Hanrahan
Cindy Henrickson, RN

Robert Lederer, MD
Marte Meyer
Cheryl Oliver, RN
Kate Paul
Connie Peterson, RN, CHES
Lynn Sauve
Emily Sharp, RN, MSN
Marti Sharp, RN, MSN
Linda Smith
Kristin Snyder
Marilyn Starrett

Ned Calonge, MD, MPH
Chief of Preventive Medicine

Tim McKay, PhD
Department of Community Medicine

Introduction

The *Healthwise Handbook* can help you improve your health and lower your health care costs. We hope it is a book you will turn to time and again as health problems arise.

The book is divided into four sections:

Self-Care Basics. What you need to know to be a wise medical consumer.

Health Problems. Prevention, treatment, and when to call a doctor for over 170 common illnesses and injuries.

Staying Healthy. Tips and techniques for dental health, fitness, stress management, nutrition, and mental wellness.

Self-Care Resources. How to manage medications and what you need to have on hand in your home to cope with health problems.

Most people will not read through the book from cover to cover in one sitting. It is more of a topic-by-topic book. Look up what you need when a problem or interest develops.

We do recommend that you read pages 1 and 2 and three special chapters right away:

Page 1, **The Healthwise Approach,** is a process to follow every time a health problem arises. Page 2, the **Ask-the-Doctor Checklist,** will help you get the most out of every doctor visit.

Chapter 2, **The Wise Medical Consumer,** offers important information you can use to improve the quality and lower the cost of the health care you need.

Chapter 3, **Prevention and Early Detection,** lists the immunizations and screening tests that are important to staying healthy and detecting health problems early.

Chapter 20, **Your Home Health Center,** lists medications, supplies, equipment, and resources you may wish to keep on hand.

The rest of the information in the book is there when you need it. We have enjoyed writing this book and keeping it up to date. We hope it will help you succeed in better managing your health problems.

The Healthwise Approach

Step 1. Observe the problem.
- When did it start? What are the symptoms? _____

  _____

  _____

  _____

  _____

- Where is the pain? Dull ache or stabbing pain? _____

  _____

  _____

- Measure your vital signs:

  Temperature:_____   Blood pressure:_____ / _____

  Pulse:_____ / minute   Breaths:_____ / minute

- Think back:

  Have you had this problem before?   Yes _____   No _____

  What did you do for it:? _____

  _____

  Any changes in your life (stress, medications, food, exercise, etc.)?

  _____

  _____

  Does anyone else at home or work have these symptoms?_____

Step 2. Learn more about it.
- *Healthwise Handbook* (note page number): _____
- Other books or articles: _____
- Advice from others (lay or professional): _____

Step 3. Make an action plan.
- Your "tentative" diagnosis: _____
- Home care plan: _____
- _____
- When to call your doctor: _____

Step 4. Evaluate your progress.
- Are your actions working? _____

Ask-the-Doctor Checklist

Before the visit:
- Complete the Healthwise Approach on page 1 and take it with you.
- Take a list of medications and record of last visit for similar problems.

During the visit:
- State your main problem first.
- Describe your symptoms (use page 1).
- Describe past experiences with the same problem.

Write down:
- Temperature: _____ Blood pressure: _____ / _____
- The diagnosis (what's wrong). _____
- The prognosis (what might happen next)._____
- Your self-care plan (what you can do at home). _____
  _____
  _____

For drugs, tests, and treatments, ask: (See pages 15 to 18.)
- What's its name?_____
- Why is it needed? _____
- What are the costs and risks? _____
- Are there alternatives? _____
- What if I do nothing? _____
- (For drugs) How do I take this? _____
- (For tests) How do I prepare? _____

At the end of the visit, ask:
- Am I to return for another visit?_____
- Am I to phone in for test results? _____
- What danger signs should I look for?_____
- When do I need to report back? _____
- What else do I need to know?_____
  _____
  _____
  _____

Good people, Good medicine.
Kaiser Permanente

Chapter 1

Using the Kaiser Permanente System

Getting the Care You Need

We are offering you the *Kaiser Permanente Healthwise Handbook* to assist you in becoming an active and informed partner in your health care, and to help you and your family stay healthy. When you or someone in your family has a medical problem, this Handbook is one source of information to help you determine what the cause of the problem might be, what you can do to treat it at home, and when to seek professional help. It also offers valuable information on preventive care, nutrition, stress reduction, and many other issues.

For those times when you or a family member need to seek professional care, we've included this chapter to help make it easier for you to understand how to obtain it.

Please note that Kaiser Permanente continues to grow and change in an effort to improve our services. As a result, some of the information in this chapter may change over time. To be sure you have the latest information on what services are available and how best to use them, please consult the most current **Member Handbook and Telephone Directory** and read **Planning for Health**, our quarterly magazine for members, both of which are mailed to you at home.

Your *Member Handbook* is an important resource to help you get care as a Kaiser Permanente member. It includes important Kaiser Permanente phone numbers, locations, and hours of operation. You will be mailed a copy of your *Member Handbook* as an insert in *Planning for Health* every spring. **We urge you to keep your Member Handbook with this book for easy reference.**

Getting Care - continued

If you don't have a copy of your *Member Handbook*, please call the Information Center at 338-3800 and we will send you one.

Questions? Problems? Suggestions? We're Here to Help

If at any time you have any questions, problems, or suggestions, please let us know. We will do everything we can to assist you.

If your question or problem is related to services you receive at our medical facilities, please talk to your personal provider, the department manager, the nursing supervisor, or the physician chief of the service in question. They are the people most able to provide you with advice and assistance.

If you're unable to resolve your problem with your provider or a manager at the facility, call the Information Center at 338-3800. Also call the Information Center if you need to report out-of-plan emergency services, change your address or telephone number, report loss of your identification card, or for answers to general questions about our services.

Our goal is to keep you both healthy and satisfied, so please let us know how we can help.

Your Personal Health Care Provider

Choosing Your Provider

When you become a Kaiser Permanente member, you can choose your personal care physician. You also may see a physician assistant or nurse practitioner as part of your physician's team at some of your appointments. Physician assistants and nurse practitioners are trained, licensed health care providers who can treat most routine medical problems.

Routine Care: Advice and Appointments

To receive medical advice or to schedule an appointment in Pediatrics, Internal Medicine, Family Practice, or OB/GYN, please call any of the telephone numbers for primary care listed in the inside front cover of this book. You can call for an appointment 24 hours a day, seven days a week; for quickest service, call between 6 a.m. and 8 p.m. For other departments, please check your *Member Handbook* for the appropriate phone number or call the Information Center for assistance.

If you would like an appointment, we will schedule one at a time convenient for you. Many times you will choose to speak with an advice nurse before scheduling an appointment. Our advice nurses are specially trained to help you with your health care needs by phone. They work closely with our medical providers, and either can give you the assistance you need over the phone or can schedule an appointment for you when you need more care.

To make your visit go more smoothly:

• Please plan to arrive at your medical facility at least 15 minutes before your appointment, so you'll have time to park and register.

- Let the receptionist know if this is your first visit or a visit for a new work-related injury. If it is, please allow a little extra time for registration.

- Please present your Kaiser Permanente identification card when registering for your appointment. Having your card with you will save you time during your visit. If you happen to forget your card, you can still be seen for your appointment, but when registering you will be asked for your name, address, and other personal information.

If you wish to reschedule or cancel an appointment, please call the same number you used to schedule your original appointment.

What to Do in an Emergency

An emergency is any sudden, serious problem requiring medical attention within minutes to several hours.

- Some problems are emergencies because they're potentially life-threatening, such as poisonings, gunshot wounds, or a sudden inability to breathe.

- Other problems are emergencies because, if not treated promptly, they may become more serious. Examples are deep cuts and broken bones.

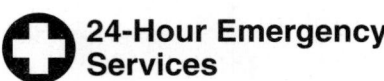 **24-Hour Emergency Services**

Emergency care is available 24 hours a day, 365 days a year at the Emergency Department at Saint Joseph Hospital in Denver, and for Boulder-area members at Boulder Community Hospital. Medical offices do not offer emergency services.

- Patients with the most urgent medical problems are treated first.

- Medical need, rather than the time of arrival, dictates the order in which patients are seen.

- An experienced emergency nurse screens patients and may direct those with less serious problems to another department.

If you have a medical problem that's not an emergency, we encourage you to call for an appointment. If you're unsure whether your problem is an emergency, you can call for advice or review the information in Chapter 15 of this Handbook, "First Aid and Emergencies," beginning on page 205, to help you decide.

Ambulance Services

If you have a life-threatening condition or other problem that requires an ambulance, call 861-3434 or 911. If you aren't sure how serious your problem is, or whether you need an ambulance, call the advice nurse for assessment.

Kaiser Permanente covers the cost of an ambulance only when:

- The transportation is medically necessary.

- A Kaiser Permanente physician or other authorized staff member orders an ambulance.

Emergency – continued

If you order an ambulance without authorization from Kaiser Permanente, and it's later determined that it was not reasonable to believe that an ambulance was medically necessary under the circumstances at the time of the call, you'll be billed for this service. For example, if you have severe chest pain and fear you may be having a heart attack, it's appropriate to call **911** for an ambulance. Kaiser Permanente would cover the cost of the ambulance service—even if it was found later that you did not suffer a heart attack—because it was reasonable to request an ambulance under the circumstances.

Health Education

As part of our commitment to helping you stay healthy, Kaiser Permanente offers a wide range of health education services. Health education specialists and registered dietitians are available in our larger facilities to provide you with support, information, and skills to help you become an active, confident partner in your health care. Individual and small group appointments are available upon request.

We urge you to take advantage of the many **Health Education programs and classes** available throughout the year. You can learn more about specific health-related topics, such as smoking cessation, diabetes, pregnancy and childbirth, heart disease, respiratory disease, staying healthy, and many more. Current classes are listed in *Planning for Health,* our quarterly magazine for members.

We are also pleased to offer you help when there are difficult medical decisions to be made. The Shared Decision Making Center, located at the 20th Avenue Medical Center, has interactive programs on topics such as breast cancer, hypertension, benign prostatic hypertrophy and screening for prostate cancer for men, hormone replacement therapy for women, and advanced directives. Call 861-3310 for more information.

To learn more about our Health Education services, call your local Health Education Department listed in your *Member Handbook* or ask your provider for information.

R_x Pharmacy Services

Your local Kaiser Permanente pharmacy provides a variety of services, including:

- Filling new prescriptions
- Transferring prescriptions from another pharmacy
- Providing refills
- Consulting about your new medications

For your convenience, our pharmacies also carry some common non-prescription medications and medical supplies. Pharmacies are located in all medical offices and are open the same hours as the medical offices.

Prescription Refills

If you need to order a refill of your prescription, the most convenient way to do it is to call the **24-Hour Refill Recorder** at the medical facility where you'd like to pick up your prescription. The number is listed in your *Member Handbook*. Be sure to leave your name, medical record number, daytime phone number, and prescription number on the recorder.

To help us help you more efficiently, please:

- Try to make your refill requests at least 24 hours before you plan to pick up your medication.

- Bring your prescription container with you when you pick up your refill.

Your Kaiser Permanente Identification Card

When you become a Kaiser Permanente member, we'll send you and each of your enrolled family members a personal ID card. This card is your "passport" to the health care benefits and services covered by your Health Plan.

Your Kaiser Permanente ID card contains important information that helps us serve you more efficiently. Please have your card handy when:

- Calling for an appointment or medical advice.

- Visiting one of our medical offices for an appointment.

- Being admitted to a Kaiser Permanente contract hospital.

- Obtaining services from laboratory, radiology, EKG, pharmacy, or other departments.

- Talking with a customer service representative

- Traveling, in case you need medical care at any of our 11 other regions in the United States.

- Hospitalized in a non-Kaiser Permanente hospital. Your ID card has the information you'll need when you notify Kaiser Permanente of your hospitalization.

Once your coverage becomes effective, you're eligible to obtain services at any of our medical facilities—even if you haven't yet received your card. If you lose your card, call the Information Center at 338-3800 and we will be happy to order a replacement card for you.

Advance Directives

Federal legislation called the Patient Self-Determination Act became effective in December 1991 and requires hospitals, health maintenance organizations, and other health agencies to inform patients about documents known as "advance directives." These include the *Durable Power of Attorney for Health Care, Living Wills,* and the *CPR Directive.* These documents permit patients to state in writing their wishes about medical care, or to designate someone to make those decisions in the event the patient is unable to do so. For more information about advance directives or how to complete them, please call the Information Center.

Receiving Care Outside the Kaiser Permanente System

You are expected to use Kaiser Permanente for all your medical care

Care Outside Kaiser – cont.

unless you are part of one of our special programs **which contain certain exceptions.** Non-emergency medical care obtained outside our Kaiser Permanente medical facilities will be covered only if it was obtained under the direction of your personal physician and after a written and approved authorization for outside medical care is issued.

If You Are Admitted to a Non-Kaiser Permanente Hospital

If you or a member of your family is admitted to a non-Kaiser Permanente hospital for emergency medical treatment, call (303) 831-6740 to notify us, so we may help coordinate your care. You may call 24 hours a day.

If you are billed for any services received from non-Kaiser Permanente providers, including 911, please call claims at 338-3600.

Health Plan Benefits Away From Home

If you are planning a trip, call the Information Center and ask us to send you a *Just in Case* packet, which includes a claim form and useful telephone numbers if you need medical care while traveling. If you become ill or injured while outside the service area, please call (303) 831-6740, as we may be able to help coordinate your care. Kaiser Permanente will pay reasonable charges you may incur for emergency and urgent care outside the service area. You pay copayments that would have been charged if the care had been received from Kaiser Permanente. For information regarding claims, call 338-3600.

Notes

Notes

You, the individual, can do more for your health and well-being than any doctor, any hospital, any drug, and any exotic medical device.
Joseph Califano

Chapter 2

The Wise Medical Consumer

The quality and the cost of medical care depend more on you than on your doctor.

To become a wise medical consumer, start with three basic principles:

- Work in partnership with your doctor.

- Take part in every medical decision.

- Become skilled at obtaining medical care.

By following these three principles, you will gain more control over the quality and cost of your health care than you have ever had before.

Work in Partnership With Your Doctor

Good partnerships are based on **a common goal, shared effort, and good communication.** If you and your doctor can make these things

happen, you will both gain from the partnership. You will get better care and your doctor will practice good medicine.

Five Ways to Be a Good Partner

1. Take good care of yourself. Both you and your doctor would prefer that you don't get sick in the first place. And if problems arise, you both want a return to good health as soon as possible.

2. At the first sign of a health problem, observe and record your symptoms. Your record of symptoms will help both you and your doctor make an accurate diagnosis. And, the better job you do recording early symptoms, the better you and your doctor can later manage the problem.

Partnership – continued

- Keep written notes on the symptoms. Record when, how long, how painful, etc., for each symptom.

- Note anything unusual that might be related to the problem.

- Measure and record vital signs. See page 32.

- Add regular updates and watch your progress. Are your symptoms getting better or worse?

3. Practice medical self-care at home. As the front-line partner, you can manage a lot of minor health problems on your own. Use this book, your own experience, and help from others to create a self-care plan.

- Learn what you can about the problem.

- Keep notes on your self-care plan and what you do.

- Note whether home treatment seems to help.

- Set a time to call a health professional if the problem continues. See page 13 for more on calling your doctor or advice nurse.

4. Prepare for office visits. Medical appointments are often scheduled for only 15 minutes per visit. The better organized you are, the more value you can get from the visit.

- Prepare an Ask-the-Doctor Checklist like the one on page 2.

- Update and bring your list of symptoms and your self-care plan.

- Write down your main concern (chief complaint) and practice describing it. Your doctor will want to hear that first.

- Write down your hunches or fears about what is wrong. These are often helpful to your doctor.

- Write down the three questions you want answered the most. (There may not be time to ask a long list of questions, so additional visits may be required.)

- Bring along a list of the medications you are taking.

5. Play an active role in the medical visit.

- State your main concern, describe your symptoms, and share your hunches and fears.

- Be honest and straightforward. Don't hold anything back because of embarrassment. If you don't intend to fill a prescription, say so. If you are getting alternative treatment such as acupuncture or chiropractic treatments, let your doctor know. To be a good partner, your doctor has to know what is going on.

- If your doctor prescribes a drug, test, or treatment, get more information. See page 14.

- Take notes. Write down the diagnosis, the treatment and follow-up plan, and what you can do at home. Then read it back to the doctor to be sure you have it right.

Calling for Advice

Is it okay to call for medical advice? Of course it is. Often a phone call to the advice nurse is all you need to manage the problem at home or determine if a visit is needed. Here's how to get the most from every call:

Prepare for your call.

• Write down a one-sentence description of your problem and why you are calling.

• Have your symptom list handy.

• Have your calendar handy in case you need to schedule an appointment.

• Be prepared to let us know times it would be best to reach you, and at which phone numbers, in case a call back is needed.

Finding the Right Doctor

If you don't have a family doctor (primary care physician), now is the time to get one. Everyone needs a regular doctor. A host of specialists working on separate health problems may not see the whole picture. In choosing a doctor there are lots of questions to ask, but these two matter the most:

• Is this doctor well-trained and experienced?

• Will this doctor work in partnership with me?

Training and Experience

For most people, a good choice for a family doctor is a board-certified family practice doctor or internist. These doctors have broad knowledge about medical problems. See page 20 for a brief description of medical specialists.

Partner Potential

During your first visit, tell your doctor that you would like to share in making treatment decisions.

Pay attention to how you feel during the visit.

• Does the doctor listen well?

• Do you think you could build a good working partnership with this doctor?

If the answers are "no," consider looking for another doctor.

The Right Doctor – continued

But I Want a Take-Charge Doctor

Not everyone wants to be a partner with their doctor. Perhaps you don't like to ask your doctor questions. Perhaps you don't want to share in any decisions. Perhaps you would rather just let your doctor tell you what is best for you. If that's what you prefer, tell your doctor. Most doctors have a lot of patients who don't want to be a partner. The doctor just needs to know what you expect.

The Advice Nurse

Advice Nurses are registered nurses who have special training to help you manage short-term illnesses, help you decide an appropriate response to symptoms, and to answer questions about your problem or concern. The Advice Nurses are easily reached by calling one of the phone numbers listed in the inside front cover of this book.

In many cases, a call to the Advice Nurse may save you the inconvenience of a trip to the clinic. In addition to being a resource for health information, the Advice Nurse works with your health care provider to monitor, support, and adjust treatment for illnesses you manage at home.

The Telephone Advice Nurse Service, pioneered by Kaiser Permanente, is available in the Departments of Medicine and Family Practice, Pediatrics, Obstetrics/Gynecology, and in many specialty areas.

Is It Time for a Change?

If you are unhappy with how your doctor treats you, it may be time for a change. Before you start looking for a new doctor, tell your current doctor how you would like to be treated. Your doctor would probably be pleased to work with you as a partner—if only you would tell him that's what you want. Otherwise, your doctor may think that you, like many patients, want the doctor to do all the work.

Take Part in Every Medical Decision

Except in an emergency, you cannot be given a treatment or test without your "informed consent." You must be informed of the risks and agree to the treatment. In a partnership, however, informed consent may not be enough. The real goal is shared decision making, where you actively participate in every medical decision.

Why should you help make decisions with your doctor? Aren't you paying him to know what to do? Well, the choices aren't always black and white. With many health problems, there is more than one option. Consider these examples:

You have moderately high blood pressure (160/95). Your doctor says that although exercise and diet might bring it down, most people don't succeed that way. Your doctor recommends that you start on medication to control it. You would rather try exercise and lose weight than take pills for the rest of your life. The best decision depends on your values.

Your three-year-old has a headache and a fever. The doctor says it's probably nothing to worry about. Then you tell the doctor your hunch that it might be meningitis. Some testing may be appropriate.

You have been suffering from carpal tunnel syndrome for several months. Your doctor is now recommending a wrist splint and a steroid injection. You would prefer trying just the splint with aspirin first. If that doesn't work, you will consider other medications. Your doctor agrees that is a good plan.

In each case, the treatment you choose will have an effect on your life. Therefore, the best medicine for you combines your doctor's medical expertise with your personal values.

Eight Ways to Share in Medical Decisions

1. Let your doctor know what you want. Tell your doctor that you want to help make decisions about what to do for your health problems.

2. Do your own research. Sometimes you need to learn things on your own before you can fully understand what your doctor is saying. Call or visit your Kaiser Permanente facility's Health Education Department for help in getting the information you need. See "Health Education Resources" on page 23.

3. Ask "why?" Always ask "why?" before agreeing to any medical test, medication, or treatment. By asking why, you will often discover another option that better meets your needs.

4. Ask about alternatives. Learn enough to understand the options your doctor thinks are feasible.

5. Consider watchful waiting. Ask your doctor if it would be risky or costly to wait a while (day, week, month) before treatment.

6. State your preferences. Tell your doctor if you prefer one option over another based on your personal desires and values.

7. Compare expectations. Tell your doctor what you are expecting from the treatment and ask if that is realistic. If appropriate, discuss side effects, pain, recovery time, long-term limitations, etc.

8. Accept responsibility. When you share decisions with your doctor, both of you must accept the responsibility for the outcomes.

Shared Decisions About Medical Tests

Medical tests are important tools, but they have limits. Some people think that the more tests they have, the better off they'll be. Wise consumers know medical tests have costs and risks as well as benefits. To help your doctor make good choices about tests for you, *you* need to:

Learn the basics.

- What is the name of the test and why do I need it?

- If the test is positive, what will the doctor do differently?

- What could happen if I don't have the test?

Take Part in Decisions – cont.
Consider the risks and benefits.

- How accurate is the test? How often does it indicate a problem exists when there is none (false positive)? How often does it say there is no problem when there is one (false negative)?

- Is the test painful? What can go wrong?

- How will I feel afterward?

- Are there less risky alternatives?

Medical Ping-Pong

Shared decision making requires two-way communication, like playing a game of ping-pong.

Ping: You describe your symptoms, main concern, and hunches.

Pong: Your doctor makes a diagnosis and describes treatment options.

Ping: You tell your doctor your personal preferences or ask about other options.

Pong: Your doctor restates the options and how they relate to your preferences.

Ping: You accept one of the recommended options or learn more about what you should do.

With good two-way discussion, the chances are better that you will end up with the treatment plan that is best for you.

Ask about costs.

- How much does the test cost?

- Is there a less expensive test that might give the same information?

Let your doctor know:

- Your concerns about the test.

- What you expect the test will do for you. Ask if that is realistic.

- Any medications you are taking.

- Whether you are pregnant or have other medical conditions.

- Your decision to accept the test.

If a test seems costly, risky, and not likely to change the recommended treatment, ask your doctor if you can avoid it. Try to agree on the best approach. **No test can be done without your permission.**

Once you agree to a test, ask what you can do to reduce the chance of errors. Ask about food, exercise, alcohol, or medications to avoid before the test. After the test, ask to review the results. Take notes for your home records. If the results are unexpected and the error rate of the test is high, consider redoing the test before basing further treatment on the results.

Shared Decisions About Medications

The first rule of medications is to know why you need each drug *before* you put it in your mouth, rub it on your skin, or whatever. The same as with medical tests, there are a few things you always need to know about medications.

Learn the basics.

- What is the name of the drug and why do I need it?
- How long does it take to work?
- How long will I need to take it?
- How do I take it (with food, etc.)?
- Are there non-drug alternatives?

Consider the risks and benefits.

- How much will this drug help?
- Are there side effects or other risks?
- Could this drug react with other drugs that I am currently taking?

Ask about costs.

- How much does it cost?
- Is a generic drug available (same formula but at a lower cost)?
- Is there a similar drug that will work almost as well and be less expensive?
- Can I start with a prescription for a few days to make sure this medication agrees with me?

Let your doctor know:

- Your concerns about the drug.
- What you expect it will do.
- All other medications (including over-the-counter drugs) you are taking.
- Whether or not you plan to fill the prescription and take the drug.

Shared Decisions About Surgery

Every surgery has risks. Only you can decide if the benefits are worth the risks. Are you willing to live with your problem or do you want to have the operation? The choice is yours.

Learn the basics.

- What is the name of the surgery?
- Get a description of the surgery.
- Why does my doctor think I need it?
- Is this surgery the common treatment for this problem? What are my other options?
- Are there alternative surgical approaches (such as using a laparoscope for some abdominal surgeries)?

Consider the risks and benefits.

- How many similar surgeries has this doctor performed?
- What is the success rate? What does success mean?
- What can go wrong? How often does this happen?
- How will I feel afterward? How long will it be until I'm fully recovered?
- How can I best prepare for the surgery and the recovery period?
- Can I avoid a general anesthetic?

Ask about costs.

- If you are considering surgery as well as other options, ask about the relative cost of surgery compared to those options.
- Can it be done on an outpatient basis, and is that less expensive?

Let your doctor know:

- How much the problem really bothers you. Are you willing to put up with the symptoms to avoid surgery?
- Your concerns about the surgery.
- If you do not want to do the surgery at this time.

Take Part in Decisions – cont.

• If you want a second opinion. Second opinions are helpful if you have any doubt that the proposed surgery is the best option for your problem. If you want a second opinion, ask your primary doctor or your surgeon to recommend another specialist. Consider getting an opinion from a different type of doctor who treats similar problems.

Once you understand the costs, risks, and benefits of surgery, the decision is yours.

Become Skilled at Obtaining Health Care

If you have ever thought that the cost of your medical care doesn't matter because your company or health plan pays the bills, think again. You do pay. Most people have to pay co-payments and deductibles. Employers pay for health care coverage by restricting wage increases. Governments pay for health care by increasing taxes or reducing other benefits.

As medical costs go up, there is less money available for housing, education, wage increases, etc. These costs do affect you. If you can help reduce health care costs, you help yourself—and everyone else.

Once you become a partner with your doctor, you can do a lot to reduce your health care costs. The goal is to get just the care you need, nothing more, and certainly, nothing less.

Nine Ways to Cut Costs (but not quality)

1. Stay healthy. Healthy lifestyles and regular preventive services are the best ways to keep costs down. See Chapter 3. Also see Chapters 17, 18, and 19 of this book for ideas on how to stay healthy your whole life long.

2. Use self-care when you can. Every time you successfully manage a health problem at home, you reduce the cost of health care for you and for others.

3. Get your professional care from a primary care provider. Family physicians, internists, pediatricians, nurse practitioners, physician assistants, and other primary care providers are the best place to start for most health problems. See page 13 for more information.

4. Reduce your medical test costs. Don't agree to expensive medical tests until you understand how they will help you. Unneeded tests are often done because "it is standard practice" or to protect doctors from possible malpractice suits. The only good reason to do a test is because the benefits to you outweigh the risks and the costs. No test can be done without your consent. See page 15 for more information.

5. Reduce your drug costs. Ask your doctor about every prescribed medication. Ask what would happen if you chose not to take a medication. Don't expect to get a prescription for every illness; sometimes self-care or non-drug remedies are all you need. See page 16 for more information.

6. Use specialists for special problems. Specialists are doctors with in-depth training and experience in a particular area of medicine. For example, a cardiologist has years of special training to deal with heart problems. Specialists generally charge more for visits than primary care doctors, and they routinely prescribe more expensive tests and treatments. Of course, they often provide the information you need to decide what to do about a major health problem.

When your primary doctor refers you to a specialist, a little preparation and good communication can help you get your money's worth. Before you go see a specialist:

- Know the diagnosis or suspected diagnosis.

- Learn about your basic treatment options.

- Know what your family doctor would like the specialist to do (take over the case, confirm the diagnosis, conduct tests, etc.).

- Make sure that any test results or records on your case have been sent to the specialist.

- Ask your regular doctor to remain involved in your case. Ask the specialist to send new test results or recommendations to both you and your regular doctor.

7. Use emergency services wisely. In life-threatening situations, modern emergency services are worth their weight in gold. However, they often cost far more for routine services. Routine services cost two to three times more in an emergency room than in a doctor's office. Also, your records are not available, so emergency room doctors have no information on your medical history.

Hospital emergency rooms are set up to handle trauma and life-threatening cases. They are not set up to care for routine illnesses, and they do not work on a first-come, first-served basis. During busy times, people with minor illnesses may wait for hours.

Use good judgment in deciding when to use emergency medical services. If you feel you can safely wait to see your regular doctor, do so. Apply home treatment in the meantime. However, if you feel that it is an emergency situation, by all means go to the emergency department.

Prepare for the emergency room:

- Call ahead, if possible, to let them know you are coming.

- If there is time, take this book and your medical records with you:

  ° Use page 1, the **Healthwise Approach,** to help you think through the problem and report symptoms to the doctor.

  ° Use page 2, the **Ask-the-Doctor Checklist,** to organize questions for the doctor.

  ° See page 15 to review the medical test checklist.

  ° Use your home medical records to discuss your medications, past test results, or treatments. Information about your allergies, medications, and conditions may be critical.

- As soon as you arrive, tell the emergency room staff why you think it is an emergency.

Who Works on What?

Cardiologist (MD): heart

Dermatologist (MD): skin

Endocrinologist (MD): diabetes and hormonal problems

Family Practitioner (MD): primary care

Gastroenterologist (MD): digestive system

Geriatrician (MD): older adults

Head and Neck Surgeon (MD): ears, nose, and throat

Internist (MD): primary care for adults

Neurologist (MD): brain and nervous system disorders

Obstetrician/Gynecologist (MD): female reproductive system and pregnancy

Oncologist (MD): cancer

Ophthalmologist (MD): eyes

Optometrist (OD): eyes when disease is not involved

Orthopedist (MD): surgery on bones, joints, muscles

Pediatrician (MD): primary care for children and teens

Podiatrist (DPM): foot care

Psychiatrist (MD): mental and emotional problems

Psychologist (PhD/PsyD): mental and emotional problems

Pulmonologist (MD): lungs

Rheumatologist (MD): arthritis and rheumatism

Urologist (MD): urinary and male reproductive systems

Obtaining Care – continued

8. Save hospitals for when you need them most. Over half of all health care costs are for hospitalizations. A stay in a modern hospital costs far more than a vacation at most luxury resorts. (And hospitals are a lot less fun.)

If you do need in-patient care, get in and out of the hospital as quickly as possible. This will reduce costs and your risk of hospital-induced infections.

Don't check in just for tests. Hospitalization is no longer needed for most medical tests. Ask if the tests can be done on an out-patient basis. If you agree to control your diet and activities, the doctor will usually support your request.

Additional days in the hospital can sometimes be avoided by bringing in extra help at home. With help available, many patients can shorten a hospital stay.

Hospitals are not the only choice for people with a terminal illness. Many people choose to spend their remaining time at home with people they know and love. Special arrangements for the needed care can be made through Kaiser Permanente's hospice care programs. Ask your doctor for a referral.

Hospital Consumer Skills

When you need to be in the hospital, good consumer skills can help improve the quality of care you receive. However, don't overdo consumerism. If you are very sick, ask your spouse or a friend to help watch out for your best interests.

• Ask "why?" Don't agree to anything unless you have a good reason. Agree only to those procedures that make sense for you.

• Provide an extra level of quality control. Check medications, tests, injections, and other treatments to see if they are correct. Your diligence can improve the quality of care that you receive.

• Kaiser Permanente patients generally do not receive itemized bills for hospital services. If you get care from providers whose services are not covered under your plan and you receive an itemized bill, check it, and ask about charges you don't understand.

• Get personal. Be friendly with the nurses and aides. Friendships increase the attention paid to your needs and speed your recovery.

• Know your rights. Most hospitals have accepted the "Patient's Bill of Rights" developed by the American Hospital Association. Ask your hospital for a copy.

9. Get smart about your medical needs. Learn as much as you can about your medical problem. Your research may turn up new options.

If you need help understanding a complicated problem, or want to learn more about your options:

Wise Use of Ambulance Services

Call 861-3434, 911, or your local emergency department of Kaiser Permanente to dispatch an ambulance if:

The person has symptoms of a heart attack: severe chest pain, sweating, shortness of breath. See page 216.

There is severe bleeding or blood loss. See page 219.

The person is unconscious or is having significant difficulty breathing.

The person is having a seizure lasting longer than seven minutes.

You suspect a spinal or neck injury.

Do not call an ambulance if:

The person is conscious, breathing without difficulty, and in stable condition.

It is not an emergency. Ambulance services are expensive and, if not needed, may not be covered by insurance.

Obtaining Care – continued

- Start by asking your doctor for any written information she might have to lend you.

- Visit your Kaiser Permanente facility's Health Education Department. See page 23.

- Review the resources on pages 307 to 311.

- If you find something interesting, make a copy for your doctor and discuss it at your next visit.

Avoid Health Fraud and Quackery

Millions of people are taken in each year by medical fraud and worthless health products.

Bogus "cures" are often advertised for chronic problems. These promotions target people with arthritis, cancer, baldness, impotence, or other problems who are ready to try anything. Unfortunately, these cures rarely help and often (one out of ten) cause harmful side effects.

Be suspicious of products that:

- Are advertised by testimonials.

- Claim to have a secret ingredient.

- Are not evaluated in prominent medical journals.

- Claim benefits that seem too good to be true.

- Are available only by mail.

Be suspicious of any doctor who:

- Prescribes medicines or gives injections at every visit.

- Promises a no-risk cure.

- Suggests something that seems unethical or illegal.

You Have the Right:

- To be spoken to in words that you understand.

- To be told what's wrong with you.

- To read your medical record.

- To know the benefits and risks of any treatment and its alternatives.

- To know what a treatment or test will cost you.

- To share in all treatment decisions.

- To refuse any medical procedure.

The best way to protect yourself is to ask questions and be observant. If you don't like what you see, find another doctor.

Trust Your Common Sense

Medicine is not as magical as we once thought. If someone takes the time to explain a problem or a treatment to us, we can usually make a pretty good decision about what is best for us.

Use your common sense to become a working partner with your doctors. The best medical tests, diagnosticians, and medical specialists are not enough. Good medical care also requires your own common sense. It will help you find the care that is right for you and avoid services (and costs) that you don't need.

If you trust your common sense, you are on your way to becoming a wise medical consumer.

Health Education Resources

You are always invited to call or stop by a Health Education Department to learn more about maintaining or improving your health, or about a medical condition or treatment. Health education specialists and registered dietitians are available in our larger medical offices. Please refer to your *Member Handbook and Telephone Directory*, or call the Information Center, to find the educator nearest you.

You may also receive counseling and educational materials from your doctor or other Kaiser Permanente health care provider as part of your office visits.

As a Kaiser Permanente member, you will also receive an award-winning quarterly magazine called *Planning for Health*. This magazine will keep you up to date on health issues, new health education programs, and changes that take place at the medical centers.

*If I'd known I was going to live this long, I'd have
taken better care of myself.*
Eubie Blake

Chapter 3

Prevention and Early Detection

Prevention works! You can save your-self and your family a lot of pain, worry, and money by avoiding health problems in the first place. If you can't prevent a problem altogether, the next best thing is to discover it early, when it is easy to treat. This chapter helps you do both.

Ten Ways to Stay Healthy

1. Immunize. Immunizations are the best bargain in health care. When you immunize, you prevent illness for your family and help prevent epidemics in your community. Immunization rec-ommendations are on page 26.

2. Seek preventive health care. See your health care provider periodically for the early detection tests and immu-nizations that are appropriate for your age and gender.

3. Keep moving. Any way you define it, fitness is essential to good health. Even moderate exercise makes a huge difference both in how you feel and what illnesses you get. For a three-part fitness plan, see page 245.

4. Eat right. Eating a well-balanced, low-fat diet of wholesome foods will keep you energetic and free of many illnesses. For more on nutrition, see Chapter 18. Consider breast-feeding your baby to help keep him or her in the best health. See page 152.

5. Control stress. Even with a hectic and hurried lifestyle, you can prevent stress from undermining your health. For a quick course on relaxation skills, see page 252.

6. Be smoke-free. Smokers who quit gain tremendous health benefits. So do people who avoid second-hand smoke. See "Quitting Smoking" on page 112.

Stay Healthy – continued

7. Avoid drugs and excess alcohol. When you say "no" to drugs and limit what you drink, you prevent accidents and illnesses and avoid a lot of problems for yourself and your family. For more on drug and alcohol problems, see page 275.

8. Put safety first. Safety at home, safety at work, safety at play, safe driving, firearm safety, and safe sex will all help keep you healthy.

9. Pursue healthy pleasures. Take naps, relax during meals, play with kids, care for a pet—they all can add to your health. See Resource 82 on page 311.

10. Avoid violence. Seek nonviolent ways of resolving conflicts at home, at school, at work, and in your community. See page 286.

Immunizations

Immunizations work by helping your immune system recognize and quickly attack diseases before they can cause problems. Some immunizations are given in a single shot while others require several shots over a period of time.

Childhood immunizations give important protection against pertussis (whooping cough), polio, measles, mumps, rubella, haemophilus influenza, and hepatitis B. Immunizations also protect against tetanus and diphtheria, although additional booster shots are needed to maintain lifelong protection.

A new vaccine can protect your children against chickenpox, although boosters may be needed and some parents may choose to let their children get the natural illness, which provides lifelong immunity.

If your children are immunized, these serious illnesses will not be a problem. Schedule your child's immunizations according to the chart on page 27. There is no need to delay childhood immunizations because of colds or other minor illnesses.

Be sure to keep good records. Children often need to show immunization records as they go through school.

Diphtheria, Pertussis, and Tetanus (DPT/DTaP)

Infectious diseases like diphtheria and pertussis were major killers before the DPT/DTaP vaccine was developed. This vaccine also protects against tetanus ("lockjaw"), a bacterial infection that can result when a wound is contaminated. The bacteria enter the body through cuts and thrive only in the absence of oxygen. So, the deeper and narrower the wound, the greater the possibility of tetanus. With proper immunization, these diseases are rare.

Childhood immunizations for these diseases are given together with a series of shots starting at age two months. Follow the DPT/DTaP guidelines on page 27.

Get a TD (tetanus and diphtheria) booster around age 15. Keeping up to date with TD boosters is important because tetanus can be fatal.

If it has been at least five years since your last shot, and you have a wound (especially a puncture wound) that is very dirty or that you suspect may be contaminated, get a TD booster.

Immunization Schedule

Immunization → / Age ↓	Diphtheria Pertussis Tetanus (DPT/DTaP)	Polio (OPV/IPV)	Measles Mumps Rubella (MMR)	Hepatitis B	*Haemophilus Influenzae* b (Hib)	Tetanus Diphtheria (TD) booster	Chickenpox (Varicella)
Birth - 2 weeks				✓			
2 months	✓	✓		✓	✓		
4 months	✓	✓			✓		
6 months	✓	✓			✓		
12 months			✓[1]		✓		discuss[2]
18 months	✓			✓			
4 - 6 years	✓	✓					
11 - 12 years			✓[3]	discuss[4]			✓[5]
14 - 16 years				discuss[4]		✓	
Adults			✓[6]	discuss[7]		✓[8]	✓[9]
Over 65	Influenza (flu) vaccine (annually)[10] Pneumococcal vaccine (at least once)[10,11]						

[1] This shot may not be given before a child's first birthday.

[2] Chickenpox or varicella vaccine will be offered for all one-year-olds. It is unknown at this time whether chickenpox vaccine boosters will be needed or how often. Parents may choose instead to allow their children to catch the natural illness, which provides lifelong immunity.

[3] This booster may be given at age four to six years instead.

[4] Hepatitis B is recommended for all adolescents who have not been previously immunized. A three-shot series is necessary for immunity.

[5] We recommend vaccination for children who have not had chickenpox by age 12.

[6] We recommend a booster for adults who did not have two shots as children and never had measles.

[7] We recommend immunization for adults who are at risk for hepatitis B and have not been previously immunized. Risk factors include multiple sexual partners, IV drug use, or occupational exposure to infected people. A three-shot series is necessary for immunity.

[8] TD boosters should be obtained at least once for adults in their 20s, at age 50, and at age 65. An alternative recommendation is to obtain boosters every 10 years.

[9] We recommend vaccination for adults who have not had chickenpox. We require that adults who wish to be immunized first have a blood test to confirm that they are not immune. A two-shot series is necessary for immunity.

[10] People younger than 65 who have chronic diseases, especially respiratory illnesses such as asthma, should also consider receiving the pneumococcal vaccine and annual flu shots.

[11] We recommend pneumonia vaccine boosters every six years for those with chronic diseases. It may be prudent for all people over 65 to consider boosters as well.

Adapted from *The Report of the Committee on Infectious Diseases,* American Academy of Pediatrics, 1994.

Immunizations – continued

Otherwise there is no need for more frequent vaccinations because this increases the risk of an uncomfortable local reaction.

Polio

Polio is a viral illness that leads to loss of mobility or even paralysis. It is rare today because of the effectiveness of polio vaccines. The first vaccine is given at age two months, and the series of immunizations gives lifelong immunity. Either the oral (OPV) or injectable (IPV) vaccine is acceptable. IPV is recommended for anyone who has an illness or takes medications that impair the immune system.

Nonimmunized adults need immunization only if they have a high risk of polio exposure. The IPV vaccine is recommended for adults.

Measles, Mumps, and Rubella (MMR)

MMR is an immunization for measles, mumps, and rubella (German measles) (see page 166). Two shots (given at 12 months and 11-12 years) are recommended. If both doses are given, no further MMR immunization is needed.

If you have a 6- to 12-month-old child in an area with a measles outbreak, call your doctor or health department to discuss an early MMR. In this case, the dose should be repeated at age 15 months for full protection.

If you don't have records showing that you received two doses of MMR vaccine, and you did not have these illnesses as a child, discuss your need for immunization with your doctor.

Hepatitis B Virus (HBV)

The hepatitis B virus causes serious and sometimes fatal liver disease. Vaccination against HBV prevents infection and its complications. Efforts to immunize only people in high-risk groups (people with many sexual partners, intravenous drug users, infants born to women who have HBV, and health care workers) have not been effective in eliminating the disease.

It is now recommended that all infants be vaccinated against HBV. This will help eliminate hepatitis B as a public health problem in the future. Three shots provide long-term immunity. Immunization is also recommended for:

• Adolescents who were not immunized as infants.

• Health care workers.

• People planning extended travel to China, Southeast Asia, and other areas where HBV infection rates are high.

Haemophilus Influenzae Type b (Hib)

Haemophilus influenzae type b does not cause the flu. It is a serious bacterial illness that causes meningitis and may lead to brain damage and death. Most serious Hib disease affects children between 6 months and 1 year of age. Every child between 2 months and 5 years should be immunized against Hib. Children over five and adults need immunizations only if they have sickle cell anemia or spleen problems.

Reactions to Childhood Immunizations

Temporary, mild reactions to immunizations are common. Babies often develop a fever after the DPT shot, and the location of the shot may be hard. A mild rash or fever may develop 10 to 14 days after the MMR vaccine is given. The rash will go away without treatment. The hepatitis B vaccines have caused nausea, low-grade fever, rash, and joint pain in some adults.

- Acetaminophen may soothe the discomfort and relieve fever. Some doctors recommend giving acetaminophen before the shot.

- Keep written notes on any reactions you observe.

- Tell your health professional if you think the reactions are excessive.

For more details, read your immunization booklet, or call your doctor.

Immunizations After Age 65

Annual influenza vaccinations are recommended for everyone age 65 and older. Younger people with chronic diseases, especially respiratory illnesses, should also consider vaccinations. The vaccines are most effective when given in the autumn.

The pneumococcal vaccine (which prevents most pneumonia) is recommended for those 65 and older. Younger people with chronic disease should also consider receiving the pneumococcal vaccine.

A booster is needed about every six years for people who have chronic diseases.

Other Immunizations

If you are in close contact with people who have an infectious disease or you are planning travel to areas where illnesses such as malaria, typhoid, and yellow fever are common, talk with your doctor or health department to ask if other immunizations are needed.

Tuberculin Test

A tuberculin test is a skin test for tuberculosis, not an immunization. A positive result does not necessarily mean that you have tuberculosis, but it does mean the bacteria have probably entered your body. Whether you should be tested depends on the prevalence of tuberculosis in your area and your risk of exposure. Once a person has a positive skin test, the test should not be repeated. Subsequent tests will always be positive and may cause more severe reactions.

Be Wise, Immunize

1. Immunizations are effective. They do prevent disease.

2. Immunizations cost very little— much less than treating the illnesses they prevent.

3. The risks are low. Reactions are usually mild and short term.

4. It's the law. In many areas children must be immunized before they can start school.

5. Immunizations reduce the risk of epidemics.

Screening and Early Detection

Another way to protect your health is to detect an illness early, while it is still easy to treat. You can do this in two ways: by getting periodic medical exams from health professionals and by becoming a good observer of your own body and health.

Periodic Medical Exams

Many doctors used to recommend a complete physical every year. Now, most doctors recommend specific medical exams based on age, gender, and risk factors. These exams are more effective than the annual physical in detecting treatable illness.

The schedule of medical exams on page 31 helps you decide which tests are valuable for you and how often you should have them.

The chart includes specific recommendations for adults age 19 and older. The chart is based on the Report of the United States Preventive Services Task Force (with a few exceptions noted). Other organizations may make different recommendations. The most appropriate schedule of preventive exams is one you and your doctor agree upon, based on your health conditions, values, and risk factors.

The recommendations apply to people of average risk in each age category. You may be at higher risk for certain diseases. Family history (whether your relatives have or had the disease), other health problems, or behaviors such as smoking all increase your risk. Talk with your doctor about whether more frequent exams are needed.

Periodic self-exams are also an important part of staying healthy. See the breast self-exam on page 169 and the testicular self-exam on page 190. If you have high blood pressure, see page 36.

For more information on cholesterol screening, see page 260.

Fecal Occult Blood Testing

The fecal occult blood test (FOBT) is a screening test for trace amounts of blood in the stool, which may be a sign of early colon cancer or other health problems. If blood is detected by this test, your doctor may recommend further testing with a flexible viewing instrument (flexible sigmoidoscopy) and/or with colon X-rays.

Having a fecal occult blood test every year between age 50 and 75 increases the likelihood of detecting colon cancer early, when it may be successfully treated. For more information, see page 306.

Other Recommended Tests and Exams

Infants

Well-baby visits are recommended at 2 weeks and at 2, 4, 6, 12, 18, and 24 months of age. Your doctor may recommend a different schedule. Babies at high risk for hearing problems may be tested during this time.

Children Age 2 to 5

Discuss the frequency of visits with your health professional. A vision test is recommended at age 3 to 4. Some childhood immunizations are also given at this age. See page 27.

Tests for Early Detection That Will Improve Your Health

Recommended Time Interval Between Tests for Adults of Average Risk
(Intervals in years unless otherwise noted.)

Test	19-49	50-64	65+	Comments
Blood pressure, p. 35	2	2	2	More often if elevated.
Cholesterol, p. 260	at least once	at least once	†	More often if elevated.
Fecal occult blood test, p. 30		1	1	Discontinue after age 75.
Vision			2	
Women				
Breast self-exam, p. 169	Monthly	Monthly	Monthly	
Pap test, p. 173	2‡	2‡	*	Women who have had a hysterectomy for non-cancer reasons may choose to stop Pap smears.
Clinical breast exam, p. 172	2(start at age 35)	2	2	
Mammogram, p. 172	**	2**	2**	May discontinue after age 75. Discuss screening before age 50 with your health care provider.

†Experts are uncertain of the benefit of routine testing for this age group.

‡Women who are at increased risk for cervical cancer should consider yearly screening. Risk factors include: 1) multiple sexual partners or sexual activity at an early age; 2) past history of abnormal Pap smear; 3) no recent Pap smear (within 3 years).

*Women who have no risk factors for cervical cancer and have had recent, normal Pap smears may choose to stop Pap smears at age 65.

**Women who have had breast cancer, have had "atypical hyperplasia" on breast biopsy, or whose mother, sister, or daughter has had breast cancer, should start annual mammography at age 40.

Experts are uncertain about approaches for people who have a family history of particular diseases, and for other higher-risk groups. If you have a family history of cancer or heart disease in close relatives, discuss it with your health care provider.

These screening test guidelines are based on the recommendations of the physicians of Kaiser Permanente (Colorado) and adapted from the U.S. Preventive Services Task Force. These recommendations are based on current scientific evidence and will be updated as additional evidence becomes available.

Other Tests and Exams – cont.

Regular blood pressure checks are recommended after age 3 and may be done during visits for other reasons.

Children Age 7 to 18

Discuss the frequency of visits with your health professional. A tetanus booster is recommended at age 15, and a series of three hepatitis B shots may also be indicated (discuss with your child's health care provider). Annual blood pressure checks are recommended and may be done during any visit.

Pap tests are recommended before age 18 if a teen girl is sexually active. See page 173.

Pregnant Women

Discuss the frequency of visits and testing with your doctor. During the first prenatal visit, blood tests, urinalysis, blood pressure, and screening for hepatitis B are recommended. Additional tests are needed during the pregnancy.

Vital Signs

With a few tools and an eye for observation, you can help detect and monitor health problems in your family. Everyone needs to know how to take a temperature and count pulse and respiration rates. It is also good to learn how to take your own blood pressure. You may even want to learn to do simple ear exams. The tools you need are inexpensive and usually come with instructions. See page 292.

Fahrenheit-Centigrade Conversion Chart		
°F		°C
98.5	=	36.9
99.0	=	37.2
99.5	=	37.5
100.0	=	37.8
100.5	=	38.1
101.0	=	38.3
101.5	=	38.6
102.0	=	38.9
102.5	=	39.2
103.0	=	39.4
103.5	=	39.7

Temperature

A normal temperature ranges from 97.6° to 99.6° and for most people is 98.6°. Temperature varies with time of day and other factors, so don't worry about minor changes.

Whenever a person feels hot or cold to your touch, it is a good idea to measure and record the person's temperature. If you have to call your doctor during an illness, knowing the person's exact temperature will be very helpful.

There are four ways to take a temperature:

• Orally (in the mouth)

• Rectally (in the anus)

• Axillary (under the armpit)

• Using an electronic oral or ear thermometer or temperature strip

Unless otherwise specified, **all temperatures in this book are oral Fahrenheit readings.** If you take a rectal or axillary temperature, adjust it accordingly. Rectal temperatures are the most accurate.

Oral temperatures are recommended for adults and children age six years and older.

- Clean the thermometer with soapy water or rubbing alcohol.

- Hold it firmly at the end opposite the bulb and shake the mercury down to 95° or lower.

- Make sure nothing hot or cold has recently been drunk.

- Place the bulb under the tongue and close the lips around it. The teeth should not bite it. Breathe through the nose and do not talk.

- Wait three to five minutes.

Rectal temperatures are recommended for children younger than six years or anyone who cannot hold the thermometer in the mouth. Use only a rectal thermometer.

- Clean the thermometer and shake it down (see above).

- Put Vaseline or other lubricant on the bulb.

- Hold the child bottom-up across your lap.

- Hold the thermometer one inch from bulb and gently insert it into the rectum no more than one inch.

Do not let go. Hold it right at the anus so that it cannot slip in further.

- Wait for three minutes.

Rectal temperature is 0.5° to 1° higher than oral temperature.

Axillary temperatures are less accurate and about 1° lower than oral. They are safer for small children who will not hold still while you use a rectal thermometer.

- Use either an oral or rectal thermometer. Shake it down below 95°.

- Place the thermometer in the armpit and have the child cross her arm across the chest and hold her opposite upper arm.

- Wait five minutes.

Electronic thermometers are convenient and easy to use. They are quite accurate, but some are expensive. Temperature strips are convenient but should only be used to measure axillary (armpit) temperature. They are inaccurate when used on the forehead.

How to Read a Thermometer

- Roll the thermometer until you can see the thin ribbon of mercury. Note that the thermometer is marked from 92° to 108°.

- Each large mark indicates one degree of temperature. Each small mark indicates 0.2°.

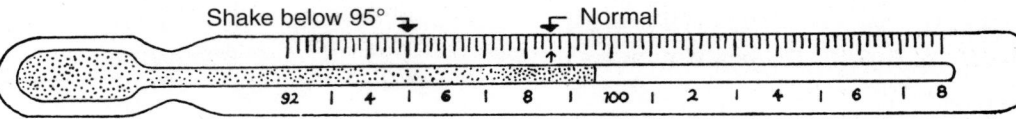

Thermometer reads 99.6°

Vital Signs – continued

Taking a Pulse

The pulse is the rate at which a person's heart is beating. As the heart forces blood through the body, a throbbing can be felt in the arteries wherever they come close to the skin surface. The pulse can be taken at the wrist, neck, or upper arm.

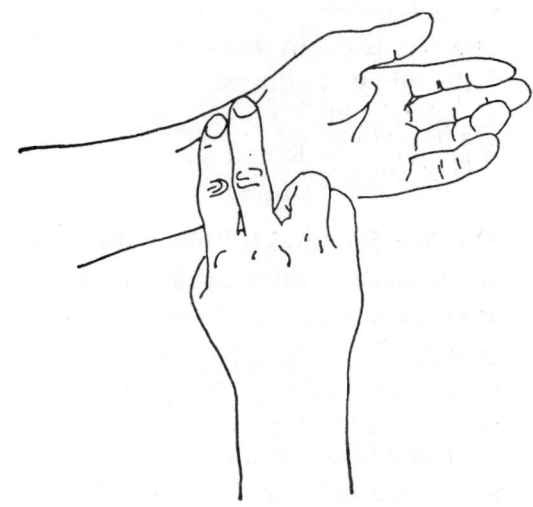

Taking a Pulse

Certain illnesses can cause the pulse to increase, so it is helpful to know your resting pulse when you are well. The pulse rate rises about 10 beats per minute for every degree of fever.

- Count the pulse after the person has been sitting or resting quietly for 5 to 10 minutes.

- Place two fingers gently against the wrist as shown (don't use your thumb).

- If it is hard to feel the pulse in the wrist, locate the carotid artery in the neck, just to either side of the windpipe. Press gently.

- Count the beats for 30 seconds, then double the result for beats per minute.

Counting Respiration Rates

Your respiration rate is how many breaths you take in a minute. The best time to count respiration is when the person is resting, perhaps after taking the pulse while your fingers are still on their wrist. The person's breathing is likely to change if they know you are counting it. Respiration rate increase with fever and some illnesses.

Normal Resting Pulse		Normal Resting Respiration	
Infant - 1 yr.	100 - 160 beats/minute	Infant - 1 yr.	40 - 60 breaths/minute
1 - 6 yrs.	65 - 140 beats/minute	1 - 6 yrs.	18 - 26 breaths/minute
7 - 10 yrs.	60 -110 beats/minute	7 - adult	12 - 24 breaths/minute
11 - adult	50 - 100 beats/minute		

- Count the rise and fall of the chest for one full minute.

- Notice whether there is any sucking in beneath the ribs or any apparent wheezing or difficulty breathing.

Measuring Blood Pressure

Blood pressure is the force of the blood pulsing against the walls of the arteries. The pressure when the heart beats is called the systolic pressure (the first number in blood pressure readings). The pressure between beats, when the heart is at rest, is called the diastolic pressure. Any blood pressure below 140/90 is considered normal for an adult over 18. See page 36 for information about high blood pressure.

Most people with good hearing can learn to measure blood pressure using a stethoscope and a blood pressure cuff (sphygmomanometer). Electronic blood pressure cuffs are also available, which do not require a stethoscope or good hearing. Most Kaiser Permanente pharmacies sell blood pressure cuffs.

- Ask your pharmacist to recommend a blood pressure kit and show you how to use it.

- Regular in-home blood pressure monitoring is recommended for anyone who has heart disease or high blood pressure.

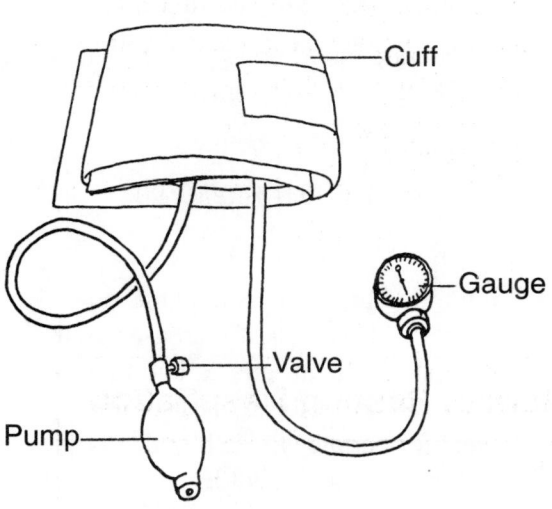

Blood pressure cuff

Fever

A fever is an abnormally high body temperature. It is a symptom, not a disease. A higher temperature is one way your body fights illness. Fever of up to 102° is generally beneficial, though it may be uncomfortable. Most healthy adults can tolerate a fever as high as 103° to 104° for short periods of time without problems.

For specific fever guidelines for children under age four, see page 163.

Home Treatment

- Drink more liquids, especially water.

- Take and record temperature every two hours and whenever symptoms change.

Fever – continued

- For fevers that cause discomfort, sponge with lukewarm water and take acetaminophen, aspirin, or ibuprofen to lower fever. Do *not* give aspirin to children or teens under age 20.

- Watch for signs of dehydration. See page 43.

- See Chapter 7 for more home treatment of colds and flu.

When to Call Kaiser Permanente

- Fever over 104° does not go down after two hours of home treatment.

- Persistent fever. Many viral illnesses, especially the flu, cause fevers of 102° or higher for short periods of time (up to 12 to 24 hours). Call a doctor if the fever stays:

  ○ 102° or higher for 2 full days

  ○ 101° or higher for 3 full days

  ○ 100° or higher for 4 full days

- Fever over 103° with dry skin, even under the armpits (possible heat stroke, see page 225).

- If fever occurs with other signs of a bacterial infection. See page 96.

- If fever occurs with the following symptoms:

  ○ Very stiff neck and headache. See "Encephalitis and Meningitis" on page 102.

  ○ Shortness of breath and cough. See Pneumonia on page 104 and Bronchitis on page 97.

  ○ Pain over eyes or cheeks. See Sinusitis on page 105.

  ○ Painful or burning urination. See Urinary Tract Infections on page 184.

  ○ Abdominal pain, nausea, and vomiting. See Stomach Flu/Food Poisoning on page 51, or Appendicitis on page 41.

- Call your doctor if fever is associated with disturbing or unexplained symptoms.

High Blood Pressure

High blood pressure (hypertension) occurs when the pressure of your blood against the artery walls is higher than normal. For more information about blood pressure, see page 35.

Doctors rate blood pressure for adults over 18 in the following categories:

- Normal: 130/85 or below

- High-normal: 131–140/86–90

- High: over 140/90

High blood pressure usually has no symptoms. However, it increases your risk of stroke, heart attack, and kidney disease. Risks of these diseases are lowest for people whose blood pressure is below 120/80.

Risk factors for high blood pressure include:

- African-American race

- Overweight

- Family history of high blood pressure

- Inactive lifestyle

- Excess alcohol intake

- Excess sodium (salt) intake

- Use of certain medications, including birth control pills, steroids, decongestants, and anti-inflammatories

In some cases, high blood pressure can be prevented. Many people with high blood pressure can control it by changing their lifestyle and may not require drugs.

Taking the following steps is especially important if you are in one of the high-risk groups listed above.

Prevention

- Lose weight. This is especially important if you tend to gain weight around the waist rather than in the hips and thighs. A weight loss of only 10 pounds can lower blood pressure. See page 266.

- Limit your alcohol intake to two drinks or less per day. Too much alcohol increases blood pressure.

- Exercise regularly. Thirty to 45 minutes of brisk walking three to five times a week help lower your blood pressure (and will also help you lose weight). See page 245.

- Reduce your salt intake. See page 265.

- Make sure you get enough potassium, calcium, and magnesium in your diet. Potassium-rich foods include orange juice and potatoes. Magnesium-rich foods include leafy green vegetables and whole grains. See page 264 for calcium-rich foods.

- Reduce the fat in your diet. Saturated fat is found in animal products (milk, cheese, and meat). Unsaturated fats are fats derived from vegetables, such as margarine and corn oil, and are found in chips, french fries, and doughnuts. Limiting these foods will help you lose weight and also lower your risk of heart disease. See page 260.

- Stop smoking. Smoking increases your risk of heart disease and stroke. See page 112 for tips on quitting.

Home Treatment

- Follow the prevention tips above even more closely if you have high blood pressure.

- Take any prescribed blood pressure medications exactly as directed.

When to Call Kaiser Permanente

- If you have had two or more blood pressure readings of 140 or higher systolic or 90 or higher diastolic. Call if either one or both numbers are high.

- To learn how to take your blood pressure at home. See page 305.

*A great step towards independence
is a good-humored stomach.*
Seneca

Chapter 4

Abdominal Problems

Abdominal problems can be hard to pin down. Stomach cramps due to gas pain, which is not often serious, can be much more painful than the early stages of appendicitis, a much more serious problem. Fortunately, most abdominal problems are minor and require only home treatment.

When you have stomach pain, it is a good idea to look carefully at your symptoms. Note whether the pain is relieved by passing gas or stools or by vomiting. Review the symptoms on page 40 and note your observations. They may help you or your doctor figure out the cause.

However, remember that abdominal pain is difficult even for a doctor to evaluate. If you have any doubts about the cause or severity of stomach pain, a call to your doctor is strongly recommended. Call any time stomach pain is severe or persistent, or if it increases over several hours.

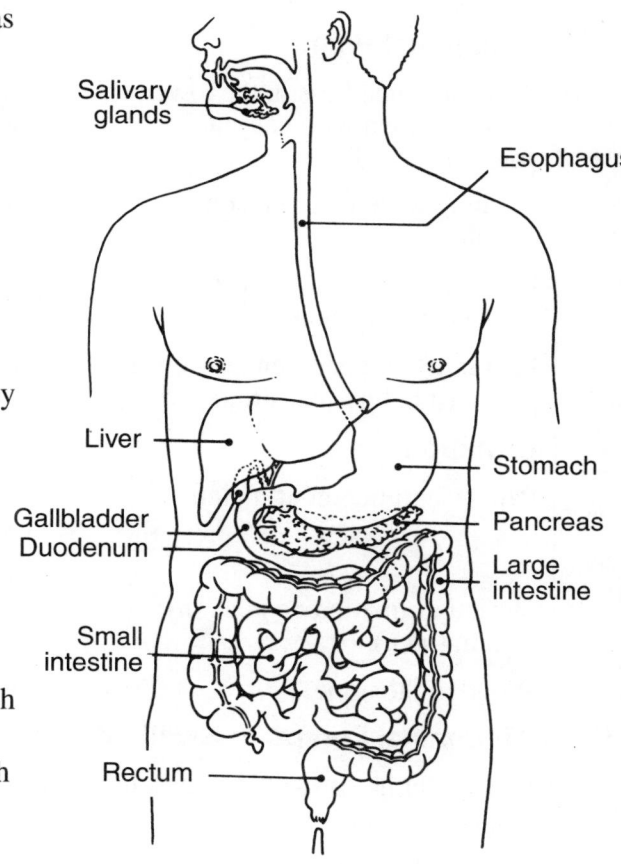

Digestive tract

Abdominal Problems

Symptoms	Possible Causes
Nausea or vomiting	See Nausea and Vomiting, p. 50. Watch for Dehydration, p. 43. Medication reaction. Call your doctor or pharmacist. See Antibiotics, p 302.
Bowel Movements	
Frequent, watery stools	See Diarrhea, p. 45; Stomach Flu and Food Poisoning, p. 51. Watch for Dehydration, p. 43. See Antibiotics, p. 302.
Stools dry and difficult to pass	See Constipation, p. 42.
Bloody or black, tarry stools	See Ulcers, p. 53.
Pain during bowel movements; bright red blood on surface of stool or on toilet paper	See Hemorrhoids, p. 47.
Abdominal Pain	
Pain and tenderness in the lower right abdomen with nausea, vomiting, and fever	See Appendicitis, p. 41; Urinary Tract Infections, p. 184.
Bloating with diarrhea, constipation, or both	Irritable Bowel Syndrome, p.48.
Burning or discomfort just below the breastbone	See Heartburn, p. 46; Ulcers, p. 53; Chest Pain, p. 98.
Pain in lower abdomen and lower back just before menstrual period	See Menstrual Cramps, p. 180.
Urination	
Pain or burning on urination	See Urinary Tract Infections, p. 180; Prostate Problems, p. 193; Sexually Transmitted Diseases, p. 199.
Difficult urination or weak urine stream (men)	See Prostate Problems, p. 193.
Blood in the urine	See p. 185.
Abdominal Lumps or Swelling	
Painless lump or swelling in groin that comes and goes	See Hernia, p. 192.
Blow to the stomach; very rigid or distended abdomen	See Blunt Abdominal Wounds, p. 212, Watch for Shock, p. 234.

Appendicitis

The appendix is a small sac extending from the large intestine. It is normally self-cleaning and does not cause problems. However, if its opening becomes blocked (usually by bowel material), bacteria can build up and the appendix may become inflamed and infected. This condition is known as appendicitis.

Appendicitis is most common in young people age 10 to 30, although it does occur in younger children and older adults. It is rare before age two. Since small children often cannot describe pain well, their cases may become quite serious before they are diagnosed.

Once appendicitis begins, it usually worsens until the appendix ruptures. If the appendix ruptures, it spreads the infection to the other abdominal organs.

However, observing the symptoms for 8 to 12 hours is usually safe and is often necessary to confirm the diagnosis. The appendix rarely ruptures within the first 24 hours. In most cases, appendicitis requires surgery.

Symptoms of appendicitis may include:

- Pain that begins around the navel or upper stomach and moves to the lower right abdomen over the course of 2 to 12 hours.

- Nausea, vomiting, loss of appetite, and constipation. Diarrhea may occur, but usually indicates the pain is due to some other cause.

- Low-grade fever (100° to 101°).

Home Treatment

- Check the vital signs. See page 32.

- Keep a careful record of the following symptoms:

  ○ Abdominal pain and tenderness

  ○ Nausea, vomiting, constipation, or diarrhea

  ○ Fever

- Keep the patient quiet and in a comfortable position.

- Try to identify or rule out other causes of abdominal pain, such as stomach flu (see page 51) or overeating.

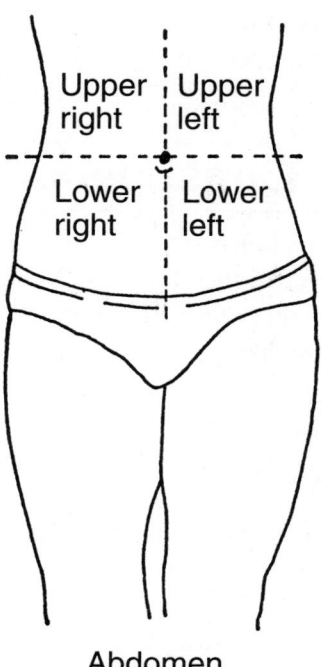

Abdomen

Appendicitis – continued

- Do not give laxatives. They can stimulate the intestine and cause the appendix to rupture sooner.

- Do not give strong pain medication. Since the location and severity of pain are diagnostic clues, strong pain relievers may mask important information.

- Do not apply heat to the abdomen.

When to Call Kaiser Permanente

- If you suspect appendicitis. Review your observations of the symptoms with your doctor.

- If there is severe, increasing, and continuous pain in the lower right abdomen for more than four hours.

- If any stomach pain localizes to a specific point in the abdomen.

Constipation

Constipation occurs when bowel movements are difficult to pass. Some people are overly concerned with frequency because they have been taught that a healthy person has a bowel movement every day. This is a misconception. Most people pass stools anywhere from three times a day to three times a week. If your stools are soft and pass easily, you are not constipated.

Constipation may be accompanied by cramping and pain in the rectum from the strain of trying to pass hard, dry stools. There may be some bloating and nausea. There may also be small amounts of bright red blood on the stool caused by slight tearing as the stool is pushed through the anus. This should stop when the constipation is controlled.

If a stool becomes lodged in the rectum (impacted), mucus and fluid will leak out around the stool, sometimes leading to fecal incontinence.

Constipation may be due to a variety of causes. Lack of fiber and inadequate water in the diet are common causes. Other causes include travel, lack of exercise, delaying bowel movements, medications, pain due to hemorrhoids, and laxative overuse. Irritable bowel syndrome (see page 48) may also cause constipation.

Children may ignore the urge to pass stools because they are involved in play or other activities. Children and adults may get constipated because they are reluctant to use toilets away from home. Stress related to toilet training may contribute to constipation in young children.

Prevention

- Eat plenty of high-fiber foods such as fruits, vegetables, and whole grains. Other ways to add fiber include:

  ○ A bowl of bran cereal with 10 grams of bran per serving.

  ○ Two tablespoons of bran added to cereal or soup.

  ○ Two tablespoons of psyllium (found in Metamucil and other bulk-forming agents).

  See page 258 for more about fiber.

- Avoid foods that are high in fat and sugar.

- Drink 1½ to 2 quarts of water and other fluids every day. (However, some people find milk constipating.)

- Exercise more. A walking program would be a good start. See page 245.

- Go when you feel the urge. Your bowels send signals when there is a need to pass stools. If you ignore the signal, the urge will go away, and the stool will eventually become dry and difficult to pass.

Home Treatment

- Set aside relaxed times for bowel movements. Urges usually occur sometime after meals. Establishing a daily routine, after breakfast, for example, may be helpful.

- Drink two to four extra glasses of water per day, especially in the morning.

- Add fruits, vegetables, and high-fiber foods, such as bran cereal, beans, or prunes, to your diet.

- If necessary, use a stool softener or very mild laxative, such as milk of magnesia. Do not use mineral oil or any other laxative for more than two weeks without consulting your doctor. See page 299.

For babies and children up to age two:

- Make sure you are adding the correct amount of water to the baby's formula.

- Give one to two ounces of water before feeding.

- After age six months, give 1/2 teaspoon to 2 ounces (increase amount slowly over time) of prune juice. At age nine months, add 1½ to 3 tablespoons of strained prunes per day.

When to Call Kaiser Permanente

- If acute constipation persists after the above treatment is followed for one week for adults or three days for infants.

- If bleeding is heavy (more than a few bright red streaks), or if the blood is dark red or brown.

- If bleeding persists longer than two to three days after constipation has improved.

- If sharp or severe pain occurs in the abdomen.

- If constipation and major changes in bowel movement patterns occur and persist longer than two weeks without clear reason.

- If you experience fecal incontinence.

- If you are unable to have bowel movements without using laxatives.

Dehydration

Dehydration occurs when your body loses too much water. When you stop drinking water or lose large amounts of fluids through diarrhea, vomiting, or sweating, the body cells reabsorb fluid from the blood and other body tissues. When too much water is lost, the blood vessels may collapse. Without medical attention, death may result.

Dehydration is very dangerous for infants, small children, and older adults. Watch closely for its early signs anytime there is an illness

Dehydration – continued

that causes high fever, vomiting, or diarrhea. The early symptoms are:

• Dry mouth and sticky saliva

• Reduced urine output with dark yellow urine

Prevention

• Prompt home treatment for illnesses that cause diarrhea, vomiting, or fever will help prevent dehydration.

  ◦ Diarrhea, page 45

  ◦ Vomiting, page 50

  ◦ Diarrhea and vomiting in children, page 161

  ◦ Stomach flu, page 51

  ◦ Fever, page 35

  ◦ Fever in children, page 163

• To prevent dehydration during hot weather and exercise, drink 8 to 10 glasses of fluids (water and/or rehydration drinks) each day. Drink extra water before exercise and every half hour during activity.

Home Treatment

• Treatment of mild dehydration involves stopping the fluid loss and gradually replacing lost fluids.

• To stop vomiting or diarrhea, stop all food for at least four hours. Take frequent, small sips of water or a rehydration drink.

• When the vomiting or diarrhea is controlled, take water or diluted broth or sports drinks a sip at a time until the stomach can handle larger amounts.

Rehydration Drinks

When you have diarrhea or are vomiting, your body can lose large amounts of water and essential minerals called electrolytes. If you are unable to eat for a few days, you are also losing nutrients. This happens faster and is more serious in infants, young children, and older adults.

A rehydration drink (Pedialyte, Lytren, Rehydralyte) replaces not only fluids, but also electrolytes in amounts that are best used by your body. Sports drinks (Gatorade, All Sport) and other sugared drinks will replace fluid, but most contain too much sugar (which can make the diarrhea worse) and not enough of the other essential ingredients. Plain water won't provide any necessary nutrients or electrolytes.

Rehydration drinks won't make the diarrhea or vomiting go away faster, but they will prevent serious dehydration from developing.

You can make an inexpensive homemade rehydration drink. However, *do not* give this homemade drink to children under age 12.

Mix:

• 1 quart water

• 1/2 teaspoon baking soda

• 1/2 teaspoon table salt

• 3 to 4 tablespoons sugar

• If available, add 1/4 teaspoon salt substitute ("Lite Salt")

• If vomiting or diarrhea lasts longer than 24 hours, sip a rehydration drink to restore lost salts and nutrients. See page 44 for a drink you can make at home. Do not give the homemade drink to children under 12.

• Watch for signs of more severe dehydration (see below).

For infants and children under four:

• Give small sips of a rehydration drink (Pedialyte, Lytren) if vomiting or diarrhea has lasted longer than two to four hours. See page 161.

When to Call Kaiser Permanente

• If, after 12 hours of no food or drink, the person cannot hold down even small sips of liquid.

• If vomiting lasts longer than 24 hours in an adult, 12 hours in a child under age four, or two to four hours in an infant under six months.

• If severe diarrhea lasts longer than two days in an adult, one day in a child under age four, or eight hours in an infant under six months.

• If the following signs of severe dehydration develop:
  ◦ Sunken eyes
  ◦ Sunken soft spot on an infant's head
  ◦ Little or no urine for eight hours
  ◦ Skin that is doughy or doesn't bounce back when pinched
  ◦ Low blood pressure and rapid heart rate
  ◦ Lethargy

Diarrhea

Diarrhea is an increase in the frequency of bowel movements and the discharge of watery, loose stools. The person with diarrhea may also have abdominal cramps and nausea.

Diarrhea occurs when the intestines push stools through before the water in them can be reabsorbed by the body. It is your body's way of quickly clearing out any viruses or bacteria.

Most diarrhea is caused by viral stomach flu (gastroenteritis). Some medications, especially antibiotics, may also upset your digestive system enough to cause diarrhea. For some people, emotional stress, anxiety, or food intolerance may bring on the condition. Irritable bowel syndrome (see page 48) may also cause diarrhea.

Drinking untreated water that contains the *giardia lamblia* parasite can also cause diarrhea that develops one to four weeks later.

Since most cases of diarrhea are viral, they will clear up in a few days with good home treatment.

For home treatment for diarrhea in infants and children under age four, see page 161.

Home Treatment

• Put your stomach at rest. Drink only clear liquids until you begin to feel better, for as long as 24 hours.

• Since diarrhea may sometimes speed recovery of the underlying problem, avoid antidiarrheal drugs

Diarrhea – continued

for the first six hours. After that, use them only if there are no other signs of illness, such as fever, and if cramping or discomfort continue. See antidiarrheal preparations on page 296.

- Begin eating mild foods, such as rice, dry toast or crackers, bananas, and applesauce the next day or sooner, depending on how you feel. Avoid spicy foods, fruit, alcohol, and coffee until 48 hours after all symptoms have disappeared. Avoid dairy products for three days.

- Take care to avoid dehydration. See page 43.

When to Call Kaiser Permanente

- If the diarrhea is black or bloody. However, Pepto-Bismol or other medications containing bismuth can cause stools to look black.

- If abdominal pain or severe discomfort accompanies diarrhea and is not relieved by passing stools or gas.

- If diarrhea is accompanied by fever of 101° or higher, chills, vomiting, or fainting.

- If signs of severe dehydration appear. See page 45.

- If severe diarrhea lasts for two days or more in an adult, one day in a child under four, or eight hours in an infant under six months.

- If mild diarrhea continues for one to two weeks without obvious cause.

- If diarrhea occurs after drinking untreated water.

Heartburn

Heartburn (indigestion) is caused by stomach acids backing up into the lower esophagus, the tube that leads from the mouth to the stomach. The medical term for heartburn is gastro-esophageal reflux disease (GERD). The acids produce a burning sensation and discomfort between the ribs just below the breastbone. Another symptom is sour or bitter fluid backing up into the throat or mouth. Heartburn can occur after overeating and sometimes in reaction to medications.

Don't be concerned if you experience heartburn now and then; nearly everyone does (25 percent of pregnant women have it every day). However, months of heartburn can injure the esophageal lining.

Prevention

Most cases of heartburn can be prevented by following the home treatment tips below.

- Stop smoking. This is especially important because smoking promotes heartburn.

- Avoid alcohol, which irritates your stomach and esophagus and may make your symptoms worse.

Home Treatment

- Eat smaller meals, and avoid late-night snacks.

- Avoid foods that bring on heartburn. Alcohol, caffeine, chocolate, orange and tomato juices, peppermint- and spearmint-flavored foods, fatty or fried foods, and carbonated drinks may make heartburn worse.

• Stop smoking. This will often completely relieve heartburn.

• If you are overweight, lose weight, even a few pounds. Being overweight can worsen heartburn.

• Avoid tight-fitting clothes, such as tight belts and waistbands.

• Raise the head of your bed six inches by placing a foam wedge or thick telephone books under the mattress or legs of the bed frame.

• Don't lie down too soon after eating. Try to stay upright for at least two to three hours after each meal. Avoid large meals and snacks before bedtime.

• Try acetaminophen rather than aspirin, ibuprofen, or other anti-inflammatory drugs, which may cause heartburn.

• Take an antacid, such as Maalox, Mylanta, TUMS, Gelusil, or Gaviscon. Ask your pharmacist for advice in choosing an antacid, and follow the manufacturer's directions.

When to Call Kaiser Permanente

• If pain occurs with shortness of breath or other symptoms that suggest heart problems. See Chest Pain on page 98.

• If heartburn persists for one to two weeks despite home treatment. Call sooner if symptoms are severe or are not relieved at all by antacids. See Ulcers on page 53.

• If stools are deep red, black, or tarry. Small amounts of bright red blood on stool or toilet paper are probably due to a scratch in the anal area.

• If you suspect that a prescribed medication is causing heartburn. Antihistamines, Valium, birth control pills, and anti-inflammatory drugs including aspirin and ibuprofen can sometimes cause heartburn.

Hemorrhoids

Hemorrhoids and piles are two terms used to describe inflammation and swelling in the veins around the anus. Hemorrhoids may develop either inside or outside the anus. Straining to pass hard, compacted stools sometimes causes these veins to become enlarged and inflamed.

The symptoms of hemorrhoids are tenderness or pain and sometimes bleeding. There may be a small lump at the opening to the anus. Hemorrhoids generally last several days and often recur.

Rectal itching is usually caused by other conditions. If the anus is not kept clean, itching may result. Skin may become irritated by any fecal seepage that comes with diarrhea. Trying to keep the area too clean by rubbing with dry toilet paper or using excess soap may also injure the skin.

Prevention

• Keep your stools soft. Include plenty of water, fresh fruits and vegetables, and whole grains in your diet. Add two tablespoons of bran or Metamucil to your diet each day. Also see Constipation on page 42.

Hemorrhoids – continued

- Avoid sitting too much, which restricts blood flow around your anus.

- Try not to strain during bowel movements. Take your time and never hold your breath.

Home Treatment

- Keep the area clean. Warm baths are soothing and cleansing, especially after a bowel movement. Try premoistened tissues (baby wipes) instead of toilet paper.

- Wear cotton underwear and loose clothing.

- Apply zinc oxide (paste or powder) or petroleum jelly to the painful area after drying. This protects against further irritation and eases the passage of stools.

- Relieve itching by using cold compresses on the anus four times a day, 10 minutes at a time.

- Sitz baths, hot baths with just enough water to cover the anal area, are soothing.

- Use medicated suppositories to relieve pain.

- The following over-the-counter preparations may help: Tucks, Balneol, or stool softeners. Avoid anal ointments with a local anesthetic compound, which can cause an allergic reaction. These will have the suffix "-caine" in the name or ingredients. Try 0.5 percent hydrocortisone cream to relieve itching.

When to Call Kaiser Permanente

- If bleeding is heavy (more than a few bright red streaks), or if the blood is dark red or brown.

- If any bleeding continues for longer than one week despite home treatment.

- If pain is severe or lasts longer than one week.

- If bleeding occurs for no apparent reason, and is not associated with straining to pass stools.

Irritable Bowel Syndrome

Irritable bowel syndrome (IBS) is one of the most common disorders of the digestive tract. Symptoms of IBS include:

- Abdominal bloating, pain, and gas

- Increase in symptoms with stress or after eating

- Mucus in the stool

- Feeling that a bowel movement hasn't been completed

- Irregular bowel habits, with constipation, diarrhea, or both

IBS is a functional bowel disorder, which means that function of the digestive tract is impaired. However, there are no physical signs of this disease and no tests that diagnose it.

IBS can persist for many years. A given episode may be milder or more severe than the one before it, but the disorder itself does not worsen over time. It does not lead to more serious diseases such as cancer.

Prevention

There is no way to prevent IBS. However, because symptoms often worsen or improve due to diet, stress, medications, exercise, or for unknown reasons, identifying those things that trigger your symptoms may help you avoid or minimize attacks.

Home Treatment

Careful attention to diet and stress management can keep your symptoms under control and perhaps even prevent them from recurring.

If constipation is the main symptom:

- Try an over-the-counter fiber supplement or bulk-forming agent that contains crushed psyllium seed or methylcellulose. Examples include Metamucil, Fiberall, and Citrucel.

- Add fiber-rich foods to the diet (add slowly so they do not worsen gas or cramps). See page 258 for a list of high-fiber foods.

- Use laxatives (e.g., Feen-A-Mint, Correctol) only on a doctor's recommendation.

If diarrhea is the main symptom:

- Avoid foods that make diarrhea worse. Try eliminating one at a time, then add it back gradually. If a food doesn't seem to be related to symptoms, there is no need to avoid it. Many people find the following foods or items worsen their symptoms:

  ○ Alcohol, caffeine, nicotine

  ○ Beans, broccoli, apples

  ○ Spicy foods

  ○ Foods high in acid, such as citrus fruit

  ○ Fatty foods, including bacon, sausage, butter, oils, and anything deep-fried

- Avoid dairy products that contain lactose (milk sugar) if they seem to worsen symptoms. However, get enough calcium in your diet from other sources. Yogurt may be a good choice, because some of the lactose has already been digested by the yogurt cultures.

- Avoid sorbitol, an artificial sweetener found in some sugarless candies and gum.

- Add more starchy food (bread, rice, potatoes, pasta) to your diet.

- If diarrhea persists, an over-the-counter medication such as loperamide (Imodium) may help. Check with your doctor if you are using it twice a month or more.

To reduce stress:

- Keep a diary or journal of your symptoms as well as life events that occur with them. This may help you see any connection between your symptoms and stressful occasions. Once you have identified certain events or situations that bring on symptoms, you can develop ways of dealing with them that are less stressful.

- Get regular, vigorous exercise such as swimming, jogging, or brisk walking to help reduce tension.

IBS – continued

- See page 250 for more tips on managing stress.

- See Resource 47 on page 309.

When to Call Kaiser Permanente

Call for an appointment:

- If you have continuous moderate to severe pain localized to any part of the abdomen accompanied by a fever not due to any other reason (such as stomach flu) of 100.5° or higher and chills or yellowing of the eyes and skin (jaundice).

- If pain is so severe that treatment is needed, or if symptoms gradually or suddenly become worse.

- If there is blood in the stool that is not obviously related to hemorrhoids that have been diagnosed by a doctor.

- If you have been diagnosed with IBS and your symptoms change significantly from their usual pattern.

If none of the more serious symptoms are present, try to rule out other causes of stomach problems (e.g., eating a new food, nervousness, stomach flu). Try home treatment for a week or two. If there is no improvement, or if your symptoms worsen, call for an appointment.

Nausea and Vomiting

Nausea is a very unpleasant feeling in the pit of the stomach. A person who is nauseated may feel weak and sweaty and produce lots of saliva. Intense nausea often leads to vomiting, which forces stomach contents up the esophagus and out the mouth. Home treatment will help ease the discomfort. Nausea and vomiting may be caused by:

- Viral stomach flu or food poisoning (see page 51)

- Medications (especially antibiotics and aspirin)

- Stress or nervousness

- Pregnancy (see page 174)

- Diabetes

- Migraine (see page 128)

- Head injury (see page 224)

Nausea and vomiting can also be signs of other serious illnesses.

Home Treatment

- For home treatment of vomiting in children under four years, see page 161.

- If vomiting is severe and persistent, take nothing by mouth for several hours, or until you are feeling better. Take frequent small sips of water or a rehydration drink (see page 44).

- Drink only clear noncarbonated liquids such as water, weak tea, diluted juice, or broth for 12 to 24 hours. Start with a few sips at a time and gradually increase.

- If vomiting lasts longer than 24 hours, sip a rehydration drink to restore lost fluids and nutrients. See page 44.

- Rest in bed until you are feeling better.

- Watch for and treat early signs of dehydration (see page 43). Infants, children, and older adults can quickly become dehydrated from vomiting.

- When you are feeling better, begin eating clear soups, mild foods, and liquids until all symptoms are gone for 12 to 48 hours, depending on how you feel. Jell-O, dry toast, crackers, and cooked cereal are good choices.

When to Call Kaiser Permanente

- If vomiting is severe or violent (it shoots out in large quantities).

- If there is blood in the vomit. It may look like red or black coffee grounds.

- If vomiting occurs with fever and increasing pain in the lower right abdomen. See Appendicitis on page 41.

- If pain localizes to one area of the abdomen rather than generalized cramping.

- If vomiting occurs with severe headache, sleepiness, lethargy, or stiff neck.

- If vomiting lasts longer than 24 hours in an adult, 12 hours in a child under age four, or eight hours in an infant under six months.

- If signs of severe dehydration develop. See page 45.

- If nausea and vomiting persist longer than two hours after a head injury, or if violent vomiting lasts longer than 15 minutes. Limited nausea or vomiting at first is usually not serious. See Head Injuries on page 224.

- If you suspect that medication is causing the problem. Antibiotics and anti-inflammatory medications (aspirin, ibuprofen, etc.) may cause nausea or vomiting. Know which of your medications can cause these symptoms.

Stomach Flu and Food Poisoning

Stomach flu and food poisoning are different ailments with different causes. However, many people confuse the two because the symptoms are so similar. Most people who get food poisoning attribute their symptoms of nausea, vomiting, diarrhea, and stomach pain to a sudden case of stomach flu, and vice versa. The disagreeable symptoms discourage you from eating until the problem clears up.

Stomach flu is usually caused by a viral infection in the digestive system, hence the medical name, viral gastroenteritis. To prevent stomach flu, you must avoid contact with the virus, which is not always easy to do.

Stomach Flu – continued

Food poisoning is caused by bacteria that grow in food that is not handled or stored properly. Bacteria can grow rapidly when certain foods, especially meats and dairy products, are not prepared carefully or are left at temperatures between 40° and 140°. The bacteria produce a poison (toxin) that causes an acute inflammation of the intestines.

Most food poisoning occurs when cold cuts, turkey, dressing, sauces, and other foods get too warm at parties or picnics.

Suspect food poisoning when symptoms are shared by others who ate the same food, or after eating unrefrigerated foods. Symptoms of food poisoning may not begin for 6 to 48 hours after eating. Nausea, vomiting, and diarrhea may last from 12 to 48 hours for common food poisoning.

Botulism is a rare but often fatal type of food poisoning. It is generally caused by improper home canning methods for low-acid foods like beans and corn. Bacteria that survive the canning process may grow and produce toxin in the jar. Symptoms include blurred or double vision, muscle weakness, and headache.

Prevention

To prevent food poisoning:

• Follow the 2–40–140 rule. Don't eat meats, dressing, salads, or other foods that have been kept for more than two hours between 40° and 140°.

• Be especially careful with large cooked meats like your holiday turkey, which require a long time to cool. Thick parts of the meat may stay over 40° long enough to allow bacteria to grow.

• Use a thermometer to check your refrigerator. It should be between 34° and 40°.

• Defrost meats in the refrigerator or quickly in the microwave, not on the kitchen counter.

• Wash your hands, cutting boards, and counter tops frequently. After handling raw meats, wash your hands and utensils before preparing other foods.

• Reheat meats to over 140° for 10 minutes to destroy any bacteria. Even then, the toxin may not be destroyed.

• Cook hamburger well done.

• Cover meats and poultry during microwave cooking to heat the surface of the meat.

• Do not eat raw eggs or sauces made with raw eggs.

• Keep party foods on ice.

• Discard any cans or jars with bulging lids or leaks.

• When you eat out, avoid rare and uncooked meats. Eat salad bar and deli items before they get warm.

• Follow home canning and freezing instructions carefully. Contact your County Agricultural Extension office for advice.

Home Treatment

- Viral stomach flu will usually go away within 24 to 48 hours. Good home care can speed recovery. See Nausea and Vomiting on page 50 and Diarrhea on page 45.

- Watch for and treat early signs of dehydration (see page 43). Infants, children, and older adults can quickly become dehydrated from diarrhea and vomiting.

- If you suspect food poisoning, check with others who may have eaten the same food. If possible, save a sample of the food for analysis in case symptoms do not improve.

When to Call Kaiser Permanente

- If vomiting lasts longer than 24 hours in an adult, 12 hours in a child under age four, or eight hours in an infant under six months.

- If severe diarrhea lasts longer than two days in an adult, one day in a child under age four, or eight hours in an infant under six months.

- If signs of severe dehydration develop. See page 45.

- If you suspect food poisoning from a canned food, or have symptoms of botulism (blurred or double vision, difficulty swallowing or breathing). If you still have it, take a food sample with you for testing.

Ulcers

An ulcer (peptic ulcer) is a sore or crater in the lining of the gastrointestinal tract. Ulcers may develop in the stomach (gastric ulcers) or in the upper part of the small intestine (duodenal ulcers). Ulcers develop when something damages the protective lining and allows stomach acid to eat away at it. Factors that increase the risk of ulcers include:

- Regular use of aspirin, ibuprofen, and other nonsteroidal anti-inflammatory drugs (NSAIDs), such as indomethacin, naproxen, clinoril, etc.

- Smoking

- Infection with bacteria called *Helicobacter pylori*

Symptoms of an ulcer may include a burning or sharp pain in the abdomen between the navel and the end of the breastbone. The pain often occurs between meals and may wake the person during the night. The pain can usually be relieved by eating something or taking an antacid. Ulcers may also cause heartburn, nausea or vomiting, and a bloated or full feeling during or after meals.

Ulcers can cause bleeding in the stomach, which may produce black or tarry bowel movements. Without treatment, ulcers may occasionally cause obstruction or break through (perforate) the stomach lining.

Bleeding and perforation are serious situations that require immediate treatment.

Ulcers – continued

Home Treatment

- Avoid foods that seem to bring on symptoms. It isn't necessary to eliminate any particular food from your diet (although milk and milk products slow healing and should be avoided).

- Eliminate alcohol, caffeine, and spicy foods if they seem to worsen symptoms.

- Try eating smaller, more frequent meals. If it doesn't help, return to a regular diet.

- Stop smoking. People who smoke are twice as likely to develop ulcers as nonsmokers. Smoking also slows healing of ulcers.

- Do not take aspirin or ibuprofen. Try acetaminophen instead.

- Antacids are usually needed to neutralize stomach acid and allow the ulcer to heal. Talk with your doctor about the best dose. You may need frequent large doses to do the job. Nonabsorbable antacids like Maalox, Mylanta, and Gelusil are often best. If you are on a low-salt diet, talk with your doctor or pharmacist before choosing an antacid. Some antacids have a high sodium content.

- Too much stress may slow ulcer healing. Practice the relaxation techniques on page 252.

When to Call Kaiser Permanente

- If pain occurs with shortness of breath or other symptoms that suggest heart problems. See Chest Pain on page 98.

- If pain localizes to one area of the abdomen.

- If increasing pain in the lower right abdomen occurs with vomiting and fever.

- If stools are deep red, black, or tarry. This usually means there is blood in the stool. Ulcers are one of many possible causes of this condition, which needs to be evaluated.

- If you have an ulcer and develop sudden severe abdominal pain that is not relieved by your usual home treatment.

- If you suspect an ulcer, and your symptoms have not improved after two weeks of home treatment. Your doctor can evaluate your symptoms and prescribe a treatment plan that may include antacids or other medications.

- To discuss your use of prescription anti-inflammatory drugs with your doctor.

Stand up straight!
Mom

Chapter 5

Back and Neck Pain

Although back and neck pain are usually preventable, most of us will suffer from one or both at some time in our lives. Fortunately, nine out of ten acute back injuries will heal on their own within 8 to 12 weeks.

By following the prevention and home treatment guidelines in this chapter, you can recover from most back and neck pain and prevent it from recurring.

Quick Reference Guide:

- First aid for back pain, page 56.
- Back pain due to arthritis, page 69.
- Neck pain, page 65.

Back Pain

Your back is made up of the bones of the spine (vertebrae that support body weight), their joints (facets that guide the direction of the movement of the spine), the discs (which separate the vertebrae and absorb shock as you move), and the muscles and ligaments that hold it all together. One or more of these structures can be injured:

- You can strain or sprain the ligaments or muscles from a sudden movement, improper movement, or through overuse.

- You can damage your discs in the same ways so that they tear or stretch. If the tear is large enough, it may press against a nerve. The nerve may also become irritated due to swelling or inflammation of the other parts of the back.

Any of these injuries can result in a two- or three-day period of acute pain and swelling in the injured tissue, followed by slow healing and a gradual reduction in pain. The pain may be felt in the low back, in the buttock, or down the leg (sometimes called sciatica). The goals of self-care are to relieve pain, promote healing, and avoid reinjury.

First Aid for Back Pain

When you first feel a catch or strain in your back, try these steps to avoid or reduce expected pain. These are the most important home treatments for the first few days of back pain. Also see Home Treatment on page 63.

First Aid #1: Ice

As soon as possible, apply ice or a cold pack to your injured back (10 to 15 minutes every hour). Cold limits swelling, reduces pain, and speeds healing.

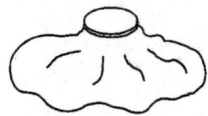

Ice

First Aid #2: Pelvic tilts

This exercise gently moves the spine and stretches the lower back.

- Lie on your back with knees bent and feet flat on the floor.

- Slowly tighten your stomach muscles and press your lower back against the floor. Hold for 10 seconds (do not hold your breath). Slowly relax.

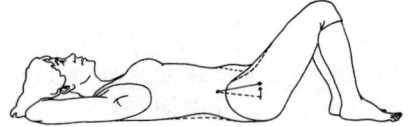

Pelvic tilt

First Aid #3: Walk

Take a short walk (three to five minutes) on a level surface (no inclines) every three hours. Walk only distances you can manage without pain, especially leg pain.

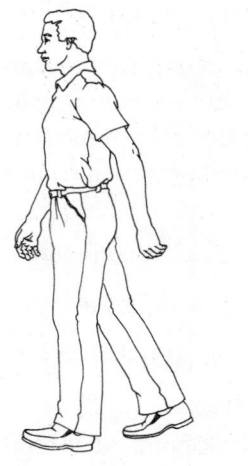

Walk

Back Pain – continued

In addition to the injuries discussed above, back pain can also be caused by other conditions that affect the bones and joints of the spine. Arthritis pain may be a steady ache, unlike the sharp, acute pain of strains, sprains, or disc injuries. If you think your back pain may be caused by arthritis, combine the self-care guidelines for back pain with those for arthritis on page 69. Osteoporosis causes weakening of the bones of the spine, which can cause bone degeneration, and lead to varying degrees of pain. See page 79.

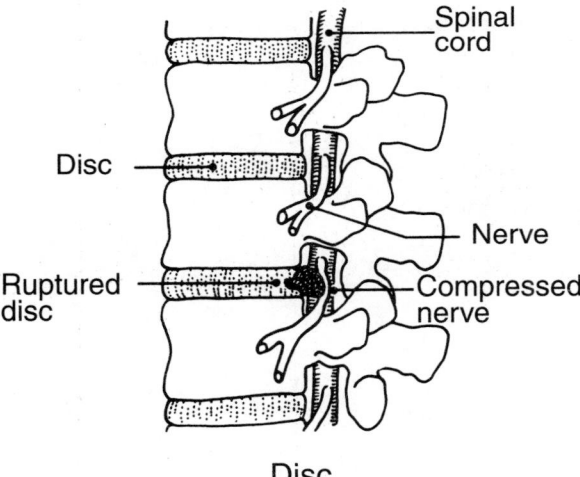

Disc

Spinal cord

Ruptured disc

Nerve

Compressed nerve

Disc

Prevention

The frequency of back pain has increased dramatically in all developed countries. The more time we spend sitting at desks, in cars, or in front of the TV, the more we must do to prevent back pain. Good posture and body mechanics will reduce the stress on your back. Exercise (stretching, strengthening, and aerobic exercise)

Sciatica

Sciatica is an irritation of the sciatic nerve, which runs from the lower back down through the buttocks and to the feet. It can result when an injured disc presses against the nerve. Its main symptom is radiating pain, numbness, or weakness that can be worse in the leg than in the back. In addition to the Home Treatment for back pain on page 63, the following may help:

- Avoid sitting if possible, unless it is more comfortable than standing.

- Alternate lying down with short walks. Increase the distance as you are able to tolerate without pain.

- An ice or cold pack will probably do the most good placed in the middle of your lower back. See page 85.

---

will help maintain your flexibility, strengthen the muscles that support your spine, and maintain your overall fitness. Maintaining an ideal body weight also reduces the load on your lower back.

Back Posture

Improper posture puts too much stress on your back and can lead to discomfort and damage. The key to good back posture is to keep the right amount of curve in your lower back. Too much curve ("swayback") or too little curve ("flat back") can result in problems. Just the right amount of curve is called the "neutral position."

Back Pain – continued

Standing and Walking

When you stand and walk with good posture, your ear, shoulder, hip, and ankle should be in a line. Do not lock your knees. Keep your low back in the neutral position.

Sitting

When you sit, keep your shoulders back and down, chin back, abdomen in, and your lower back supported in the neutral position. Slouching can stress the ligaments and muscles in your lower back.

• Avoid sitting in one position for more than one hour at a time. Get up or change positions often.

• If you must sit a lot, the exercises on page 61 are particularly important.

• If your chair doesn't give enough support, use a small pillow or rolled towel to support your lower back.

• See the illustration of proper sitting posture on page 66.

• To rise from a chair, keep your back in the neutral position and scoot forward to the edge of the chair. Use your leg muscles to stand up without leaning forward at the waist.

• For driving, pull your seat forward so that the pedals and steering wheel are within comfortable reach. Your forearms should be parallel to the floor. Stop often to stretch and walk around.

Sleeping

A firm bed is better than a soft mattress or waterbed. Sleep so that your back is in the neutral position.

• If you sleep on your back, you may want to use a towel roll to support your lower back or a pillow under your knees.

• If you sleep on your side, try placing a pillow between your knees.

• To rise from bed, lie on your side, bend both knees, and drop your feet over the side of the bed as you push with both arms to sit up. Scoot to the edge of the bed and position your feet under your buttocks. Stand up, keeping your back in the neutral position.

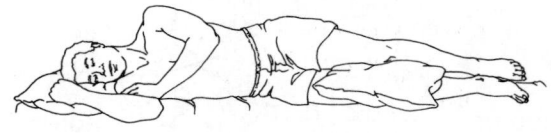

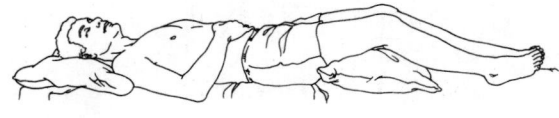

Sleeping positions

Body Mechanics

Good body mechanics means practicing good posture during daily activities. Use good body mechanics all the time, not just when you have back pain.

- Keep your back in the neutral position.

- When doing activities that require you to stay in one position for long periods, take regular breaks to stretch and restore the neutral position of your back.

- For prolonged standing activities, stand with one foot on a small stool.

Lifting

- Bend your knees and use your legs to lift. Tighten your buttocks and abdomen to further support your back. Let your arms and legs do the work. Do not bend forward from the waist to lift.

- Keep your upper back straight and your lower back in the neutral position.

- Keep the load as close to your body as possible, even if it is light.

- Avoid turning or twisting your body while holding a heavy object. Turn your feet, not your back.

- Never lift a heavy object above shoulder level.

- Get close to objects you are reaching for. Use a stool or ladder for items that are above your head. Keep the ladder or stool close to what you are doing.

- Use a hand truck or ask someone to help with heavy or awkward objects.

Exercises to Prevent Back Pain

Both the exercises in this chapter and general aerobic exercise (such as walking, swimming, cycling) are important to prevent back injury and pain. They will also speed your recovery from injuries and decrease chronic pain.

These exercises are *not recommended* for use during a back pain attack or spasm. Instead, see First Aid for Back Pain on page 56.

- You do not need to do every exercise. Stick with the ones that help you most.

- If any exercise causes increasing or continuing back pain, stop the exercise and try something else. Stop any exercise that causes the pain to radiate away from your spine into your buttocks or legs, either during or after the exercises.

- Start with five repetitions three to four times a day, and gradually increase to 10 repetitions. Do all exercises slowly.

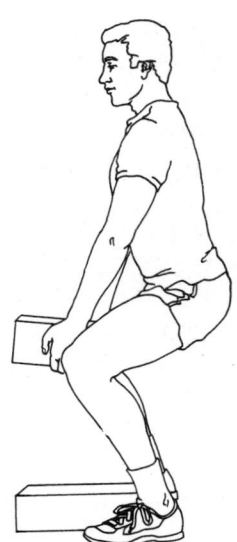

Proper lifting posture

Back Pain – continued

The basic types of exercises that can help your back include: flexion, extension, and stretching and strengthening.

Flexion exercises stretch the lower back muscles and strengthen the stomach muscles.

Extension exercises strengthen your lower back muscles and stretch the stomach muscles and ligaments.

Flexion Exercises

1. Curl-ups

Curl-ups strengthen your abdominal muscles, which work with your back muscles to support your spine.

- Lie on your back with knees bent (60° angle) and feet flat on the floor, arms crossed on your chest. Do not hook your feet under anything.

- Slowly curl your head and shoulders up until your shoulder blades barely rise from the floor. Keep your lower back pressed to the floor. To avoid neck problems, remember to lift your shoulders and do not force your head up or forward. Hold for 5 to 10 seconds (do not hold your breath), then curl down very slowly.

2. Knee-to-Chest

The knee-to-chest exercise stretches the low back and hamstring muscles and relieves pressure on the bone facets where the vertebrae come together.

- Lie on your back with knees bent and feet close to buttocks.

- Bring one knee to your chest at a time, keeping the other foot flat on the floor, or the other leg straight, whichever feels better on your lower back. Hold for 5 to 10 seconds.

- Relax and lower knees to starting position.

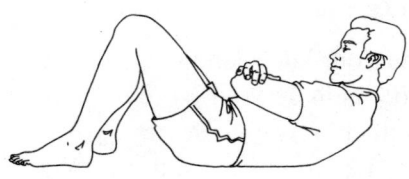

1. Curl-ups

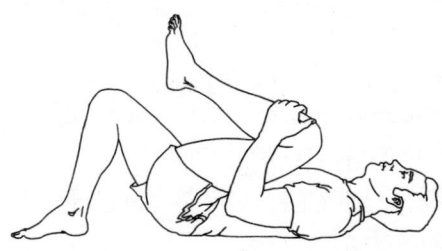

2. Knee-to-chest

Extension Exercises

3. Press-ups

Begin and end every set of exercises with a few press-ups (see illustration).

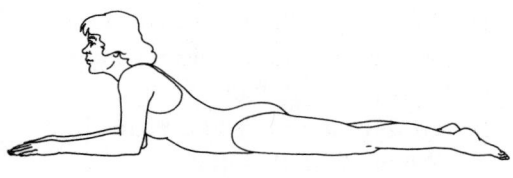

3. Press-ups

- Lie face down with hands at shoulders, palms flat on floor.

- Prop yourself up on your elbows, keeping lower half of body relaxed. If it's comfortable, press your chest forward.

- Keep hips pressed to the floor. Feel the stretch in your lower back.

- Lower upper body to the floor. Repeat 3 to 10 times, slowly.

4. Shoulder Presses

Shoulder presses strengthen the back muscles that support the spine.

- Lie on your back with your arms beside your body, head supported by a small pillow.

- Press your head and arms straight into the floor as much as you can without pain. Don't hold your breath.

5. Backward Bend

Practice the backward bend at least once a day and whenever you work in a bent-forward position.

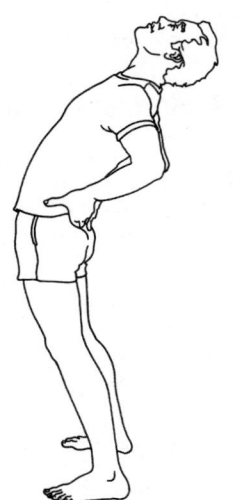

5. Backward bend

- Stand upright with your feet slightly apart. Back up to a counter top for greater support and stability. See illustration.

- Place your hands in the small of your back and gently bend backward. Keep your knees straight (not locked) and bend only at the waist.

- Hold the backward stretch for one to two seconds.

Back Pain – continued

Strengthening and Stretching Exercises

6. Prone Buttocks Squeeze

This exercise strengthens the buttocks muscles, which support the back and aid in lifting with the legs.

- Lie flat on your stomach with your arms at your sides.

- Slowly tighten your buttocks muscles. Hold for 5 to 10 seconds (do not hold your breath). Slowly relax.

- You may need to place a small pillow under your stomach for comfort.

7. Pelvic Tilts

See illustration on page 56.

8. Hamstring Stretch

This stretches the muscles in the back of your thigh that allow you to bend your legs while keeping your back in the neutral position. See illustration.

- Lie on your back in a doorway with one leg through the doorway on the floor and the leg you want to stretch straight up with the heel resting on the wall next to the doorway.

- Keep the leg straight and slowly move your heel up the wall until you feel a gentle pull in the back of your thigh. Do not overstretch.

- Relax in that position for 30 seconds, then bend the knee to relieve the stretch. Repeat with the other leg.

9. Hip Flexor Stretch

This stretches the muscles in the front of your hip, which avoids "swayback" caused by tight hip muscles. See illustration.

- Kneel on one knee with your other leg bent and foot in front of you. Keep your back in the neutral position.

- Slowly shift your weight onto your front foot, maintaining your back in the neutral position. Hold for 10 seconds. You should feel a stretch in the groin of the leg you are kneeling on. Repeat with the other leg.

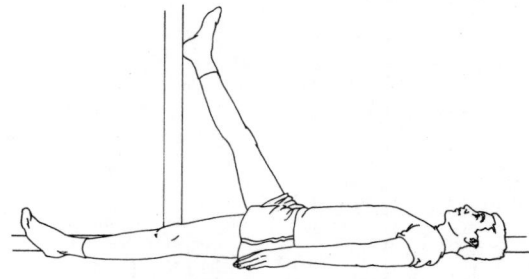

8. Hamstring stretch

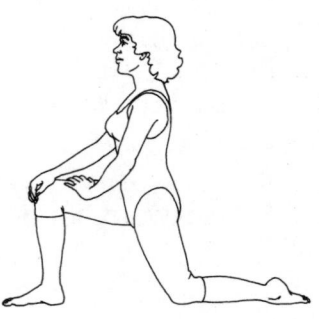

9. Hip flexor stretch

Exercises to Avoid

Many common exercises actually increase the risk of low back pain. Avoid the following:

- Straight leg sit-ups

- Bent leg sit-ups during acute back pain (may be safe if back is kept neutral)

- Leg lifts (lifting both legs while lying on your back)

- Lifting heavy weights above the waist (military press, biceps curls while standing)

- Any stretching done while sitting with the legs in a V

- Toe touches while standing

Home Treatment

For the first two to three days: Immediately after an injury and for the next few days, the most important home treatment includes:

- Get in a comfortable position and apply cold to the injured area. See the icing guidelines on page 85. Apply cold packs or ice for 15 to 20 minutes three to four times a day or up to once an hour for at least the first three days. Cold decreases inflammation, swelling, and pain.

- Sit or lie in positions that are most comfortable and reduce your pain, especially any leg pain.

- Do not sit up in bed, and avoid soft couches and twisted positions. Avoid positions that worsen your symptoms, such as sitting for long periods of time. Follow the posture and body mechanics guidelines discussed earlier.

- Do the first aid exercises on page 56 three to four times a day.

- Bed rest can help relieve back pain but may not speed healing. Stick with what makes you feel better. Unless you have severe leg pain, one to three days of rest should relieve pain. More than three days is not recommended and could actually delay healing. Try one of the following positions: (see illustrations on page 58.)

   ○ Lie on your back with your knees bent and supported by large pillows, or on the floor with your legs on the seat of a sofa or chair.

   ○ Lie on your side with your knees and hips bent and a pillow between your legs.

Back Pain – continued

- Take aspirin or ibuprofen regularly as directed (call your doctor if you've been told to avoid anti-inflammatory medications). Acetaminophen may also be used. Take these medications sensibly; the maximum recommended dose will reduce the pain. Masking the pain completely might allow movement that could lead to reinjury.

- Take short walks (three to five minutes every three hours) on level surfaces (no inclines) as soon as you can to keep your muscles strong. Only walk distances that you can manage without pain, especially leg pain.

- Relax your muscles. See page 252 for progressive muscle relaxation.

- See Resources 19 and 20 on page 308.

After two to three days of home treatment:

- Continue daily walks (increase to 5 to 10 minutes three to four times a day) and the exercises above.

- Try swimming, which is good for your back. It may be painful immediately after a back injury, but lap swimming or kicking with swim fins is often helpful to prevent back pain from recurring.

- When your pain has improved, begin easy exercises that do not increase your pain. One or two of the exercises in the Prevention section (pages 59 to 62) may be helpful. Start with 5 repetitions twice a day and increase to 10 repetitions as you are able.

When to Call Kaiser Permanente

- If you have loss of bowel and/or bladder control. Although constipation and frequent or urgent urination are common in people with low back pain, any new problems with bowel or bladder control should be discussed with your doctor.

- If you have new numbness in the genital or rectal area.

- If you have leg weakness that is not solely due to pain. Many people with low back pain say their legs feel weak. However, significant leg weakness should be evaluated, especially if you are unable to bend your foot upward, get out of a chair, or climb stairs.

- If you have new or increased back pain with unexplained fever and/or painful urination or other signs of urinary tract infection. See page 184.

- If you have a dramatic increase in your chronic back pain, especially if it is unrelated to a new or changed physical activity.

- If you have a history of cancer or HIV infection and develop a new or increased back pain.

- If you have new back pain that does not improve after one week of home treatment, contact your doctor for advice.

- If you develop a new, severe pain in your lower back that does not increase with movement and is not related to stress or muscle tension.

- If chronic back pain does not improve after two weeks of home treatment.

Back Surgery

Doctors recommend back surgery much less often now than in the past. Rest, posture changes, and exercise can relieve 90 percent of back problems, even disc problems.

Surgery is often appropriate for certain conditions that do not improve with the usual treatment. If you do plan to have surgery, the posture and body mechanics guidelines and exercises in this chapter are still important. A strong, flexible back is important to a quick recovery after surgery.

Medical Doctors

In addition to diagnosing the cause of back pain and evaluating back injuries, a medical doctor may also:

• Help you develop an individualized exercise and home care plan or modified work plan if needed.

• Prescribe muscle relaxants, anti-inflammatory drugs, and pain relievers. Note: If you do get a strong painkiller or muscle relaxer, take special care to avoid postures and activities that could reinjure your back.

• Suggest physical therapy.

• Recommend back surgery.

Physical Therapists

After the initial first-aid actions, a physical therapist with training in orthopedic treatment can help you:

• Identify specific muscle or disc problems.

• Provide other therapies if you aren't improving.

• Help you improve your posture and customize an exercise program for recovery and long-term protection.

Other Professionals

Chiropractors, acupuncturists, massage therapists, and others may also provide short-term relief.

Neck Pain

Neck pain and stiffness are usually caused by strain or spasm of the neck muscles or inflammation of the neck joints. It may occasionally be due to arthritis or damage to the discs between the neck (cervical) vertebrae. Neck movement may be limited, usually more to one side than the other. Headaches often come with neck problems.

Neck pain and headaches are sometimes related to tension in the trapezius muscles, which run from the back of the head across the back of the shoulder. When you have neck pain, you may also notice that these muscles feel tight and painful.

Neck problems often cause pain in the shoulder, upper back, or down the arm.

Neck muscle strain may be due to:

• Forward head posture

• Sleeping on a pillow that's too high, too flat, or doesn't support your head

• Sleeping on your stomach or with the neck twisted or bent

Neck Pain – continued

- Extended periods of the "thinker's pose" (resting your forehead on your upright fist or arm)

- Watching TV or reading lying down with the neck in an awkward position

- Stress

- Workstation that puts the neck in an awkward position

- Other pressures on the neck muscles

- Injury that causes sudden movement of the head and neck (whiplash) or a direct blow to the neck

- Strenous activity with the upper body and arms

Meningitis is a serious illness that causes a severe stiff neck with headache and fever. If these three symptoms occur together, see a doctor promptly.

Prevention

Good posture, body mechanics, and exercise are important to preventing neck pain. Most neck pain that isn't due to arthritis or an injury is completely avoidable.

If pain is worse at the **end of the day**, evaluate your posture and body mechanics during the day.

- Sit straight in your chair with your low back supported. Avoid sitting for long periods without getting up or changing positions. Take mini-breaks several times each hour to stretch your neck muscles.

- If you work at a computer, adjust the monitor so that the top of the screen is at eye level. Use a document holder that puts the copy at the same level as the screen.

- If you use the telephone a lot, consider a headset or speaker phone.

- Adjust your car seat to a more upright position that supports your head and lower back.

If neck stiffness is worse **in the morning**, check your sleeping posture (and your activities the day before).

- Improve your sleeping support. A hard mattress or special neck support pillow may solve the problem (try before buying). Or, you can fold a towel lengthwise into a four-inch wide pad, wrap it around your neck, and pin it for good support.

- Avoid pillows that force your head forward when you are sleeping on your back.

- When sleeping on your side, make sure your nose is in line with the center of your body.

- If stress is a factor, practice the progressive muscle relaxation exercises on page 252.

- Strengthen and protect your neck by doing neck exercises once a day. See page 68.

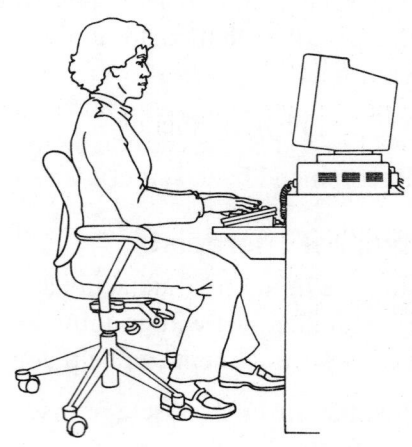

Proper sitting posture

Home Treatment

Much of the home treatment for back pain is also helpful for neck pain, including the guidelines on posture, body mechanics, and ice. Also see page 63.

- Place a cold pack over painful muscles for 10 to 15 minutes at a time. Do this as often as once an hour. It will help decrease any pain, muscle spasm, or swelling. If the problem is near the shoulder or upper back, it will usually help more to ice the back of the neck.

- Keep your head and neck in the neutral position over your body. Avoid slouching or forward head posture.

- Aspirin, ibuprofen, or acetaminophen can help relieve pain.

- Walking is also helpful in relieving and preventing neck pain. The gentle swinging motion of your arms often relieves pain. Start with short walks of 5 to 10 minutes, three to four times a day.

- The exercises on page 68 will help maintain your flexibility and strength. Start with 5 repetitions twice a day. Gradually increase to 10 repetitions.

- If neck pain occurs with headache, see Tension Headaches on page 129.

- Once the pain subsides, do the prevention exercises every two to three hours. Stop doing any exercise that causes pain.

- See Resource 62 on page 310.

When to Call Kaiser Permanente

- Call *immediately* if stiff neck occurs together with headache and fever. Also see "Encephalitis and Meningitis" on page 102.

- If the pain extends or shoots down one arm, or you have numbness or tingling in your hands.

- If you develop new weakness in the arms or legs.

- If a blow or injury to the neck (whiplash) has caused new pain.

- If you are unable to manage the pain with home treatment.

- If the pain has lasted two weeks or longer without improvement despite home treatment.

Neck Exercises

Stop any exercise that increases pain. Start with five repetitions twice a day. Do each exercise slowly.

1. Dorsal glide: Sit or stand tall, looking straight ahead (a "palace guard" posture). Slowly tuck your chin as you glide your head backwards over your body. Hold for a count of five, then relax. Repeat 6 to 10 times. This stretches the back of the neck. If you feel pain, do not glide so far back. Some people find this exercise easier while lying on their back with ice on the neck.

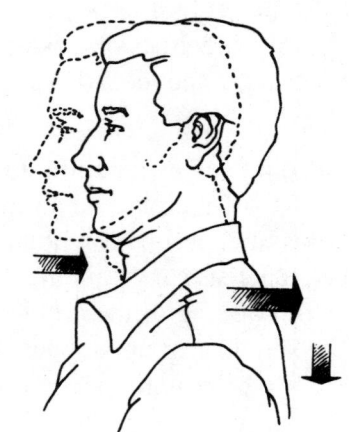

Dorsal glide

2. Move your head backward, forward, and side to side against gentle pressure from your hands, holding each position for several seconds. Repeat 6 to 10 times.

3. Chest and shoulder stretch: Sit or stand tall and glide your head over your body as in exercise 1. Raise both arms so that your hands are next to your ears. As you exhale, lower your elbows down and back. Feel your shoulder blades slide down and together. Hold for a few seconds. Relax and repeat.

4. Do 6 to 10 shoulder presses as described on page 61.

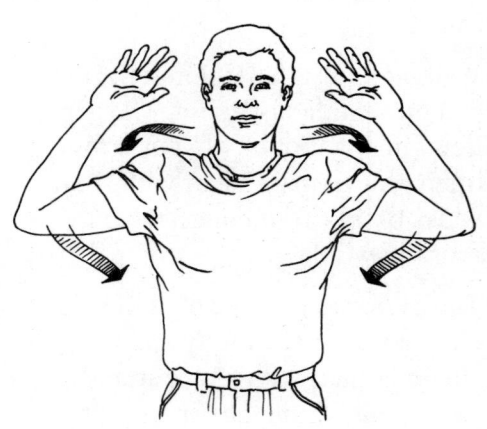

Chest and shoulder stretch

I don't deserve this award, but then I have arthritis
and I don't deserve that either.
Jack Benny

Chapter 6

Bone, Muscle, and Joint Problems

Our aches and pains remind us that life isn't always easy. But pain can be managed. This chapter covers pain from arthritis to ankle sprains. The focus is less on reducing pain and more on limiting its impact on our quality of life. As with most chapters in this book, we hope you rarely have to refer to these pages. But when you do, we hope these guidelines will make your life more comfortable.

Arthritis

Arthritis refers to a variety of joint problems that cause pain, swelling, and stiffness. Simply put, arthritis means inflammation of a joint. Arthritis can occur at any age, but it affects older people the most.

There are over 100 different types of arthritis, each with its own specific symptoms. Little is known about what causes most types. Some seem to run in families; others seem to be related to imbalances in body chemistry or immune system problems.

The chart on page 70 describes the three most common kinds of arthritis. Osteoarthritis is the most common type and can usually be successfully managed at home. Rheumatoid arthritis and gout will improve with a combination of self-care and professional care.

Prevention

It may not be possible to prevent arthritis, but you can prevent a lot of pain by being kind to your joints. This is especially important if you already have arthritis.

Arthritis – continued

- Avoid repeated jarring activities, such as high-impact aerobic activities.

- Control your weight.

- Exercise regularly.

While repeated jarring activities can increase joint pain, regular exercise can relieve or prevent it. Exercise is needed to nourish the joint cartilage and remove waste products. It also strengthens the muscles around the joint. Strong muscles support the joint and reduce injuries caused by fatigue. Stretching maintains your range of pain-free motion.

Home Treatment

- Rest sore joints. Avoid activities that put weight or strain on the joint for a few days. Take short rest breaks from your regular activities through-out the day.

- Put each of your joints gently through its full range of motion one to two times each day.

- If the joint is not swollen, apply moist heat for 20 to 30 minutes two to three times a day. Do not apply heat to a swollen, inflamed joint. A warm shower or bath may help relieve morning stiffness. Try to avoid sitting still after a warm shower or bath.

Common Types of Arthritis

Type	Cause	Symptoms	Comments
Osteoarthritis	Breakdown of joint cartilage	Pain, stiffness, and swelling; common in fingers, hips, and knees.	Most common type for both women and men between the ages of 45 and 90.
Rheumatoid Arthritis	Inflammation of the membrane lining the joint	Pain, stiffness, swelling in multiple joints; joints may be "hot" and red; common in hands, wrists, and feet.	Occurs most often around age 30 to 40; more common in women.
Gout	Build-up of uric acid crystals in the joint fluid	Sudden onset of burning pain, stiffness, and swelling; common in big toe, ankle, knee, wrist, elbow.	Most common in men over 40; may be aggravated by alcohol and organ meats.

- Apply cold packs to inflamed, swollen joints for 10 to 15 minutes, once an hour. Cold will help relieve pain and reduce inflammation (although it may be uncomfortable for the first few minutes).

- Regular exercise is important to help maintain strength and flexibility in the muscles and joints.

- Strengthening exercises protect against the muscle decline that leads to loss of function. Try low-impact activities, such as swimming, water aerobics, biking, or walking.

- Acetaminophen can provide safe pain relief for osteoarthritis. Aspirin or ibuprofen also help ease pain, but can cause stomach upset. Do not use anti-inflammatory medications (aspirin, ibuprofen, naproxen, etc.) together. See page 300 for dosage information and the symptoms of aspirin overdose.

- Enroll in an arthritis self-management program. Participants usually have less pain and fewer limitations on their activities. See Resource 16 on page 308.

When to Call Kaiser Permanente

- If you have fever or skin rash along with severe joint pain.

- If the pain is so great that you cannot use the joint.

- If there is sudden, unexplained swelling, redness, or pain in any joint.

- If there is severe pain and swelling in multiple joints.

- If you experience sudden back pain that occurs with numbness in the legs or loss of bowel or bladder control.

- If the problem continues for over six weeks and home treatment is not helping.

- If you experience side effects of large doses of aspirin or other arthritis medication (stomach pain, nausea, persistent heartburn, or dark tarry stools). Do not exceed recommended doses of over-the-counter medications without your doctor's advice.

Bunions and Hammertoes

A **bunion** is a swelling of the joint at the base of the big toe. The big toe may bend toward and overlap the other toes. A **hammertoe** is a toe that bends up permanently at the middle joint. Both conditions are usually irritated by wearing shoes that are too short or narrow. These problems sometimes run in families.

Prevention

- Wear shoes with no heel (or a low heel) and a roomy toe box. Tennis or basketball court shoes are often best. Make sure that your shoes fit properly. Tight or high-heeled shoes increase the risk of bunions and hammertoes and irritate them if they are already present.

Bunions – continued

Home Treatment

Once you have a bunion or hammertoe, there is usually no way to completely get rid of it. Home treatment will help keep it from getting worse.

- Wear low-heeled, roomy shoes that have good arch support.

- Cut out the area over the bunion or hammertoe from an old pair of shoes to wear around the house, or wear comfortable sandals that don't press on the area.

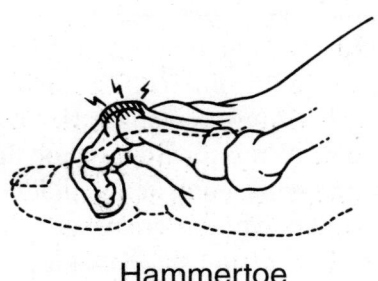

Hammertoe

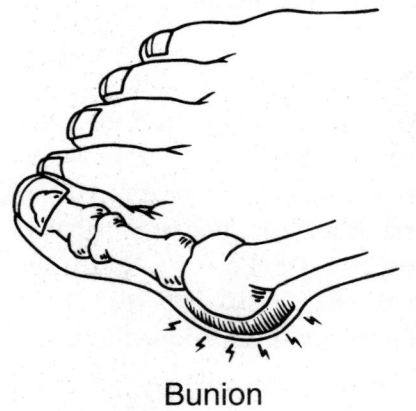

Bunion

- Cushion the bunion or hammertoe with moleskin or donut-shaped pads to prevent rubbing and irritation.

- Try aspirin, ibuprofen, or acetaminophen to relieve pain. Ice or cold packs may also help.

When to Call Kaiser Permanente

- If severe pain in the big toe came on suddenly, and you have not been diagnosed with gout.

- If pain does not respond to home treatment in two to three weeks.

- If severe pain interferes with walking or daily activities.

- If the big toe begins to overlap the second toe.

- If you have diabetes, poor circulation, or peripheral vascular disease. Irritated skin over a bunion or hammer toe can easily become infected in people with these conditions.

Bursitis and Tendinitis

A bursa is a small sac of fluid that helps the muscles slide easily over other muscles or bones. Injury or overuse of a joint or tendon may result in pain, redness, heat, and inflammation of the bursa, a condition known as bursitis. Bursitis often develops quickly, over just a few days, often after a specific injury or excessive use (overuse).

Tendons are tough, rope-like fibers that connect muscles to bones. Injury or overuse may cause pain, tenderness, and inflammation in the tendons or the tissues surrounding them, a condition known as tendinitis. Both bursitis and tendinitis can also be related to job, sports, or household activities that require repeated twisting or rapid joint movements.

Bursitis and tendinitis can occur at several different places in the body, and both can occur at the same time in a single area. The same home treatment is good for both problems.

Prevention

Regular warm-ups and stretching may help prevent bursitis or tendinitis. Warm up well before exercising, gradually increase the intensity of the activity, and stretch afterwards. See below for additional joint-specific prevention tips.

Home Treatment

Bursitis or tendinitis will usually go away or at least subside in a few days or weeks if you avoid the activity that caused it.

The most common mistake in recovery is thinking that your problem is gone when the pain is gone. Chances are, bursitis or tendinitis will recur if you do not take steps to strengthen and stretch the muscles around the joint, and change the way you do some activities.

- Rest the inflamed area. Change the way you do the activity that causes pain so that you can do it without

---

> **Bone, Muscle, and Joint Problems**
>
> In many cases, you can determine the cause of bone, muscle, or joint problems by thinking back to how the pain started.
>
> Traumatic injuries (turning an ankle or twisting a knee) usually cause **Strains, Sprains, or Fractures.** See page 82.
>
> A single episode of overuse or repeated heavy use of a joint can cause **Bursitis or Tendinitis.** See page 72.
>
> Joint pain that comes on gradually and seems unrelated to any specific injury may be due to **Arthritis** (see page 69) or poor posture (see page 57).

pain. See below for joint-specific guidelines. To maintain fitness, substitute activities that don't stress the inflamed area.

- As soon as you notice pain, apply ice or cold packs for 10-minute periods, once an hour for 72 hours. Continue applying ice (15 to 20 minutes, three times a day) as long as it relieves pain. See page 85. Although heating pads or hot baths may feel good, ice or cold packs will relieve inflammation and speed healing.

- Aspirin or ibuprofen may help ease pain and inflammation, but don't use medication to relieve pain while you continue overusing a joint. See page 300 for dosage.

Bursitis and Tendinitis – cont.

- Gently move the joint through as full a range of motion as you can without pain several times a day to prevent stiffness. As the pain subsides, continue stretching and add exercises to strengthen the affected muscles.

- Warm up before and stretch after the activity. Apply ice to the injured area after exercise to prevent pain and swelling.

- Gradually resume the activity at a lower intensity. Increase slowly and only if pain does not recur.

In addition to the general prevention and home treatment information for bursitis and tendinitis above, the following tips will be useful if you have a specific joint problem:

Wrist pain may be due to tendinitis in the wrist. See the home treatment for Carpal Tunnel Syndrome on page 76.

Tennis elbow and **golfer's elbow** are due to tendinitis in the forearm muscle tendons. Tennis elbow causes pain on the outside of the elbow where the muscles that bend the wrist back attach. Golfer's elbow causes pain on the inside of the elbow where the muscles that bend the wrist down attach.

- Strengthen the wrist, arm, shoulder, and back muscles to help protect the elbow.

- A brace or elbow sleeve may help relieve pain.

- Use tools with larger handles.

- Use a two-handed tennis backhand and a midsize, more flexible racquet.

- Avoid hitting divots in golf.

- Avoid side-arm pitching and throwing curve balls.

- Support a sore elbow with a sling for one to two days. Do not use a sling for more than two days. Do range-of-motion exercises daily to prevent stiffness.

Shoulder pain that occurs on the outside of the upper arm is often due to tendinitis or bursitis in the shoulder joint. Pain on the top of the shoulder closer to the neck is often due to tension in the trapezius muscles, which extend from the back of the head down to the tip of the shoulders. See Neck Pain on page 65.

- Use proper throwing techniques for baseball and football.

- Use a different swim stroke: breast stroke or sidestroke instead of the crawl or butterfly.

- Do not rest a sore shoulder with a sling for more than two days. Keep the elbow at your side, not in front of your body. Do range-of-motion exercises 10 times daily to prevent stiffness.

Hip pain: Tendinitis or bursitis in the hip can cause pain at the side of the hip when rising from a chair and for the first few steps, while climbing stairs, or while driving. If pain is severe, sleeping on your side may also be painful. Hip pain may also be due to arthritis. See page 69.

- Wear well-cushioned shoes and avoid high heels.

- Walk up and down stairs one at a time, leading with your strong leg, until the pain is gone.

- Avoid activities that force one side of the pelvis higher than the other, such as running in only one direction on a track or working sideways on a slope. Keep the pelvis level.

- Sleep on your uninjured side with a pillow between your knees, or on your back with pillows beneath your knees.

- See the hip stretches on page 62. Stretch after activity, when your muscles are warm.

Knee pain may be caused by bursitis or tendinitis. See Knee Problems on page 77.

Heel or foot pain may be due to plantar fasciitis or to Achilles tendinitis. See page 80. Shin-splints will cause pain in the front of the lower leg. See page 78.

When to Call Kaiser Permanente

- If there is fever, rapid swelling, and redness, or an inability to use a joint.

- If severe pain continues when the joint is at rest and you have applied ice.

- If the problem is severe and you can think of no injury or activity that might have caused it.

- If the pain persists for two weeks or longer despite home treatment. Your doctor or physical therapist can help you develop a specific exercise and home treatment plan. Medication may be used for severe cases. Ask about the risks and alternatives before agreeing to any treatment.

Carpal Tunnel Syndrome

The carpal tunnel is a narrow passageway of bone and ligament in your wrist. The nerve that controls sensation in your fingers and some muscles in the hand passes through this tunnel along with some of the finger tendons. Repeated motion or use of the hand or wrist may cause the tendons to become inflamed and press the nerve against the bone. Pressure on the nerve causes pain and numbness in the hand and fingers. This is known as carpal tunnel syndrome (CTS).

The symptoms of CTS include:

- Numbness or tingling in one or both hands that involves all but the little finger.

- Wrist pain that may affect your fingers and radiate up your arm.

- Hand or wrist pain that is often greater at night and early morning.

Carpal tunnel syndrome can be caused by anything that causes swelling against the nerve; for example, a cyst on the tendon or rheumatoid arthritis. Most often, CTS is caused by inflammation due to overuse of the tendons from repetitive finger and hand movements in a bent-wrist position. Pregnancy, diabetes, underactive thyroid, and birth control pills increase the risk of CTS.

Carpal Tunnel – continued

Prevention

- Avoid repetitive hand motions with a bent wrist. Keep wrist straight for the following:

  ○ Writing, typing, drawing

  ○ Driving

  ○ Using power tools, pliers, or scissors

  ○ Playing piano or other musical instruments

  ○ Knitting, crocheting, needlepoint

- Take frequent breaks (five minutes each hour) from repetitive hand motions. Stretch your fingers and thumb and change your grip often.

- Learn to type with a soft touch.

- Maintain good posture. Avoid rounding your shoulders or slouching. See page 57.

Home Treatment

- Don't ignore wrist pain. If possible, stop the activity that triggered the problem. If the symptoms decrease, resume the activity gradually with a greater effort to keep the wrist straight.

- If you cannot stop the activity, try to change the way you do it so that your wrist is not stressed. Alternate tasks so that you don't spend more than one to two hours doing an activity involving your hands.

- Gently warm up your hands before starting work. Do some wrist circles and stretch your fingers and wrists. Repeat every hour.

- Use a wrist rest pad with your computer keyboard to help maintain the straight alignment of your wrist, but don't lean on it continuously.

- Use aspirin, ibuprofen, or acetaminophen to decrease pain.

- Apply ice or a cold pack to the palm side of the wrist. See "Ice and Cold Packs" on page 85.

- A wrist splint that keeps your wrist straight or slightly extended (no more than 15 degrees) may help relieve pain. Try to combine a splint with a real effort to change the activities that cause you pain. Wear the splint at night and when doing heavy lifting. You can buy a splint in some pharmacies and in hospital supply stores.

- When the pain is gone, begin arm and upper body strengthening exercises so you can maintain good posture and a straight wrist without the splint.

- Some people find that 50 mg of vitamin B6 taken twice a day helps relieve wrist pain. (Talk with your doctor before taking B_6.)

- Reducing the salt in your diet (see page 265) may help reduce water retention and relieve swelling in the wrist.

- Avoid sleeping on your hands.

When to Call Kaiser Permanente

A health professional can confirm the diagnosis, properly fit you with a splint or, in severe cases, recommend a surgical solution. Call a health professional:

- If the pain or numbness is severe and is not relieved by rest, changing positions, ice, or a normal dose of aspirin, ibuprofen, or acetaminophen.

- If your hand grip becomes weak.

- If minor symptoms do not improve after one month of prevention and home treatment.

- If any numbness remains after one month of home treatment. Long-term numbness can lead to *permanent* loss of some hand function.

Knee Problems

The knee is a vulnerable joint. It is basically just two long leg bones held together with ligaments and muscles. Problems develop when we put too much stress on the joint. The three most common knee problems are:

- Strained or sprained ligaments and muscles caused by a blow to the knee, forcing it in a direction that it does not normally bend. See Strains, Sprains, and Fractures on page 82.

- Kneecap pain, also known as patellofemoral pain. This problem causes pain around or behind the kneecap when running downhill,

going up or down stairs, or after sitting for long periods of time.

- Patellar tendinitis, also known as jumper's knee, is an inflammation of the tendon that attaches the kneecap (patella) to the shinbone (tibia). It is common in basketball and volleyball players.

Prevention

- The best way to prevent knee problems is to strengthen and stretch the leg muscles. Exercises that strengthen and stretch the hamstring and thigh muscles (quadriceps) are especially helpful. See page 248.

- Avoid deep knee bends.

- Avoid running downhill unless you are fully conditioned.

- Avoid shoes with cleats in contact sports.

- Wear shoes with good arch support. Replace running shoes every 300 to 500 miles.

- Avoid high-heeled shoes.

- Also see Bursitis and Tendinitis on page 72.

Home Treatment

- Apply ice to your knee. See "Ice and Cold Packs" on page 85.

- Reduce the activities that cause pain by at least half.

- A brace or elastic or neoprene sleeve or band with a hole for the kneecap that holds the kneecap in place may help ease pain during activity. You can buy one at a pharmacy or sporting goods store.

Growing Pains

Children age 6 to 12 often develop harmless "growing pains" in their legs at night. The cause is unknown. A heating pad, acetaminophen, or gentle massage of the legs may help.

Knee Problems – continued

- Stretch the front and back of your thigh (quadriceps and hamstring) muscles after exercise, when they are warm. See page 248.

- Also see Sprains on page 82 and Bursitis and Tendinitis on page 72.

- If knee pain is not due to a recent or past injury or related to exercise, see Arthritis on page 69.

When to Call Kaiser Permanente

- If the knee wobbles from side to side or "gives out."

- If you felt or heard a "pop" during a knee injury which was followed by immediate swelling.

- If you are unable to straighten the knee, or if the joint "locks."

- If knee is red, hot, swollen, and painful to touch.

- If pain is severe or does not substantially improve within two to five days.

Muscle Cramps and Leg Pain

Leg and muscle cramps ("charley horse" or "stitch") are common. They often occur during exercise, especially during hot weather, or at night. Dehydration or low levels of potassium in the body may cause cramps, as can using a muscle that is not stretched well.

Pain in the front of the lower leg may be due to shinsplints, especially if you have recently increased your exercise.

Arthritis can also cause leg pain (see page 69). Leg pain that runs from the buttocks down the back of the leg and into the foot may be due to sciatica. See page 57.

Phlebitis, an inflammation of a vein, also causes leg pain, usually in one leg. This condition can be serious if blood clots formed in the vein break loose and lodge in the lungs. It is most common after surgery or prolonged bed rest. Hardening of the arteries (atherosclerosis) in the leg can also cause pain that is worse during activity and is relieved by rest.

Prevention

- Warm up well and stretch before any activity. Stretch after exercise to keep hot muscles from shortening and cramping.

- Drink extra water before and during exercise, especially during hot or humid weather.

- Include plenty of potassium in your diet. Bananas, orange juice, and potatoes are good sources.

- To avoid stomach cramps ("stitches") during exercise, do side stretches before exercising and learn to breathe with your lower lungs. See page 252.

- If cramps wake you at night, take a warm bath and do some stretching exercises before bed. Keep your legs warm while sleeping.

Home Treatment

If there is pain, swelling, or heaviness in the calf of one leg only, or other symptoms that cause you to suspect phlebitis (see When to Call Kaiser Permanente below), call your doctor before attempting home treatment.

• Follow the prevention guidelines.

• Gently stretch the cramping muscle. Rub or massage the cramp.

• Straighten your leg, grab the foot, and pull it toward you to stretch the calf.

• Drink some extra water. Cramps are often related to dehydration.

• The best treatment for shin-splints is ice, aspirin, ibuprofen, or acetaminophen, and a week or two of rest followed by a gradual return to exercise. If healing is slow, consider the home treatment advice for stress fractures on page 84.

When to Call Kaiser Permanente

• If you have the following symptoms:

  ○ Pain deep in the leg or calf

  ○ Heat, redness, or pain along the course of a leg vein

  ○ Swelling of one leg

  ○ Leg is white or blue and cold

  ○ Shortness of breath or chest pain

• If leg cramps worsen or persist in spite of the prevention and home treatment.

• If cramps or leg pain occur repeatedly during even mild exercise, such as walking, even if relieved by rest.

Osteoporosis

Osteoporosis or "brittle bones" is a condition that affects 25 percent of women over age 60. It is much less common and not as severe in men. Osteoporosis is caused by loss of bone mass and strength. It is more common during menopause, when estrogen levels decline. Bones weakened by osteoporosis are easily broken. Risk factors for osteoporosis include thin body frame, Asian or Caucasian race, family history, and inactivity. Women who smoke or drink are also at greater risk.

Osteoporosis is a silent disease; there may be no symptoms until a bone breaks and the condition is recognized after X-rays. The first sign may be hip or low back pain, or painful swelling of a wrist after a fall.

Prevention

Start to build sturdy bones in childhood. Peak bone mass is reached during your twenties and thirties. These steps can help you build and keep strong bones throughout your life.

• Get regular weight-bearing exercise, such as walking. Exercise helps keep bones strong. See Chapter 17.

• Get plenty of calcium in your diet. The average American diet contains about 500 mg per day, but 1,000 mg are recommended. Pregnant women or mothers who are breast-feeding should get about 1,200 mg per day. After menopause, 1,000 to 1,500 mg are recommended. The best source of calcium is low-fat dairy products. See page 264.

Osteoporosis – continued

- If you are unable to get all the calcium you need from your diet, take two to three calcium carbonate tablets (TUMS) each day with meals or with milk. Don't take more than four to six tablets per day, and drink lots of water, since they can cause constipation.

- Don't smoke, and drink alcohol only in moderation (one drink per day), if at all.

When to Call Kaiser Permanente

- If you are at risk of osteoporosis and are nearing menopause, talk with your doctor about estrogen or hormone replacement therapy. It is the most effective way to prevent osteoporosis. See page 178.

- If a fall causes hip pain or if you are unable to get up after a fall.

- If you have sudden, unexplained back pain that does not improve after two to three days of home treatment.

Plantar Fasciitis

Plantar fasciitis is a condition that occurs when the thick, fibrous tissue that covers the bottom of your foot (plantar fascia) becomes inflamed and painful. Athletes (particularly runners), middle-aged people, and those who are overweight tend to develop plantar fasciitis. Repetitive exercises such as running and jumping sports can lead to heel pain and plantar fasciitis.

An excessive inward rolling of the foot during walking (called over-pronation) can also cause heel pain and plantar fasciitis. Overpronation can be due to poor arch support, worn-out shoes, tight calf muscles, or by running downhill or on uneven surfaces.

Achilles tendinitis can cause pain in the back of the heel.

A **heel spur** is a calcium buildup that may occur where the plantar fascia attaches to the heel. It does not change the treatment of plantar fasciitis.

Prevention

- Stretch your Achilles tendon and calf muscles several times a day (see page 248). Stretching is important for both athletes and nonathletes.

- Maintain a reasonable weight for your height.

- Wear good athletic shoes with well-cushioned soles and good arch supports. Replace shoes every few months because padding wears out.

- Establish good exercise habits. Increase mileage slowly, limit your running and training on uphill terrain, and run on softer surfaces (grass or dirt) rather than concrete.

- Cross-train by alternating running with different sports.

Home Treatment

Treating the first symptoms of plantar fasciitis with rest and ice can help prevent your heel pain from becoming chronic.

- Reduce all weight-bearing activities to a pain-free level.

- Apply ice to your heel. See "Ice and Cold Packs" on page 85.

- You may wish to try an over-the-counter arch support (Spenco).

- Do not go barefoot until the pain is completely gone. Support your arches during all weight-bearing activities, even going to the bathroom during the night. Wear shoes or arch-supporting sandals.

- For short-term pain relief, take aspirin or ibuprofen.

- Stretch the calf muscles. See page 248.

- For achilles tendinitis, try putting heel lifts in both shoes. Use them only until the pain is gone (continue other self-care).

- Avoid "running through the pain." Reduce your activity to a level that does not cause pain. Try low-impact activities such as cycling or swimming to speed healing.

- Do not return to high-impact activity until you have been pain-free for one week. When you do return, start slowly and ice your heel afterward. Continue for as long as the pain recurs.

When to Call Kaiser Permanente

- If heel pain occurs with fever, redness or heat in your heel, or if there is numbness or tingling in your heel.

- If pain continues when you are not standing or bearing any weight on your heel.

- If heel pain persists for one to two weeks despite home treatment.

Sports Injuries

Injuries are common among physically active people. Most sports injuries are due to either traumatic injury or overuse and can be avoided by proper conditioning, training, and equipment.

Traumatic injuries:

Strains, Sprains, and Fractures, page 82.

Stress fractures, page 83.

Turf toe, page 83.

Overuse injuries:

Tennis or golfer's elbow, page 74.

Patellar tendinitis, page 77.

Bursitis and Tendinitis, page 72.

Achilles tendinitis, page 80.

Plantar fasciitis, page 80.

Prevention

- Warm up before exercise. Cold, stiff muscles and ligaments are more susceptible to injury. Cool down and stretch after activities. See page 248.

- Increase the intensity and duration of activities and exercise gradually. As your fitness level improves, you will be able to do increasingly strenuous exercise without injury.

- Use proper sports techniques and equipment. For example, wear supportive, well-cushioned shoes for running, aerobics, and walking; use

Sports Injuries – continued

a two-handed tennis backhand stroke; wear protective pads for rollerskating. Make sure that your bicycle's seat and handlebars are adjusted properly for your body.

- Alternate hard workouts with easier ones to let your body rest. For example, if you run, alternate long, hard runs with shorter, easier ones. If you lift weights, don't work the same muscles two days in a row.

- Cross-train (do several activities regularly) to rest your muscles. Alternate days of walking with biking, running, or swimming.

- Don't ignore aches and pains. A few days of reduced activity or rest when you feel the first twinge of pain may help you avoid more serious problems.

Home Treatment

The biggest home treatment challenge for most sports injuries is to get enough rest to allow healing without losing overall conditioning. This approach is called relative rest.

- Keep the rest of your body fit by cross-training with activities that don't stress the injured area: swimming or biking for sore ankles or feet; walking or biking for sore shoulders or elbows; do floor exercises.

- Don't hurry the return to the activity that caused the injury. Cross-training can maintain your level of fitness.

- Resume your regular activity gradually. Start with a slow, easy pace and increase only if you have no pain.

- Break your sport down into components. If you can throw a ball a short distance without pain, try increasing the distance. If you can walk comfortably, try jogging. If jogging seems fine, work up to running.

- Also see Bursitis and Tendinitis on page 72.

- See below for tips on deciding whether a bone is broken.

Strains, Sprains, and Fractures

A **strain** is an injury caused by over-stretching a muscle.

A **sprain** is an injury to the muscle and the ligaments, tendons, or soft tissues around a joint.

A **fracture** is a broken bone.

All three injuries cause pain and swelling. Unless a broken bone is obvious, it may be difficult to tell if an injury is a strain, sprain, or fracture. Rapid swelling often indicates a more serious injury. Injuries often involve all three.

Most minor strains and sprains can be treated at home, but severe sprains and fractures need professional care. Apply home treatment while you wait to see your doctor.

You may have a severe sprain or broken bone if:

- The injured area is visibly swollen.

- The injured area is twisted or bent out of shape or a bone is poking through the skin.

• The injured area is black and blue.

• The pain from the injury prevents normal use of the limb, such as walking.

A **stress fracture** is a weak spot or small crack in a bone caused by repeated overuse. Stress fractures in the small bones of the foot are common during intensive training for basketball, running, and other sports. The main symptom is persistent foot pain and tenderness that increases during use. There may be no visible swelling.

Turf toe or "jammed toe" is a sprain caused by bending or a blow to the toe. Fingers can also be "jammed" or sprained.

Splinting

Splinting immobilizes a suspected fracture to prevent further injury. There are two ways to immobilize a fracture: tie the injured limb to a stiff object, or tie the limb to some other part of the body.

For the first method, tie rolled-up newspapers or magazines, a stick, a cane, or anything that is stiff to the injured limb with a rope, a belt, or anything else that will work.

Position the splint so the injured limb cannot bend. A general rule is to splint from a joint above the fracture to a joint below it. For example, splint a broken forearm from above the elbow to below the wrist.

For the second method, tape a broken toe to the next toe or immobilize an arm by tying it across the victim's chest.

Prevention

• Don't climb stairs with both hands full. Make sure you can always see where you are walking.

• Don't carry objects that are too heavy.

• Use a stepstool. Do not stand on chairs or other objects.

See prevention tips for Sports Injuries on page 81.

Home Treatment

Generally speaking, if the injury is to a muscle, ligament, tendon, or bone, the basic treatment is the same. It is a two-part process: **RICE** (rest, ice, compression, elevation) to treat the acute pain or injury; and **MSA** (movement, strength, alternate activity) to help the injury heal completely and to prevent further problems.

Begin the RICE process immediately for most injuries. If you suspect a fracture, splint the affected limb to prevent further injury.

If the sprain is to a finger or part of the hand, remove all rings immediately. See page 86.

R. Rest. Do not put weight on the injured joint for at least 24 to 48 hours.

• Use crutches to support a badly sprained knee or ankle.

• Support a sprained wrist, elbow, or shoulder with a sling. The inconvenience is justified by the faster healing of the injury.

• Rest a sprained finger or toe by taping it to a healthy one.

Strains, Sprains – continued

Injured muscle, ligament, or tendon tissue needs time and rest to heal itself. Stress fractures need rest for two to four months to heal.

I. Ice. Cold will reduce pain and swelling and promote healing. Heat feels nice, but it does more harm than good until all of the swelling is gone.

• Apply ice or cold packs immediately to prevent or minimize swelling. For difficult-to-reach injuries, a cold pack works best. See "Ice and Cold Packs" on page 85.

C. Compression. Wrap the injury with an elastic (Ace) bandage or compression sleeve to immobilize and compress the sprain. Don't wrap it too tightly; this can cause swelling beyond the injury. Loosen the bandage if it gets too tight. A tightly wrapped sprain may fool you into thinking you can keep using the joint. With or without a wrap, the joint needs total rest for one to two days.

E. Elevation. Elevate the injured area on pillows while you apply ice and anytime you are seated or lying down. Try to keep the injury at or above the level of your heart to help minimize swelling.

• Aspirin or ibuprofen may help ease inflammation and pain. Do not use drugs to mask the pain while you continue to use the injured joint. Do not give aspirin to children or teens under age 20. Review aspirin guidelines on page 299.

• The use of heat (hot water bottle, warm towel, heating pad) after 48 hours of cold treatments is controversial. Some experts think it will increase swelling; others think it may speed healing. If you use heat, do not apply anything that is uncomfortably warm.

Begin the **MSA** process as soon as the initial pain and swelling have subsided. This may be in two days or up to a week or longer, depending on the location and severity of the injury. Resume sports and activities slowly. Consider any increased pain as a sign to rest a while longer.

M. Movement. Resume a full range of motion as soon as possible after an injury. After one to two days of rest, begin moving the joint. If an activity causes pain, continue resting the joint. Gentle stretching during healing will ensure that scar tissue formed as the injury heals will not limit movement later.

S. Strength. Once the swelling is gone and range of motion is restored, begin gradual efforts to strengthen the injured part.

A. Alternate activities. After the first few days, but while the injured part is still healing, phase in regular exercise using activities or sports that do not place a strain on the injured part. See page 82.

Ice and Cold Packs

Ice can relieve pain, swelling, and inflammation. When you have an injury, be consistent and thorough in applying ice. Continue for as long as you have symptoms. Use either a commercial cold pack or one of the following:

• Ice towel: Wet a towel with cold water and squeeze it until it is just damp. Fold the towel, place it in a plastic bag, and freeze it for 15 minutes. Remove the towel from the bag and place on the affected area.

• Ice pack: Put about a pound of ice in a plastic bag. Add water to barely cover the ice. Squeeze the air out of the bag and seal it. Wrap the bag in a wet towel and apply to the affected area.

• Homemade cold pack: See instructions on page 291.

Ice the area at least three times a day. For the first 72 hours, ice for 10 minutes once an hour. After that, a good pattern is to ice for 15 to 20 minutes three times a day: In the morning, late afternoon after work or school, and about one-half hour before bedtime. Also ice after any prolonged activity or vigorous exercise.

Always keep a damp cloth between your skin and the cold pack, and press firmly against all the curves of the affected area. Do not apply ice for longer than 15 to 20 minutes at a time, and do not fall asleep with the ice on your skin.

When to Call Kaiser Permanente

• If you suspect a severe sprain or fracture (see page 82), call for an urgent-care or same-day appointment. After you have splinted the injury and applied ice, a short delay in professional care will not affect the outcome.

• If a sprained joint is very unstable, won't support your weight, or wobbles from side to side.

• If pain is still severe after two days of home treatment.

• If a sprain does not improve after four days of home treatment.

Weakness and Fatigue

Weakness is a physical inability or difficulty in moving an arm or leg or other muscle due to lack of strength.

Fatigue is a feeling of tiredness, exhaustion, or lack of energy.

Unexplained muscle weakness is usually more serious. It may be due to metabolic problems such as diabetes (see page 269), thyroid problems, kidney problems, or stroke. Call your doctor immediately.

Fatigue, on the other hand, can usually be treated with self-care. Most fatigue is caused by lack of exercise, stress or overwork, poor sleep, depression, worry, or boredom. Colds and flu may sometimes cause fatigue and weakness, but the symptoms disappear as the illness runs its course.

Removing a Ring

If you did not remove a ring before a sprained finger started to swell, try the following method to remove it:

- Stick the end of a slick piece of string, such as dental floss, under the ring toward the hand.

- Starting at the knuckle side of the ring, wrap the string snugly around the finger toward the end of the finger, wrapping beyond the knuckle. Each wrap should be right next to the one before.

- Grasp the end of the string that is stretched under the ring and start unwrapping it, pushing the ring along in place of the unwrapped string until the ring passes the knuckle.

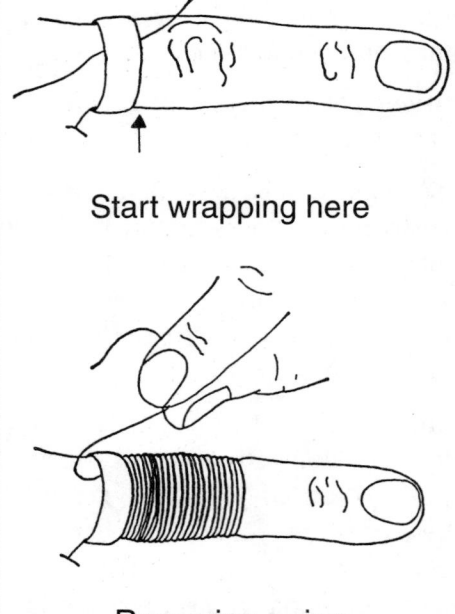

Start wrapping here

Removing a ring

Weakness and Fatigue – cont.

Prevention

- Regular exercise is your best defense against fatigue. If you feel too tired to exercise vigorously, try a short walk.

- Eat a well-balanced diet. See Chapter 18.

- Improve your sleeping habits. See page 284.

- Deal with feelings of depression. See page 280.

Home Treatment

- Follow the prevention guidelines above and be patient. It may take a while to feel energetic again.

- Listen to your body. Alternate rest with exercise.

- Limit drugs that might contribute to fatigue. Tranquilizers and cold and allergy medications are particularly suspect.

- Reduce your use of caffeine, nicotine, and alcohol.

- Cut back on television. Replace it with friends, new activities, or travel to break the fatigue cycle.

When to Call Kaiser Permanente

- If you have unexplained muscle weakness in one area of the body.

- If you experience sudden, unplanned weight loss.

- If, in spite of home treatment, you are unable to do your usual activities.

- If you do not feel more energetic after six weeks of home treatment.

Chronic Fatigue Syndrome

Chronic fatigue syndrome (CFS) is a flu-like illness that causes severe fatigue lasting longer than six months. Other symptoms include mild fever, sore throat, painful lymph glands, muscle weakness and pain, headaches, and sleep problems.

CFS is difficult to diagnose. There is no definitive lab test. Many other illnesses, such as depression, thyroid disorder, or mononucleosis, cause similar symptoms. A CFS diagnosis is made only after fatigue and other symptoms continue for at least six months and other possible causes have been ruled out.

The fatigue and other symptoms usually develop quickly in a previously healthy person. Treatment is focused on adequate rest, balanced diet, and mild exercise. No medications are known to cure CFS. Treatment of the individual symptoms can be effective. For treatment of depression, which develops in about half of CFS patients, see page 280.

Call Kaiser Permanente if unexplained fatigue is severe, persistent, and interferes with your activities for a week or more in spite of home treatment.

Life is made up of sobs, sniffles, and smiles,
with sniffles predominating.
O. Henry

Chapter 7

Chest and Respiratory Problems

Chest problems can be as simple as a minor cold or as life-threatening as a heart attack. For most chest problems, this chapter will help you decide what to do at home and when to call your doctor. Because allergies, colds, sore throats, sinusitis, and tonsillitis are often related to chest and respiratory problems, they are included as well.

Start this chapter with a look at the chart on the next page. From asthma to pneumonia and from heart attack to heartburn, the chart will lead you to the information you need the most. If you don't find what you are looking for, please try the index.

Allergies

Allergies come in many forms. Hay fever, with its symptoms of itchy, watery eyes, sneezing, runny, stuffy, or itchy nose, temporary loss of smell, headache, and tiredness, is the most common allergy. Dark circles under the eyes ("allergic shiners") or post-nasal drip may also accompany hay fever. A child with allergies may snore, wake with a sore throat, breathe through the mouth, and frequently rub the nose. Allergy symptoms are often like cold symptoms, but usually last longer.

The most common causes of allergies are particles in the air, such as pollen, house dust mites, mold or mildew, and animal dander. Allergies seem to run in families. Parents with hay fever often have children with allergies. Hay fever usually develops in the early teens, but can occur at any age.

You can often discover the cause of an allergy by noting when symptoms occur. Symptoms that occur at the same time each year (especially during spring, early summer, or early fall) are often due to grass, weed, or tree pollen. Allergies that seem

Chest, Respiratory, Nose, and Throat Problems

Chest or Respiratory Symptoms	Possible Causes
Wheezing or difficulty breathing	See Allergies, p. 89; Asthma, p. 93; Bronchitis, p. 97; Pneumonia, p. 104.
Rapid, shallow, labored breathing	See Pneumonia, p. 104.
Chest pain with cough, fever, and yellow-green or grey sputum	See Bronchitis, p. 97; Pneumonia, p. 104.
Burning, pain, or discomfort behind the breastbone	See Heartburn, p. 46; Chest Pain, p. 98.
Chest pain with sweating or rapid pulse	Possible heart attack. Call for help. See CPR, p. 206.
Coughing	See Coughs, p.101.

Nose and Throat Symptoms	Possible Causes
Stuffy or runny nose with watery eyes, sneezing	See Allergies, p. 89; Colds, p. 99.
Cold symptoms with fever, headache, body aches	See Influenza, p. 103.
Thick green, yellow, or grey discharge with fever and facial pain	See Sinusitis, p. 105.
Foul odor from nose; swollen, inflamed nasal tissue	See Objects in the Nose, p. 230; Sinusitis, p. 105.
Pale, bluish nasal tissue	See Allergies, p. 89.
Sore throat	See Sore Throat, p.106; Tonsillitis, p. 109.
Sore throat with white spots on tonsils, swollen glands, fever of 101° or higher	See Strep Throat, p. 107.
Swollen tonsils, sore throat, fever	See Tonsillitis, p. 109.
Swollen lymph nodes in the neck	See Swollen Glands, p. 108; Tonsillitis, p. 109.
Hoarseness, loss of voice	See Laryngitis, p. 103.

Allergies – continued

to persist all year long may be due to dust mites in household dust, mold spores, or animal dander. Animal allergies are often easy to detect; staying away from the animal clears up the symptoms.

Severe, Life-Threatening Allergies (Anaphylaxis)

A few people have severe allergies to insect stings or certain foods or drugs, especially penicillin. For these people, the allergic reaction is sudden and severe, and may cause difficulty breathing and a drop in blood pressure (anaphylactic shock).

An anaphylactic reaction is a medical emergency and prompt care is needed. If you have had a severe allergic reaction, doctors suggest that you carry an epinephrine syringe (Epi-pen, Ana-kit) designed to self-administer a shot that will decrease the severity of the reaction. If you have had an allergic reaction to a drug, wear a medical identification bracelet that will tell health professionals about your allergy if you cannot.

Prevention

- There is no practical prevention for hay fever. Avoiding the substance that causes allergy attacks will help. See page 268 for more information on food allergies.

- If you or your spouse have a history of allergies, consider breast-feeding your infants. There is some evidence that solely feeding breast milk during the first six months of life may reduce a child's risk of developing food allergies.

Home Treatment

If you can discover the source of your allergies, avoiding that substance is the best treatment. Keep a record of your symptoms and the plants, animals, foods, or chemicals that seem to trigger them.

If your symptoms are seasonal and seem to be related to pollen:

- Keep your house and car windows closed. Keep bedroom windows closed at night.

- Limit the time you spend outside when pollen counts are high. Dogs and other pets may bring large amounts of pollen into your house.

If your symptoms are year-round and seem to be related to dust:

- Keep the bedroom as dust-free as possible, since most of your time is spent there.

- Avoid carpeting, upholstered furniture, and heavy draperies that collect dust. Vacuuming doesn't pick up dust mites.

- Cover your mattress and box spring with dust-proof cases and wipe them clean weekly. Avoid wool or down blankets and feather pillows. Wash all bedding weekly in hot water.

- Consider using an air conditioner or air purifier with a special HEPA filter. Rent one before buying to see if it helps.

If your symptoms are year-round and worsen during damp weather, they may be related to mold or mildew:

- Keep the house well ventilated and dry. Keep the humidity below 50 percent. Use a dehumidifier during humid weather.

Allergies – continued

- Use an air conditioner, which removes mold spores from the air. Change or clean heating and cooling system filters regularly.

- Clean bathroom and kitchen surfaces often with bleach to reduce mold growth.

If you are allergic to a pet:

- Keep the animal outside, or at least out of the bedroom.

- If your symptoms are severe, the best solution may be to get rid of the pet.

General information on avoiding irritants:

- Avoid yardwork (raking, mowing), which stirs up both pollen and mold. If you must do it, wear a mask and take an antihistamine beforehand.

- Avoid smoking and inhaling other people's smoke.

- Eliminate aerosol sprays, perfumes, room deodorizers, cleaning products, and other substances that may add to the problem.

- Antihistamines and decongestants may relieve some allergy symptoms. Use caution when taking these drugs. See page 296.

- For more information on allergies, including immunotherapy, call the Allergy Department of your local Kaiser Permanente facility.

What About Immunotherapy?

Immunotherapy involves a series of shots given to desensitize your body to an allergen. It requires regular treatments lasting up to three to four years. Because of the time and expense involved, you need a realistic idea of the benefits before agreeing to the treatment.

Immunotherapy is 98 percent effective for allergies to bee stings and other insect venoms. For most people, it is effective against grass, tree, and weed pollens, as well as house dust, the house dust mite, and dog and cat dander. Treatment is effective only if the specific allergen has been identified by sensitivity testing.

The following factors make it more likely that immunotherapy will be worthwhile for you:

1. Your symptoms have bothered you a lot for at least two years.

2. You have tried home treatment without success.

3. You have tried both prescription and nonprescription medications without relief.

4. Immunotherapy is effective for allergens identified by skin tests.

When to Call Kaiser Permanente

- Go to the Emergency Room *immediately* if signs of a severe allergic reaction develop, especially soon after taking a drug, eating a food, or being stung by an insect:

  ◦ Wheezing or difficulty breathing

  ◦ Swelling around the lips, tongue, or face, or significant swelling around the site of the insect sting (e.g., entire arm or leg is swollen)

  ◦ Skin rash, itching, feeling of warmth, or hives

- If symptoms worsen over time, and your home treatment doesn't help. Your doctor can recommend stronger medication or desensitizing shots. Allergy shots may help reduce sensitivity to some allergens. See page 92.

Asthma

Asthma is the Greek word for panting. A person having an asthma attack is literally panting for breath. Asthma is a condition that causes inflammation and obstruction of the airways. The muscles surrounding the air tubes (bronchial tubes) of the lungs go into spasm, the mucous lining swells, and secretions build up. Breathing becomes quite difficult.

Asthma usually occurs in attacks or episodes. During an attack, the person may make a wheezing or whistling sound while breathing, cough a great deal, and spit up mucus.

Many things can trigger asthma, including allergens, such as dust, pollen, mold, and animal dander. In general, infections are the most common triggers of asthma. Other triggers include exercise; cigarette or wood smoke; changes in weather; colds or the flu; chemical vapors from household or workplace products; analgesics (especially aspirin); food preservatives and dyes; and emotional stress.

Asthma usually develops in childhood but may also begin later in life. Often, the first episode follows a cold or the flu. It is more common in children who are exposed to cigarette smoke in the home. Many children outgrow asthma as they get older but will still be at risk for it in adulthood.

Most children and adults can control their asthma by avoiding triggers that cause attacks and using medications to manage symptoms. Severe attacks can usually be treated with inhaled or injected medications. Asthma attacks are rarely fatal if they are treated promptly.

Prevention

Discover and avoid the things that cause your asthma attacks:

- Review the home treatment for allergies on page 91.

- Avoid smoke of all kinds. Stop smoking and avoid exposure to secondhand smoke. Eat, work, travel, and relax in smoke-free areas. Stay away from wood-burning stoves.

- Avoid air pollution. Stay indoors when the air pollution is high.

Asthma – continued

- Avoid strong odors, fumes, and perfume.

- Avoid breathing cold air. In cold weather, breathe through your nose and cover your nose and mouth with a scarf or cold weather mask. Masks are available at most drug stores.

- Pets that stay outdoors, or pets such as fish or turtles, may be less troublesome.

- Reduce your risk of colds and flu by washing your hands often and getting a flu shot each year.

Build up the strength of your lungs and airways:

- Get regular exercise. Swimming or water aerobics may be good choices because the moist air is less likely to trigger an attack. If vigorous exercise triggers asthma attacks, talk with your doctor. Adjusting your medication and your exercise routine may help.

- Practice roll-breathing as described on page 252.

Home Treatment

- Learn to use a peak-flow meter to monitor your ability to exhale. Used regularly, this device measures your progress as you improve your ability to breathe. It also helps you tell when an attack may be coming on so you can take appropriate steps.

- If you have significant asthma, ask your doctor for a written care plan to guide you in adding medication as needed.

How to Use an Inhaler and Spacer

1. Shake the inhaler well for five seconds. Remove the protective cap and insert the mouthpiece of the inhaler into one end of the spacer. Hold the inhaler with your index finger on top and your thumb supporting the bottom.

2. Breathe out as much as possible to empty the lungs. Tilt your head back and place the mouthpiece of the spacer tube in your mouth. Close your lips around the mouthpiece.

3. Press down on the top of the inhaler to release a puff of medication. Breathe in slowly and deeply, filling your lungs with as much air as possible. If you hear a musical sound, you are inhaling too fast. Hold your breath for at least 10 seconds, then breathe out.

4. With your lips still closed around the mouthpiece, take two or three more deep breaths, holding each for 10 seconds. To get the maximum effectiveness, wait a minute or two before taking the next puff.

5.Wash the inhaler mouthpiece, spacer, and protective caps weekly with mild soapy water and allow to air dry.

- If your child has an asthma attack, remain calm. Give the recommended medication and help the child relax. Make sure your child—and his teachers or childcare providers—know what to do in case of an attack.

- Learn to use a metered-dose inhaler. Inhalers help get the right amount of medication to the airways. However, it takes some skill to use the inhaler correctly. A device called a spacer is now recommended for use with an inhaler. Ask your doctor to watch you use your inhaler and spacer to make sure you are doing it right.

- Ask your doctor about anti-inflammatory inhalers.

- People with asthma usually do better in warm, moist air than in cold, dry air. If you're feeling "tight," stand or sit in a warm shower for 5 to 10 minutes.

- Increase your fluid intake to thin bronchial mucus.

- Aspirin and ibuprofen can cause severe reactions in some people with asthma. Use them with caution and discuss them with your doctor. If you find that these medications bother you, avoid using them.

- Do not use over-the-counter cold and cough medicines unless your doctor tells you to do so.

- Practice the relaxation exercises on pages 252 to 254.

- Follow the prevention tips above.

- Work in partnership with your doctor to maximize your control over your asthma.

- To get information on managing asthma, contact your local Kaiser Permanente facility's Pediatrics or Family Practice Department, or Health Education Department.

When to Call Kaiser Permanente

- If acute asthma symptoms have occurred for the first time.

- If asthma symptoms fail to respond to your usual treatment, or if the attack is severe (peak flow less than 50 percent of best).

- If sputum becomes discolored, particularly green, yellow, or bloody. This may be a sign of a bacterial infection.

- If a person with asthma or other family members have not been educated about treatment, or if the medication required is not immediately at hand.

- To learn exactly what to do when an attack begins. With proper training, medication, and confidence, a person with asthma can often handle acute episodes without professional help.

- If you begin to use your asthma medication more often than usual. This may be a sign that your asthma is worsening.

- To discuss allergy shots, which may be helpful in preventing asthma attacks. See page 92.

- To get a referral to a support group. Talking with others who have asthma can help you gain information and confidence in dealing with prevention and treatment.

Bacterial Infections

Upper respiratory infections caused by bacteria are often hard to distinguish from those caused by viruses. In particular, a bad case of the flu may be hard to distinguish from a bacterial infection. Bacteria will sometimes attack the weakened system of a person with a cold or the flu. (Bacterial infections sometimes follow viral infections.)

The most common bacterial infections are ear infections and strep throat. Bronchitis, sinusitis, and pneumonia may also be caused by bacteria.

Symptoms of a bacterial infection may include:

- Fever of 104° or higher that does not reduce with two hours of home treatment.

- Persistent fever. Many viral illnesses, especially the flu, cause fevers of 102° or higher for short periods of time (up to 12 to 24 hours). Call a doctor if the fever stays high:
  - 102° or higher for 2 full days
  - 101° or higher for 3 full days
  - 100° or higher for 4 full days

- Nasal discharge that changes from clear to colored (yellow, green, grey, rust-colored) after five to seven days of a cold or flu, with other worsening symptoms. If sputum is yellow or green at the start of a cold, call a doctor if it persists longer than 7 to 10 days.

Viral or Bacterial?

Viral Infections

- Usually involve different parts of the body: sore throat, runny nose, headaches, muscle aches. In the abdominal area, viruses cause nausea and/or diarrhea.

- Typical viral infections: cold, flu, stomach flu.

- Antibiotics *do not* help.

Bacterial Infections

- May follow a viral infection that does not improve.

- Usually localized at a single point in the body: sinuses, ear, lungs.

- Typical bacterial infections: strep throat, ear infection.

- Antibiotics *do* help.

- Cough that lingers more than 10 to 14 days after other symptoms have cleared, especially if it is productive.

- Ear pain that is more than just stuffiness, especially only on one side, that lasts more than 24 hours. See page 118.

- Localized sinus pain that persists despite two to four days of home treatment, especially if nasal discharge is colored rather than clear. See page 105.

- Cold symptoms that last more than two weeks without improvement.

Antibiotics cannot prevent complications of a viral infection. They are effective against bacterial infections only after they have developed. However, antibiotics are sometimes used to prevent recurrent sinus and ear infections. Most doctors will not prescribe antibiotics until a bacterial infection is confirmed. For important information about antibiotics, see page 302.

When to Call Kaiser Permanente

Bacterial infections need to be diagnosed and treated by a doctor. Call if symptoms of a bacterial infection develop.

Bronchitis

Bronchitis is an inflammation and irritation of the bronchial tubes in the lungs. It is most often caused by viruses or bacteria, but may also be caused by cigarette smoke or air pollution. It often occurs after a cold or an upper respiratory infection that does not heal completely.

The inflamed bronchial tubes secrete a sticky mucus, which is difficult for the hairs (cilia) on the bronchi to clear out of the lungs. The productive cough that comes with bronchitis is the body's attempt to get rid of the mucus. Other symptoms include discomfort or tightness in the chest, tiredness, low fever, sore throat, runny nose, and sometimes wheezing. Severe cases may lead to pneumonia.

Bronchitis can become chronic, especially among people who smoke or who work in polluted air. Seventy-five percent of people with chronic bronchitis have a history of heavy smoking.

Chronic bronchitis may occur with emphysema or chronic asthma. Any combination of these conditions is known as chronic obstructive pulmonary disease (COPD).

Prevention

- Give proper home care to minor respiratory problems such as colds and flu. See pages 99 and 103.

- Stop smoking. People who smoke and those who live with them have more frequent bouts of bronchitis.

- Avoid polluted air.

Home Treatment

Self-care for bronchitis focuses on getting rid of the mucus in your lungs. Here is what you can do at home to speed healing.

- Increase your fluid intake to as much as 8 to 12 glasses per day (until you are urinating more than usual). Liquids help thin the mucus in the lungs so your cough can clear it out.

- Stop smoking and avoid others' smoke. Smoke irritates the lungs and slows healing.

- Breathe moist air from a humidifier, hot shower, or a sink filled with hot water. The heat and moisture will liquefy mucus and help the cough bring it up.

Bronchitis – continued

- Get some extra rest. Let your energy go to healing.

- Have someone massage your chest and back muscles. The massage increases blood flow to the chest and helps you relax.

- Take aspirin or acetaminophen to relieve fever and body aches.

- If a dry, unproductive cough keeps you awake, take a cough syrup containing dextromethorphan. Avoid products containing more than one active ingredient. See page 298.

When to Call Kaiser Permanente

- If cough lasts longer than two weeks without improvement.
- If signs of a bacterial infection develop. See page 96.
- If there is difficulty in breathing, wheezing, or shortness of breath.
- If the sick person is an infant, an older adult, or is chronically ill, especially with lung problems

Chest Pain

CALL 861-3434, 911, OR OTHER EMERGENCY SERVICES IMMEDIATELY if chest pain is crushing or squeezing, increases in intensity, or occurs with any of the symptoms of a heart attack:

- **Sweating**

- **Shortness of breath**

- **Pain radiating to the arm, neck, or jaw**

- **Nausea or vomiting**

- **Dizziness**

- **Rapid and/or irregular pulse**

Chest pain is a key warning sign of a heart attack, but it may also be caused by other problems.

Pain that increases when you press on the site is probably chest wall pain, which may be caused by strained muscles or ligaments in the chest wall. A shooting pain that lasts a few seconds, or a quick pain at the end of a deep breath, is usually not a cause for concern. Hyperventilation (see page 226) can also cause chest pain.

Chest pain can be associated with other disorders. With pleurisy or pneumonia (see page 104), the pain will get worse with a deep breath or cough; heart pain will not. An ulcer (see page 53) can cause chest pain that is worse on an empty stomach. Gallbladder pain may worsen after a meal or in the middle of the night. Heartburn or indigestion can also cause chest pain. See page 46.

Angina is pain, pressure, heaviness, and/or numbness behind the breastbone and/or across the chest. It is caused by poor circulation to the heart muscle. The symptoms of angina may radiate to the neck, jaws, shoulders, arms, or wrists. It may be brought on by stress or exertion and is relieved by rest. Angina lasts from just a few to 20 minutes and usually *does not* occur with sweating, nausea, or shortness of breath.

A **heart attack** (myocardial infarction) is caused by blocked blood flow to the heart muscle. The symptoms of a heart attack are similar to those of angina, but they are more severe and last longer than 20 minutes. The symptoms above may also be present. Unlike angina, heart attack symptoms are not relieved by rest.

Some medical and lifestyle factors may increase your risk of a heart attack. These factors include:

• Smoking

• Inactive lifestyle

• High blood pressure

• High cholesterol

• High stress levels

• Diabetes

Contact the Health Education Department of your local Kaiser Permanente facility to learn more about these risk factors.

Home Treatment

For chest wall pain caused by strained muscles or ligaments:

• Use pain relievers such as aspirin, ibuprofen, or acetaminophen.

• Ben-Gay or Vicks VapoRub may soothe sore muscles.

• Avoid the activity that strains the chest area.

When to Call Kaiser Permanente

CALL 861-3434, 911, OR EMER-GENCY SERVICES IMMEDI-ATELY if symptoms of a heart attack are present (see page 98). See CPR on page 206.

• If your chest pain has been diagnosed by a doctor and he has prescribed a home treatment plan, follow it. Call 861-3434, 911, or emergency services if the pain worsens or any of the signs on page 98 develop.

• If you suspect angina and your symptoms have not been diagnosed, call your doctor immediately.

• If symptoms of angina do not respond to your prescribed treatment, or if the pattern of your angina changes.

If minor chest pain occurs without the symptoms of a heart attack, call a health professional:

• If the person has a history of heart disease or blood clots in the lungs.

• If chest pain is constant, nagging, and not relieved by rest.

• If chest pain occurs with symptoms of pneumonia. See page 104.

• If any chest pain lasts 48 hours without improvement.

Colds

The common cold is caused by any one of 200 viruses. The symptoms of a cold are a runny nose, red eyes, sneezing, sore throat, dry cough, headache, and general body aches. There is a gradual one- or two-day onset. As a cold progresses, the nasal mucus may thicken. This is the stage just before a cold dries up. A cold usually lasts about one or two weeks.

Colds – continued

Colds occur throughout the year, but are most common in late winter and early spring. The average child has six colds a year; adults have fewer.

Using a mouthwash will not prevent a cold and antibiotics will not cure one. In fact, there is no cure for the common cold. If you catch one, treat the symptoms.

Sometimes a cold will lead to more serious complications. A bacterial infection (see page 96) such as bronchitis or pneumonia may develop after a cold. Good home treatment of colds can help prevent these complications.

If it seems you or your child has a cold all the time, or if cold symptoms last two weeks or more, suspect allergies (see page 89) or sinusitis (see page 105).

Prevention

- Eat well and get plenty of sleep and exercise to keep up your resistance.
- Wash your hands often, particularly when you are around people who have colds.
- Keep your hands away from your nose, eyes, and mouth.
- Stop smoking.
- Consider breast-feeding your baby. Breast-fed babies seem to have fewer, less severe colds.

Home Treatment

Home treatment for a cold will help relieve symptoms and prevent complications.

- Get extra rest after work or school. Slow down just a little from your usual routine. It isn't necessary to stay home in bed, but take care not to expose others.

Description and Treatment of Coughs

Type of Cough	Possible Causes
Loud cough like a seal's bark	See Croup, p. 160.
Dry cough in the morning that gets better as day goes on	Dry air; cigarette smoking. Increase fluids. Humidify the bedroom. Stop smoking. See Coughs, p. 101.
Hacking, dry, nonproductive cough	Postnasal drip; cigarette smoking. Increase fluids. Try a decongestant. Stop smoking. See Coughs, p. 101.
Productive cough following a cold or flu	See Sinusitis, p. 105; Bronchitis, p. 97; Pneumonia, p. 104.
Dry, sudden-onset cough after a choking episode, most often in an infant or toddler	Foreign object in the throat. See Choking, p. 216.

- Drink plenty of liquids. Hot water, herbal tea, or chicken soup will help relieve congestion.

- Take aspirin or acetaminophen to reduce fever and relieve aches and pains. Do not give aspirin to children and teens under age 20. See page 299 for precautions.

- Humidify the bedroom and take hot showers to relieve nasal stuffiness.

- Watch the back of your throat for postnasal drip. If streaks of mucus appear, gargle to prevent a sore throat.

- Use disposable tissues, not handkerchiefs, to reduce the spread of virus to others.

- If your nose is red and raw from rubbing with tissues, put a bit of petroleum jelly on the sore area.

- Avoid "cold" remedies that combine drugs to treat many different symptoms. These products often combine decongestants, antihistamines, and pain relievers. Treat each symptom separately. Take a decongestant for stuffiness, a cough medicine for a cough. See Home Treatment for coughs on page 102.

- Avoid antihistamines. They are not an effective treatment for colds.

- Use nasal decongestant sprays for only three days or less. Continued use may lead to a "rebound" effect, when the mucous membranes swell up more than before using the spray. See page 298 for nose drops you can make at home.

When to Call Kaiser Permanente

- If signs of a bacterial infection develop. See page 96.

- If signs of strep throat develop. See page 106.

Coughs

Coughing is the body's way of removing foreign material or mucus from the lungs. Coughs have distinctive traits you can learn to recognize.

Productive coughs produce phlegm or mucus that comes up with the cough. This kind of cough generally should not be suppressed; it is needed to clear mucus from the lungs.

Nonproductive coughs are dry coughs that do not produce mucus. A dry, hacking cough may develop toward the end of a cold or after exposure to an irritant, such as dust or smoke.

Prevention

- Don't smoke. A dry, hacking "smoker's cough" means your lungs are constantly irritated.

- Increase fluid intake to as much as 8 to 10 glasses of water every day. You are drinking enough if you are urinating more often than usual.

Coughs – continued

Home Treatment

- Drink lots of water. Water helps loosen phlegm and soothe an irritated throat. Dry, hacking coughs respond to honey in hot water, tea, or lemon juice. (Do not give honey to children under one year of age.)

Encephalitis and Meningitis

Encephalitis is an inflammation of the brain that may occur following a viral infection, such as chicken pox, flu, measles, mumps, or cold sores (herpes simplex). A serious type of encephalitis is spread by mosquitoes in the eastern and southeastern U.S.

Meningitis is a viral or bacterial illness that causes inflammation around the tissues surrounding the brain and spinal cord. It may follow an infection, such as an ear or sinus infection, or a viral illness.

Encephalitis and meningitis are serious illnesses with similar symptoms. Both require immediate medical attention. Call a health professional if the following symptoms develop, especially following a viral illness or a mosquito bite:

- Severe headache with stiff neck, fever, nausea, and vomiting

- Drowsiness, lethargy, confusion, or delirium

- Bulging soft spot on an infant's head (when the baby is not crying)

- Cough drops can soothe irritated throats, but most have no effect on the cough-producing mechanism.

- Expensive medicine-flavored cough drops are not any better than inexpensive candy-flavored ones or hard candy.

- Coughs that follow viral illnesses may last up to several weeks and often get worse at night. Elevate your head with extra pillows at night.

- Use an over-the-counter cough suppressant containing dextromethorphan to help quiet a dry, hacking cough so you can sleep. If you have a productive cough, don't suppress it so much that you are no longer bringing up mucus. See Cough Preparations on page 298.

- For coughs caused by inhaled irritants (smoke, dust, or other pollutants), avoid exposure or wear a face mask.

When to Call Kaiser Permanente

- If sputum becomes thick, green, or brown, or if blood is coughed up.

- If the cough involves wheezing, shortness of breath, difficulty breathing, or tightness in the chest. See Pneumonia on page 104.

- If signs of a bacterial infection develop. See page 96.

- If a productive cough lasts longer than 7 to 10 days without improvement. Dry, hacking coughs can last several weeks after a viral illness.

Influenza

Influenza, or flu, is a viral illness that commonly occurs in the winter. The flu often affects many people at once (epidemic). (The name "influenza" comes from the Italian word for "influence.")

Influenza has symptoms similar to a cold, but they are usually more severe and come on quite suddenly.

The flu is commonly thought of as a respiratory illness, but the whole body can be affected. Symptoms include weakness, fatigue, muscle aches, headaches, fever (101° to 102°), chills, sneezing, and runny nose. Symptoms may last five to seven days. Most other viruses, such as colds, have less severe symptoms that don't last as long.

Although a person with the flu feels very sick, it seldom leads to more serious complications. The illness is usually dangerous only for infants, older adults, and people with chronic diseases.

Prevention

- Get a flu shot each autumn if you are over 65, if you have a chronic illness, such as asthma, heart disease, or diabetes, or if you are a health care worker who is either exposed to people with the flu or who might expose patients to the flu if you catch it.

- Keep up your resistance to infection with a good diet, plenty of rest, and regular exercise.

- Avoid exposure to the virus. Wash your hands often and keep your hands away from your nose, eyes, and mouth.

Home Treatment

- Get plenty of rest.

- Drink extra fluids, at least one glass of water or juice every waking hour.

- Take acetaminophen, aspirin, or ibuprofen to relieve fever and head and muscle aches. (Do not give aspirin to children and teens under age 20.)

When to Call Kaiser Permanente

- If signs of a bacterial infection develop. See page 96.

- If the person seems to get better, then gets worse again.

- If flu-like symptoms or a red rash occur four days to three weeks after being bitten by a tick. See page 148.

Laryngitis

Laryngitis is an infection or irritation of the voice box (larynx). The most common cause is a viral infection or a cold. It can also be caused by allergy, excessive talking, singing, or yelling cigarette smoke, or reflux of acid from the stomach into the throat. Symptoms include hoarseness or loss of voice, the urge to clear your throat, fever, tiredness, pain in the throat, and coughing. Heavy drinking or smoking can lead to chronic laryngitis.

Laryngitis – continued

Prevention

- To prevent hoarseness, stop shouting as soon as you feel minor pain. Give your vocal cords a rest.

Home Treatment

- Laryngitis will usually heal in 5 to 10 days. Medication does little to speed recovery.

- If hoarseness is caused by a cold, treat the cold (see page 99). Some hoarseness may last up to a week after a cold.

- Rest your voice by not shouting and by talking as little as possible. Do not whisper, and avoid clearing your throat.

- Stop smoking and avoid other people's smoke.

- Humidify the air with a humidifier, or take a hot shower.

- Drink lots of liquids.

- To soothe the throat, gargle with warm salt water (one teaspoon in eight ounces of water) or drink honey in hot water, lemon juice, or weak tea.

- If you suspect problems with stomach acid may be contributing to your laryngitis, refer to the remedies on page 46.

When to Call Kaiser Permanente

- If signs of a bacterial infection develop. See page 96.

- If hoarseness persists for three to four weeks.

Pneumonia

Pneumonia is an infection or inflammation of the smallest air passages in the lungs (alveoli). These passages fill up with pus or mucus, preventing oxygen from reaching the blood. It can be caused by a variety of bacteria or viruses.

Pneumonia may follow or accompany a cold, flu, or bronchitis. Symptoms may include:

- Fever and shaking chills

- Pain in the chest, especially when coughing or taking a deep breath

- Labored, shallow, or rapid breathing

- Cough that produces greenish-yellow or reddish-brown sputum, especially if sputum changes from clear to colored

- Sweating and flushed appearance

- Loss of appetite or upset stomach

- Generalized fatigue that is worse than you would expect from a cold

Prevention

- Keep up your resistance to infection with a good diet, plenty of rest, and regular exercise.

- Take care of minor illnesses. Don't try to "tough them out." See home treatment for colds on page 99 and flu on page 103.

- Avoid smoke and other irritants.

- If you are over age 65, or if you have chronic lung disease (asthma, COPD), get a pneumococcal vaccination. See page 29.

Home Treatment

Call a health professional if you suspect pneumonia. After pneumonia is diagnosed, follow the home treatment below.

• Increase your fluid intake to 8 to 12 glasses of water a day. Extra fluids are necessary to keep the mucus thin. You are drinking enough if you are urinating more than usual.

• Get lots of rest. Don't try to rush recovery.

• Take the entire course of all prescribed medications.

• Stop smoking.

When to Call Kaiser Permanente

• If you suspect pneumonia.

• If there is rapid or labored breathing during any respiratory illness.

• If signs of a bacterial infection develop after any viral illness. See page 96.

The key symptom of sinusitis in adults is pain in the cheekbones and upper teeth, in the forehead over the eyebrows, or around and behind the eye. In children, a chronic stuffy nose is a common symptom. There may also be headache, fever (if the sinuses are infected), mucus running down the back of the throat (postnasal drip), and sore throat or cough. Sinus headaches may occur on rising and get worse in the afternoon or when bending over.

If there is a bacterial infection, antibiotics may be needed.

Prevention

• Treat colds promptly. Blow your nose gently. Do not close one nostril when blowing your nose.

• Drink plenty of extra fluids when you have a cold, to help keep mucus thin and draining.

• Stop smoking. Smokers are more prone to sinusitis.

Sinusitis

Sinusitis is an inflammation or infection of the sinuses. The sinuses are cavities, or hollow spaces, in the head that are lined with mucous membranes. The sinuses usually drain easily unless there is an inflammation or infection. Sinusitis may follow a head cold and is often associated with hay fever, asthma, or any air pollution that causes inflammation. It can develop in infants and children but is more common in adults.

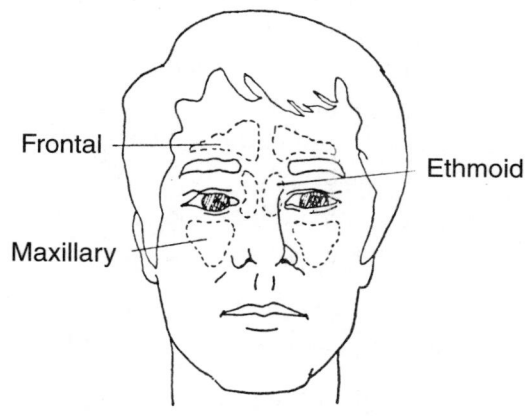

Sinus cavities

Sinusitis – continued

Home Treatment

The goal of home treatment is to get your sinuses draining normally again.

• Drink extra fluids to keep mucus thin. Drink a glass of water or juice every waking hour.

• Breathe moist air from a humidifier, hot shower, or sink filled with hot water.

• Increase home humidity, especially in the bedrooms

• Take an oral decongestant or use a decongestant nasal spray (see page 297). Do not use a nasal spray for more than three days. Avoid products containing antihistamines.

• Take aspirin, acetaminophen, or ibuprofen for headache.

• Check the back of your throat for postnasal drip. If streaks of mucus appear, gargle with warm water to prevent a sore throat.

• Elevate your head at night.

• Salt water (saline) irrigation helps wash mucus and bacteria out of the nasal passages. Use an over-the-counter saline nasal spray or a homemade solution (see page 298 for instructions):

   ○ Use a bulb syringe and squirt the solution gently into the nose.

   ○ Snuff the solution from the palm of your hand one nostril at a time.

   ○ Blow the nose gently afterward. Repeat two to four times a day.

When to Call Kaiser Permanente

• If symptoms of a cold last longer than 10 to 14 days or worsen over time.

• If there is a severe headache, different from a "normal" headache, that is not relieved by acetaminophen, aspirin, or ibuprofen.

• If there is increased facial swelling or blurring or changes in vision.

• If signs of a bacterial infection develop. See page 96.

• Some nasal stuffiness and facial pressure are common with a cold and often respond to home treatment. Call a health professional if facial pain, especially in one sinus area or along the ridge between the nose and lower eyelid, persists after two to four days of home treatment.

• If sinusitis symptoms persist after you have taken a full course of antibiotics.

Sore Throat and Strep Throat

Most sore throats are caused by viruses and sometimes accompany a cold. A mild sore throat is often due to low humidity, smoking, air pollution, or perhaps yelling. People who have allergies or stuffy noses may breathe through their mouths while sleeping, causing a mild sore throat.

Another common cause of sore throat is stomach acid that refluxes into the throat. Although this is often associated with heartburn or an "acid" taste in the mouth, sometimes the only symptom is a sore throat.

Strep throat is a sore throat caused by strep bacteria. It is more common in children age 4 to 11, and is less common in older children and adults. Symptoms of strep throat include sore throat with two of these three:

- Fever of 101° or higher (fever may be lower in adults)
- White or yellow coating on the tonsils
- Swollen glands in the neck

In children, other symptoms may include general body aches, headache, stomachache, nausea, vomiting, runny nose, or listlessness. Strep throat is treated with antibiotics.

If a sore throat is accompanied by runny or stuffy nose and or cough, it is probably due to a virus, not to strep throat, and antibiotics will not help.

Another cause of persistent sore throat is **mononucleosis** (mono or "the kissing disease"), a viral infection. It is most common in older teens and young adults. In addition to a severe sore throat and fatigue, mono symptoms often include weakness, aches, dizziness, swollen lymph nodes in the neck, and an enlarged spleen. It is diagnosed by a blood test for the Epstein-Barr virus.

Mono may last for several weeks and is usually not severe. Symptoms can recur for several months, and it is normal for the lymph nodes to remain enlarged for up to a month. There is no specific treatment except rest, plenty of fluids, and aspirin or acetaminophen for body aches.

Prevention

- Increase your fluid intake to as much as 8 to 12 glasses of water a day (until you are urinating more often than usual).
- Identify and avoid irritants that cause sore throat (smoke, fumes, yelling, etc.). Don't smoke.
- Avoid contact with people who have strep throat.
- If you have mono, don't share eating or drinking utensils and avoid kissing to keep from spreading the virus.

Home Treatment

Home care is usually all that is needed for viral sore throats. If you are taking antibiotics for strep throat, these tips will also help you feel better.

- Gargle with warm salt water (one teaspoon of salt in eight ounces of water). The salt reduces swelling and discomfort.
- If you have postnasal drip, gargle frequently to prevent more throat irritation.
- Drink more fluids to soothe a sore throat. Honey and lemon or weak tea may help.
- Stop smoking and avoid others' smoke.
- Acetaminophen, aspirin, or ibuprofen will relieve pain and reduce fever. Do not give aspirin to children and teens under age 20.

Sore Throat – continued

- Some over-the-counter throat lozenges have a local anesthetic to deaden pain. Dyclonine hydrochloride (Sucrets Maximum Strength) and benzocaine (Spec-T and Tyrobenz) are safe and effective. Regular cough drops or hard candy may also help.

- If you suspect problems with stomach acid may be contributing to your sore throat, refer to the remedies on page 46.

When to Call Kaiser Permanente

- If the following symptoms develop:

  ○ Excessive drooling in a small child (more than the usual amount)

  ○ Difficulty swallowing

  ○ Labored or difficult breathing

- If sore throat develops after exposure to strep throat.

- If a sore throat occurs with two of these three symptoms of strep throat:

  ○ Fever of 101° or higher (may be lower in adults)

  ○ White or yellow coating on the tonsils

  ○ Swollen glands in the neck

- If a rash occurs with sore throat. Scarlet fever is a rash that may occur when there is a strep throat infection. Like strep throat, scarlet fever is treated with antibiotics.

- If you cannot trace the cause of a sore throat to a cold, allergy, smoking, overuse of your voice, or other irritation.

- If a mild sore throat lasts longer than two weeks.

Swollen Glands

The lymph nodes are small glands in the body. The most noticeable nodes are those in the neck. The lymph nodes swell as the body fights minor infections from colds, insect bites, or small cuts. More serious infections may cause the glands to greatly enlarge and become very firm and tender.

Swelling in the glands on either side of the neck is common with a cold or sore throat. The lymph nodes in the groin may swell if there is a cut or sore on the leg or foot, or if there is a vaginal or other pelvic infection.

Once lymph nodes harden, they may remain hard long after the initial infection is gone. This is especially true in children, whose glands may get smaller but remain hard and visible for several weeks.

Home Treatment

- There is no specific home treatment for swollen lymph glands. Continue treating the cold or other infection that is causing the glands to swell.

- Small hardened glands that follow a child's cold or minor infection and are not tender can be observed without professional help. Report swollen glands at your next regular visit to a doctor.

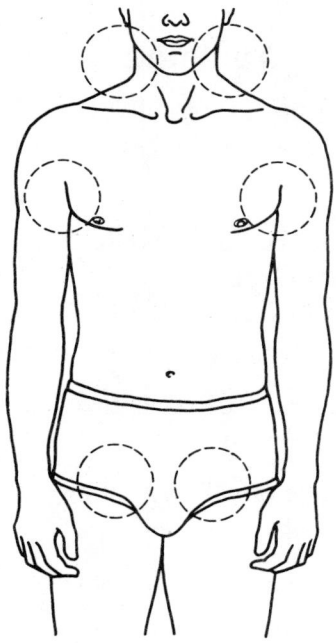

Common sites of
swollen lymph nodes

When to Call Kaiser Permanente

- If the glands are large, very firm, red, and very tender.

- If enlarged glands are associated with other signs of infection in a cut or sore:

  ○ Fever over 100° or higher with no other cause

  ○ Swelling and tenderness

  ○ Discharge from the cut

  ○ Red streaks extending from the area

- If enlarged glands continue to get bigger, or appear without apparent cause and persist two weeks or longer.

- If enlarged glands appear in areas other than the ones shown above.

Tonsillitis

The tonsils and adenoids are lymph tissues in the throat. The tonsils can be seen on either side of the throat at the back of the mouth. The adenoids are higher in the throat and usually cannot be seen. They assist in the production of antibodies to fight infections.

Inflammation of the tonsils (tonsillitis) and adenoids (adenoiditis) is common in children and may occur separately or together. Symptoms of tonsillitis or adenoiditis are sore throat, fever, and tiredness. It may be painful to swallow, and the tonsils are often bright red, spotted with pus, and swollen. The lymph glands in the neck may also swell. Adenoiditis can also cause headache and vomiting.

If the adenoids are chronically inflamed, the child may breathe through the mouth, snore, and have a nasal or muffled voice. Inflamed adenoids can block the eustachian tubes, contributing to ear infections. See page 118.

Tonsillitis and adenoiditis are usually caused by a virus, but can also be caused by strep throat infection. See page 107 for signs of strep throat, which needs antibiotic treatment.

Surgical removal of the tonsils (tonsillectomy) or adenoids (adenoidectomy) used to be common operations for children who had frequent sore throats. Now it is thought that this lymph tissue may be helpful in filtering infection and should not be removed unless necessary. These surgeries are not without risk, and should be done only for valid reasons and after discussion with your doctor. See page 110.

Tonsillectomy and Adenoidectomy

It was once common to remove children's tonsils and adenoids. Today, in recognition of the risks, costs, and limited benefits, tonsillectomy and adenoidectomy are performed much less frequently. They should only be done when the benefits greatly outweigh the risk, inconvenience, and pain.

Tonsillectomy may be recommended if at least one of the following criteria is met:

- If there have been *at least* four to six severe strep tonsillitis infections in the past year despite treatment with at least two different antibiotics.

- If the enlarged tonsils cause severe breathing difficulty or sleep disturbance.

- If there are deep pockets of infection in the tonsils that haven't responded to drug treatment.

Adenoidectomy may be recommended if at least one of the following criteria is met:

- If the enlarged adenoids are obstructing the airway, causing breathing difficulty and sleep disturbance.

- If the adenoids are believed to cause persistent ear infections despite antibiotic treatment.

If surgery is recommended without meeting one of the above criteria, a second opinion may be advisable. See page 18.

Tonsillitis – continued

Home Treatment

- Tonsillitis can usually be treated like any viral sore throat. See page 106.

When to Call Kaiser Permanente

- If sore throat occurs with two of these three signs of strep throat:

  - Fever of 101° or higher (may be lower in adults)

  - White or yellow coating on the tonsils

  - Swollen glands in the neck

- If sore throat or tonsillitis develop after exposure to strep.

- If there are repeated bouts of tonsillitis, especially more than four or five per year.

- If a child has persistent mouth breathing, snoring, or very nasal or muffled voice.

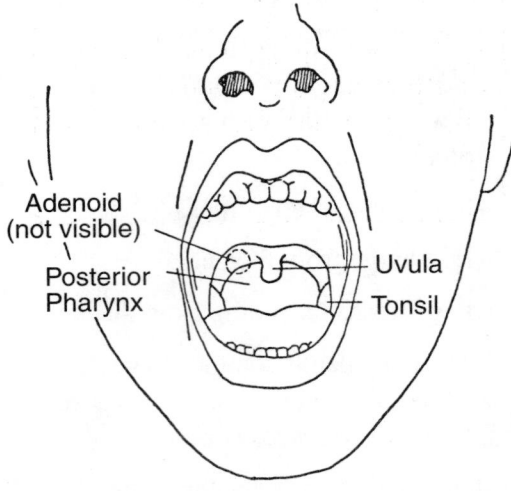

Location of tonsils

The Nicotine Patch

The nicotine patch is an adhesive patch that releases nicotine into the bloodstream through the skin. Used together with a smoking cessation program, it may help some smokers gradually withdraw from nicotine addiction by supplying smaller and smaller amounts of nicotine.

First try to stop smoking without the patch. Many people succeed without it.

The patch is most useful for people who have had serious withdrawal symptoms (headaches, anxiety, depression, difficulty concentrating, insomnia) when they try to quit smoking. Generally, it is prescribed only to those who smoke more than a pack a day.

Using the patch alone is not always successful. By combining the patch with a good smoking cessation program, your chances of success can be greatly increased.

For information on all our smoking cessation program options, including the nicotine patch, call 344-7891.

Quitting Smoking

Before You Quit

- **Set a quit date.**
- List your reasons for quitting: for you and your family's health, to save money, to prevent wrinkles, or whatever.
- Figure out why you smoke. Do you smoke to relax? To pep yourself up? To deal with anger or other negative feelings? Do you like the ritual of smoking?
- Plan healthful alternatives to smoking.
    - How will you deal with stress or anger?
    - How will you keep your hands or mouth busy?
    - What other rituals can you substitute?
- Plan an activity for when the urge to smoke hits. Urges don't last long—take a walk, brush your teeth, have a mint, or chew gum.
- Choose a reliable smoking cessation program. Good programs have at least a 20 percent success rate after one year; great programs, 50 percent. Higher numbers may be too good to be true. Call 344-7891 for all our smoking cessation program options.
- Plan a regular, healthful reward for quitting smoking. Take the money you save by not buying cigarettes and spend it on yourself.

After You Quit

- Know what to expect. The worst will be over in just a few days, but physical withdrawal symptoms may last one to three weeks. After that, it is all psychological. See Chapter 17 for relaxation tips.
- Remove all reminders of smoking from your surroundings. Do things that are incompatible with smoking, like bicycling or going to a movie.
- Get help and support. Ask an ex-smoker to help you.
- Think of yourself as an ex-smoker. Be positive.
- For the first few weeks, avoid situations and settings that you associate with smoking.
- Drink plenty of water to help flush the nicotine out of your system. Keep alcohol to a minimum, if any.
- Keep low-calorie snacks handy for when the urge to munch hits. Your appetite may perk up, but most people gain less than 10 pounds when they quit smoking. A healthy, low-fat diet and regular exercise will help you resist the urge to smoke and avoid unwanted pounds.
- Be prepared for slip-ups. It often takes several tries to quit smoking permanently. If you do smoke, forgive yourself and learn from the experience. You will not fail as long as you keep trying.
- **Good luck!**

You can observe a lot just by watching.
Yogi Berra (naturally)

Chapter 8

Eye and Ear Problems

From earaches to earwax and dry eyes to pinkeye, your ears and eyes can cause you trouble. With home care and patience, most of these problems will clear up. This chapter will explain what you can do at home and when to get professional help.

Conjunctivitis

Conjunctivitis, or pinkeye, is an inflammation of the delicate membrane (conjunctiva) that lines the inside of the eyelid and the surface of the eye. It can be caused by bacteria, viruses, allergies, pollution, or other irritants.

The symptoms are redness in the whites of the eyes, red and swollen eyelids, lots of tears, a sandy feeling in the eyes, and sensitivity to light. There may be a discharge that causes the eyelids to stick together during sleep.

Prevention

- Wash your hands thoroughly after treating pinkeye.

- Do not share towels, handkerchiefs, or washcloths with an infected person.

- If a chemical or object gets into your eye, immediately flush it with water. See page 215 and page 229.

Home Treatment

Although most cases of conjunctivitis will clear up in five to seven days on their own, viral pinkeye can last many weeks. Conjunctivitis due to allergies or pollution will last as long as you are exposed to the irritating substance. Good home care will speed healing and bring relief.

- Apply cold or warm compresses several times a day to relieve discomfort.

Eye and Ear Problems

Eye Symptoms	Possible Causes
Red, itchy, watery eyes	See Allergies, p. 89. Think about allergy to eye care products, make-up, smoke; contact lens irritation. Remove lenses. See p. 115.
Excessive discharge from eye; red, swollen eyelids; scratchy/sandy feeling	See Conjunctivitis, p. 113. Possible contact lens irritation. See p. 115.
Pimple or swelling on eyelid	See Styes, p. 122.
Pain in the eye	See Chemical Burns to the Eye, p. 215; Migraine Headaches, p.128; Cluster Headaches, p. 129; Objects in the Eye, p. 229; consider contact lens irritation, p. 115; Glaucoma, p. 121.
Severe eye pain, blurred vision, reddened eyeball	Possible iritis. See a doctor now!
Red spot on white of eye	See Blood in the Eye, p. 116.
Blow to eye	See Bruises (black eye), p. 213.
Dry, scratchy eyes	See Dry Eyes, p. 118.

Ear Symptoms	Possible Causes
Pain in ear (earache); pulling at ears by infants and small children, especially with inconsolable crying	See Ear Infections, p. 118.
Pain while chewing; headache	See TMJ Syndrome, p. 243.
Pain when ear is wiggled; itching or burning in ear	See Swimmer's Ear, p. 123.
Discharge from ear	See Swimmer's Ear, p. 123; eardrum rupture, p. 118.
Feeling of fullness in ear; with runny or stuffy nose, cough, fever	See Colds, p. 99; Ear Infections, p. 118.
Feeling of something in ear; as if ear is "bumping around"	See Objects in the Ear, p. 229.
Hearing loss; inattentiveness	See Earwax, p. 120; serous otitis media, p. 118.
Ringing or noise in the ears	See Tinnitus, p. 121.

Conjunctivitis – continued

- Gently wipe the edge of the eyelid with moist cotton or a clean wash-cloth and water to remove encrusted matter.

- Don't wear contact lenses or eye makeup until the infection is gone. Discard eye makeup after an eye infection.

- If eye drops are prescribed, insert as follows:

  ○ For older children and adults, pull the lower lid down with two fingers to create a little pouch. Put the drops there. Close the eye for several minutes to let the drops move around.

  ○ For younger children, ask the child to lie down with eyes closed. Put a drop in the inner corner of the eye. When the child opens the eye, the drop will run in.

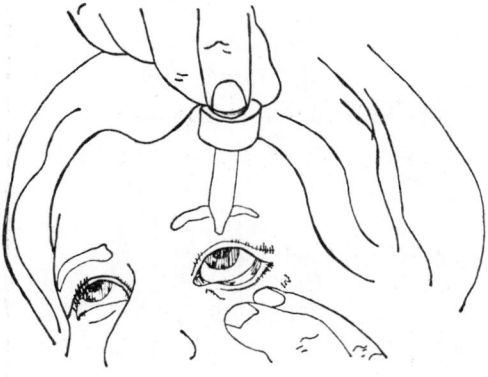

Inserting eye drops

Contact Lenses

If you wear contact lenses, these tips will help you avoid problems.

- Follow the cleaning instructions for your lenses. Keep your lenses and anything that touches them (hands, storage containers, solution bottles, makeup) very clean. Wash your hands before handling your contacts.

- Use a commercial saline solution. Homemade solution is easily contaminated with bacteria. (Generic brands are just as good as name brands.)

- Insert your contacts *before* applying eye makeup. Replace eye makeup every three to six months to reduce the risk of contamination. Do not apply makeup to the inner rim of the eyelid.

- When worn for long periods of time, extended-wear lenses are more likely to cause severe eye infections. If you choose to wear them, follow the wearing and cleaning schedule your doctor recommends.

- Symptoms of a possible problem with your contacts include unusual redness, pain or burning in the eye, discharge, blurred vision, or extreme sensitivity to light. Remove your lenses and disinfect them. If symptoms persist longer than two to three hours after removing and cleaning your contacts, call your eye care professional.

- Visit your eye care professional once a year to check the condition of your lenses and the health of your eyes.

Conjunctivitis – continued

- ○ Be sure the dropper is clean and does not touch the eye, eyelid, or any surface. Eye drops are washed out by normal tearing, so they will need to be replaced at least three times a day.

- Putting antibiotic ointment in the eye can be tricky, especially with children. If you can get it on the eyelashes, it will melt and get into the eye.

- Make sure any over-the-counter medicine you use is *ophthalmic* (for eyes), not *otic* (for ears).

When to Call Kaiser Permanente

- If there is pain in the eye (rather than irritation), blurring, or loss of vision, not cleared even momentarily with blinking.

- If eye is painfully sensitive to light.

- If you feel there is a foreign object in the eye.

- If the eye is red and there is a thick, greenish-yellow discharge.

- If there is an abnormal difference in size of pupils.

- If the problem continues for more than seven days.

Blood in the Eye

Sometimes, blood vessels in the whites of the eyes break and cause a red spot or speck. This is called a subconjunctival hemorrhage. The blood may look alarming, especially if the spot is large. It is usually not a cause for concern, and will clear up in two to three weeks.

However, if your eye is bloody and painful, if there is blood in the colored part of the eye, or if the bleeding followed a blow to the eye, call a health professional. Also call if bleeding in the eye occurs often, or occurs after you begin taking blood thinners (anti-coagulants).

Dizziness

Dizziness or **lightheadedness** is usually not due to a serious problem; in fact, it is common to feel lightheaded ocassionally. It is often due to a momentary drop in blood pressure and blood flow to the head that occurs when you get up too quickly from a seated or lying position. This is called orthostatic hypotension and is most often caused by medications or dehydration.

Other causes of dizziness include side effects of medications, stress, anxiety or drinking alcohol. Another less common cause is an abnormality in your heart rhythm. This usually causes recurrent spells of lightheadedness over a period of a few days.

Vertigo is a sensation that your body or the world around you is spinning. It may occur with nausea and vomiting. It may be impossible to walk while you are experiencing severe vertigo. Benign positional vertigo, the most common form, is triggered by changes in the position of the head, such as when you move your head from side to side or lean your head back to look up. Vertigo may also be caused by inflammation in the part of the inner ear that controls balance (called labyrinthitis). Labyrinthitis is usually caused by a viral infection and sometimes occurs following a cold or the flu.

Home Treatment

Dizziness is not usually a cause for concern unless it is severe, persistent, or occurs with other symptoms.

- When you feel dizzy, sit down for a minute or two and take some deep breaths. Stand up again slowly.

- Sit up or stand up slowly to avoid the changes in blood flow to the head that can make you feel dizzy.

Floaters and Flashers

Floaters are spots, specks, and lines that "float" across the field of vision. They are caused by stray cells or strands of tissue that float in the vitreous humor, the gel-like substance that fills the eyeball. Floaters can be annoying, but are not usually serious. However, if you see floaters or flashes of light for the first time, call the Ophthalmology Advice Nurse for an appointment. If you have had floaters for some time, or if you have occasional flashes, call for a routine eye exam.

- Avoid head positions or changes in position that bring on vertigo. However, some experts suggest that practicing these positions may help overcome the problem.

- If you have vertigo, avoid lying flat on your back. Prop yourself up slightly to relieve the spinning sensation.

When to Call Kaiser Permanente

- If dizziness is accompanied by headache, confusion, loss of hearing or changes in vision, weakness in the arms or legs, or numbness in any part of the body.

- If you feel like you might faint or if there is a complete loss of consciousness.

- If you suspect dizziness may be a side effect of a medication.

- If dizziness lasts more than three to five days and interferes with your daily activities.

- If you experience vertigo (sensation that room is spinning around you) that is severe or persists for more than three days, has not been diagnosed, or is significantly different from previous episodes.

- If you have repeated spells of lightheadedness over a few days.

- If your pulse when you are feeling lightheaded is less than 50 or more than 130 beats per minute.

Eye Twitches

Eye twitches or muscle spasms around the eye are most often associated with fatigue and/or stress. Twitches will usually stop on their own in a short time, and they will improve with rest or reduced stress.

Call a health professional if twitches occur with redness, swelling, discharge from the eye, or fever, or if the eye twitch lasts longer than one to two weeks.

Dry Eyes

Eyes that don't have enough moisture in them may feel dry, hot, sandy, or gritty. Dry eyes may be due to low humidity, smoke, the natural aging process, or certain medications such as antihistamines, decongestants, and birth control pills.

Home Treatment

• Try an over-the-counter artificial tear solution, such as Akwa-Tears, Duratears, or Hypotears. These are different from drops like Visine, which reduce eye redness rather than dryness.

• Call Kaiser Permanente if dry eyes are persistent and artificial tears do not help.

Ear Infections

A middle ear infection (otitis media) is caused by bacteria and often requires antibiotic treatment. It usually starts when a cold causes the eustachian tube between the ear and throat to swell and close. When the tube closes, fluid seeps into the ear and bacteria start to grow. As the body fights the infection, pressure builds up, causing pain. The pressure can cause the eardrum to rupture.

A single eardrum rupture (perforation) is not serious and does not cause hearing loss. Repeated ruptures may cause hearing loss. Antibiotic treatment stops bacterial growth, relieving pressure and pain.

Young children get more ear infections because their eustachian tubes are more easily blocked, and also because they get more colds.

Symptoms of a bacterial ear infection include earache, dizziness, ringing or fullness in the ears, hearing loss, fever, headache, and runny nose.

Serous otitis media is a collection of fluid in the ear (effusion) without infection. Usually the only symptoms are temporary hearing loss or a full feeling in the ear. These symptoms are not usually a cause for concern unless they last more than 10 days.

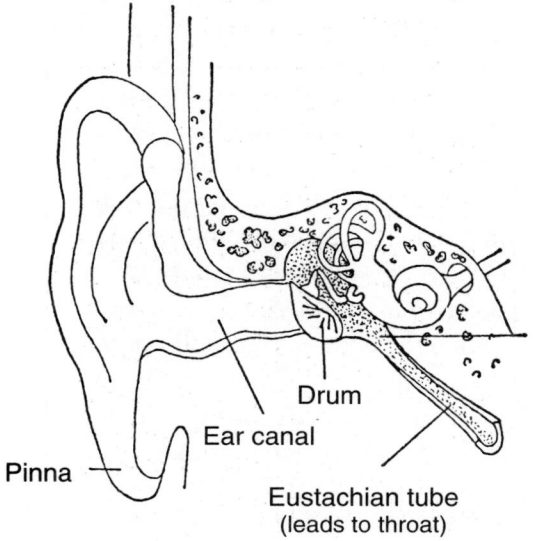

Pinna

Ear canal

Drum

Eustachian tube
(leads to throat)

Ear

Prevention

- Teach your children to blow their noses gently. This is a good idea for adults, too.

- Breast-feed your baby. Breast-fed babies have fewer ear infections.

- Feed infants in a relatively upright position to prevent milk from getting into the eustachian tubes. Do not allow infants to fall asleep with a bottle. (Nursing infants may fall asleep at the breast.)

- Avoid exposing children to cigarette smoke, which is associated with more frequent ear infections.

- Limit your child's contact with other children who have colds.

Home Treatment

- Apply heat to the ear to ease the pain. Use a warm washcloth or a heating pad set on low. Don't leave a child alone with a heating pad.

- Rest. Let your energy go to fighting the infection.

- Increase clear liquids.

- Aspirin or acetaminophen will help relieve earache. Do not give aspirin to a child or a teen under 20. See dosage on page 300.

- If dizziness occurs, see page 116.

When to Call Kaiser Permanente

- Anytime an ear infection is suspected. If the exam confirms an infection, antibiotics may be prescribed.

- If a severe earache lasts longer than one hour or any earache lasts longer than 12 to 24 hours. If the pain is severe at night, call the next morning even if the pain has stopped. The infection may still be present.

- If a child has an earache and fever and appears ill.

- If a headache, fever, and stiff neck are also present, which may be signs of meningitis.

Ear Infections – continued

- If home otoscope exam shows redness in the ear of a small child who cannot describe ear pain. See page 292.

- If you suspect an eardrum rupture. Look for a white, yellow, or bloody discharge from the ear.

- If there is no improvement after three to four days of antibiotics.

- If stuffy ears or hearing loss persist without other symptoms more than 10 days after a cold has cleared up. Some infections are painless.

Earwax

Earwax is a protective secretion, similar to mucus or tears, that filters dust and keeps the ear clean. Normally, earwax is liquid, self-draining, and does not cause problems. Occasionally, the wax will build up, harden, and cause some hearing loss. Poking at the wax with cotton swabs, fingers, or other objects will only further compact the wax against the eardrum. Professional help is needed to remove tightly packed wax. You can handle most earwax problems by avoiding cotton swabs and following the home treatment tips below.

Children have a lot of earwax. It seems to taper off as they grow older. You should be concerned only if the earwax causes ringing or a full feeling in the ears, or some hearing loss.

Recurrent Ear Infections

Some children have repeated ear infections despite treatment. If your child has at least three ear infections in a six-month period, or has more than two infections before age six months, prophylactic antibiotics may be recommended. This is a low dose of antibiotics taken daily throughout the season when the child is especially prone to ear infections. It is effective in reducing the frequency of ear infections. Antibiotics don't always prevent fluid in the ear (effusion) or infection.

If infection persists after one month or fluid persists after three months of continuous treatment (with at least two different antibiotics), or if there is significant persistent hearing loss, your doctor may suggest inserting ear tubes (tympanostomy) through the eardrum to drain the fluid. The tubes remain in the eardrum for 6 to 12 months and help prevent ear infections.

Continued long-term use of antibiotics may be just as effective in preventing infection and clearing fluid from the ear. If ear tubes are recommended without trying antibiotics first, consider asking for a second opinion. See page 18.

Home Treatment

- Warm mineral oil helps loosen wax. Wash the wax out with an ear syringe and warm mineral oil. (Cold fluid may make you dizzy.) Use very gentle force. Do not do this if there is discharge from the ear, if you suspect an ear infection or that the eardrum is ruptured, or if you have ear tubes.

- If the warm mineral oil does not work, use an over-the-counter wax softener, followed by gentle flushing with an ear syringe, each night for a week or two. Do not use it if you suspect infection or eardrum rupture.

When to Call Kaiser Permanente

- If the above procedures do not work and the wax build-up is hard, dry, and compacted.

- If you suspect that earwax is causing a hearing problem.

- If the ear is sore or bleeding.

Glaucoma

Glaucoma is an eye disorder caused by too much pressure within the eyeball. Pressure builds up when the fluid within the eye is unable to drain normally. If the pressure is not relieved, it may eventually cause damage to the optic nerve and result in blindness. Untreated glaucoma is one of the leading causes of blindness among older adults.

Tinnitus

Almost everyone has experienced an occasional ringing (or hissing, buzzing, or tinkling) in their ears. The sound usually lasts only a few minutes. If it becomes persistent, you may have tinnitus.

Tinnitus is usually caused by damage to the nerves in the inner ear from prolonged exposure to loud noise. Other, more treatable causes include: excess earwax, ear infection, dental problems, and medications, especially antibiotics and large amounts of aspirin. Drinking excessive alcohol can also cause tinnitus.

To protect your hearing and relieve tinnitus, limit or avoid exposure to loud noises, such as music, power tools, gunshots, and industrial machinery.

Other tips to relieve tinnitus:

- Cut back or eliminate caffeine, nicotine, and alcohol.

- Try to relax. Stress and fatigue seem to make it worse.

- Limit your use of aspirin and products containing aspirin.

Call Kaiser Permanente:

- If tinnitus becomes persistent and interferes with your daily activities or sleep.

- If ringing occurs with dizziness, loss of balance, vertigo, nausea, or vomiting.

- If tinnitus persistently affects only one ear.

Glaucoma – continued

Glaucoma is normally painless and without any noticeable symptoms. A person cannot sense whether his eye pressure is high or not. Glaucoma typically develops slowly over several years without being detected.

Risk factors for developing glaucoma include:

• Family history of the disorder

• African-American race

• Diabetes or nearsightedness

• Taking corticosteriod drugs (e.g., prednisone)

A rare form of the disorder, called closed-angle glaucoma, comes on suddenly and can lead to blindness within hours. This attack commonly occurs at night. It is marked by severe eye pain, blurred vision, and a red-dened eyeball. This is a medical emergency.

Prevention

The goal is to detect glaucoma before significant nerve damage occurs. If you are age 40 to 64, have a glaucoma test every five years. If you are at increased risk (which includes all African Americans), screening is recommended more often.

Home Treatment

Use the eyedrop medications pre-scribed for glaucoma regularly and consistently. Return to your eye doctor at recommended intervals to determine if the treatment is effective.

When to Call Kaiser Permanente

• If you have sudden blurred vision, loss of vision, or pain in the eye.

Styes

A sty is a noncontagious infection of the eyelash follicle. It looks like a small, red bump, much like a pimple, either in the eyelid or on the edge of the lid. It comes to a head and breaks open after a few days.

Styes are very common and are not a serious problem. Most will resolve on their own and don't require removal.

Home Treatment

• Do not rub the eye, and do not squeeze the sty.

• Apply warm, moist compresses for 10 minutes, five to six times a day until the sty comes to a head and drains. Styes respond very well to warm compresses and time.

When to Call Kaiser Permanente

• If the sty interferes with vision.

• If the sty gets worse despite your home treatment.

• If the redness centered on the sty spreads to involve the entire lid.

Swimmer's Ear

Swimmer's ear (otitis externa) is an infection of the outer ear canal. It often develops after water has gotten into the ear, especially after swimming. Sand or other debris that get into the ear canal may also cause swimmer's ear. Scratching the ear or injury from a cotton swab or other object may also irritate the ear canal.

Symptoms include pain, itching, and a feeling of fullness in the ear. The ear canal may be swollen. A more severe bacterial infection may cause increased pain, a discharge from the ear, and possibly some hearing loss. Unlike a middle ear infection (otitis media), swimmer's ear pain is worse when you chew and when you press on the "tag" in front of the ear or wiggle the earlobe.

Prevention

- Keep your ears dry. After swimming or showering, shake your head to remove water from the ear canal. Gently dry your ears with the corner of a tissue or towel, or use a blow-dryer on its lowest setting held several inches from the ear.

- Put a few drops of rubbing alcohol or alcohol mixed with an equal amount of white vinegar in the ear after swimming or showering. Wiggle the outside of the ear to let the liquid enter the ear canal, then tilt your head and let it drain out. You can also use over-the-counter drops (Star-Otic, Swim-Ear) to prevent swimmer's ear.

- Avoid cleaning the ears with cotton swabs or other objects. See page 120 for tips on removing excess earwax. Remove dirt or sand that gets into the ear while swimming by using a bulb syringe or gentle warm shower directed into the ear.

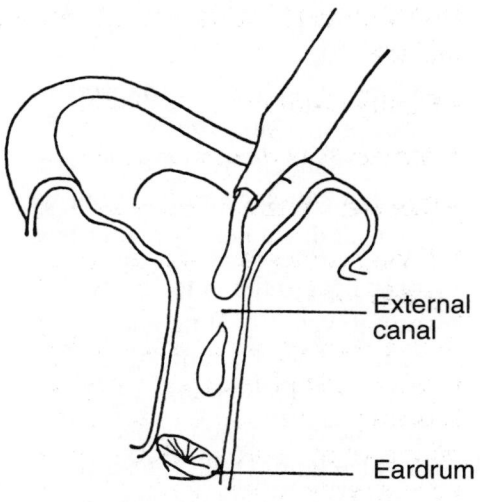

External canal

Eardrum

Inserting eardrops

Home Treatment

- Make sure there isn't an object or insect in the ear. See Objects in the Ear on page 229.

- Gently rinse the ear using a bulb syringe and saline solution or a half-and-half solution of white vinegar and warm water.

- Avoid getting water in the ear until the irritation clears up. Cotton coated with petroleum jelly can be used as an earplug. Do not use plastic earplugs.

- If your ear is itchy, try over-the-counter swimmer's eardrops (see above). Use them before and after swimming or getting your ears wet.

Swimmer's Ear – continued

- To insert eardrops, have the person lie down, ear facing up. Warm the drops first by rolling the container between your hands. Place drops on the wall of the ear canal in small quantities so air can escape and drops can get into the ear. Wiggling the outer ear will help.

- You may find it easier to insert eardrops in a small child in the following manner: Hold the child on your lap with legs around your waist and head down between your legs.

- Apply heat to the outer ear with a warm towel or heating pad set on low to relieve discomfort. Don't leave a child alone with a heating pad. Acetaminophen or aspirin may also help. Don't give aspirin to children or to teens under age 20.

When to Call Kaiser Permanente

- If ear pain and itching persist or worsen despite five days of home treatment.

- If the ear canal is swollen, red, and very painful, or if there is a discharge from the ear.

- If the earache follows a cold. See page 118.

I'm very brave generally, only today I happen
to have a headache.
Tweedledum in *Alice in Wonderland*

Chapter 9

Headaches

Headaches are one of the most common health complaints. They can be caused by tension, infection, allergy, injury, hunger, changes in the flow of blood in the vessels of the head, or exposure to chemicals. **See page 224 for information on head injuries.**

Most headaches that occur without other symptoms will respond well to self-care. The information in this chapter will help you treat common headaches at home, as well as provide tips on how you may be able to prevent them.

The majority of headaches—over 90 percent—are caused by tension and respond well to prevention and home care. See page 129.

You can usually discover the cause of and treat a headache at home. The chart on the next page can help.

An unusual headache that is very different from any you have had before is a cause for concern. See "Headache Emergencies." However, if you have had similar headaches before and your doctor has recommended a treatment plan for them, emergency care may not be needed.

Headache Emergencies

Call for care now if you have:

- A severe headache that strikes suddenly without apparent cause or is very *different* from previous headaches.

- Severe and stabbing head pain.

- Severe headache that occurs with a stiff neck, fever, nausea, and vomiting.

- Headache pain that increases when you try to touch your chin to your chest with mouth closed.

- Headache accompanied by one-sided weakness, numbness, speech or vision problems, confusion, or loss of coordination.

- A blow to the head that causes severe pain, enlarged pupils, lethargy, confusion, or vomiting.

Possible Headache Causes

If headache occurs:	Possible causes
On awakening.	See Tension Headaches, p. 129; Allergies, p. 89; Sinusitis, p. 105. May also be due to low humidity.
In jaw muscles or in both temples.	See TMJ, p. 243; Tension Headaches, p. 129.
Each afternoon or evening; after hours of desk work; with sore neck and shoulders.	See Tension Headaches, p. 129.
On one side of the head.	See Migraine Headaches, p. 128; Cluster Headaches, p. 129.
After a blow to the head.	See Head Injuries, p. 224.
After exposure to chemicals (paint, varnish, insect spray, cigarette smoke).	Chemical headache. Get into fresh air. Drink water to flush poisons.
With fever, runny nose, or sore throat.	See Sinusitis, p. 105; Flu, p. 103; Sore Throat, p. 106.
With fever, stiff neck, nausea, and vomiting.	See Encephalitis and Meningitis, p. 102.
With runny nose, watery eyes, and sneezing.	See Allergies, p. 89.
With fever and pain in the cheek or over the eyes.	See Sinusitis, p. 105.
On mornings when you drink less caffeine than usual.	Caffeine withdrawal headache. Cut back slowly. See p. 129.
Following a stressful event.	See Tension Headaches, p. 129.
At the same time during menstrual cycle.	See Premenstrual Syndrome, p. 182.
With new medication.	Drug allergy. Contact doctor.
With severe eye pain.	Acute glaucoma. See doctor now!

Headaches in Children

Children's headaches rarely indicate a serious problem. They are more frequent in children whose parents often discuss their own headaches. Children tend to imitate their parents, so it is wise to mention headaches as infrequently as possible.

Emotional tension is the most common cause of headache in children. Often, a parent can discover the cause of stress and help relieve it. Many times, just talking about a problem may help a child. Some children try to do too much, or are pushed by family or school to do too much. Even fun activities can be overdone and cause fatigue and headaches. Encourage your children to talk openly about problems and stress at school.

Tension headaches (see page 129) are common in teens, and are generally caused by emotional stress related to school, sports, or relationships.

Hunger can also cause headaches in children. A daily breakfast and a nutritious after-school snack may prevent them. Eyestrain may also cause headaches. Headache is also common with viral illnesses that cause fever, such as colds.

Home Treatment

- Talk to your child. Try to discover the source of the headache and deal with it. Let the child know you care. Tension headaches are sometimes "attention" headaches.

- Play quietly with the child, or read stories together.

- If the headache is still present, have the child lie down in a darkened room with a cool cloth on the forehead.

- With quiet time and extra attention, most tension headaches in children can be managed without pain relievers. If non-drug treatments do not relieve the pain, try acetaminophen. See page 300 for the proper dosage. Avoid creating the pattern of using a pill for every pain. Do not give aspirin to children.

When to Call Kaiser Permanente

- If a headache is severe and is not relieved by relaxation or acetaminophen.

- If a severe headache occurs with signs of encephalitis or meningitis (see page 102), especially following a viral illness.

- If a child's headaches occur two to three times a week or more, or if you are using pain relievers to control headaches more than once a week.

- If you cannot discover a reasonable cause. A child may share problems with someone other than a parent.

- If headaches awaken the child at night or are worse early in the morning.

- Also see "Headache Emergencies" on page 125.

Migraine Headaches

Migraine headaches have very specific symptoms. Migraines are also called vascular headaches, because they are believed to be caused by changes in the flow of blood in the vessels of the head.

Symptoms of a migraine include throbbing pain on one or both sides of the head and sensitivity to light or noise. Because migraines may also cause nausea or vomiting, they are sometimes called "sick" headaches.

Although the headache comes on quite suddenly, it is sometimes preceded by visual disturbances, such as zig-zagged lines, called an aura. Dizziness and numbness on one side of the body may also precede a migraine. The headaches last from a few hours to a few days, and recur from several times a week to once every few years.

Migraines are more common in women. The headaches may begin during childhood, but most begin during the teens and early twenties.

Prevention

Keep a diary of your headache symptoms. See "Tracking Your Headaches" on page 130. Once you know what events, foods, medications, or activities bring on a headache, you may be able to prevent or limit their recurrence.

Some women find that their headaches improve if they stop taking birth control pills. Experiment with a nonhormonal form of birth control. See page 198.

Home Treatment

- Lie down in a darkened room at the first sign of a migraine. Relax the entire body, starting with the forehead and eyes and working down to the toes. See page 252.

- Many people find aspirin, acetaminophen, or ibuprofen helps relieve a migraine.

- If a doctor has prescribed medication for your migraines, take the recommended dose at the first sign that a migraine is starting.

- If you use over-the-counter or prescription headache medications too often, they may actually make the headaches more frequent or severe. If this occurs, call your doctor for advice.

- Most migraine headaches will require professional diagnosis and treatment.

When to Call Kaiser Permanente

- If you suspect your headaches are migraines. Professional diagnosis and treatment can help decrease the impact of migraines on your life. Discuss relaxation and biofeedback techniques, which help many people prevent migraines.

- Also see "Headache Emergencies" on page 125.

Tension Headaches

More than 90 percent of headaches are caused by tension. Tension headaches are often caused by tight muscles in the neck, back, and shoulders. Both emotional stress and physical stress, such as sitting at a computer too long, can cause muscle tension. A previous neck injury or arthritis in the neck can also cause tension headaches.

A tension headache may cause pain all over the head, pressure, or a feeling of having a band around the head.

Cluster Headaches

Cluster headaches are sudden, very severe, sharp, stabbing headaches that occur on one side of the head, usually in the temple or behind the eye. The eye and nostril on the affected side may be runny.

The pain often begins at night, and may last from 30 minutes to a few hours. The headache may recur several times a day. Attacks may last 4 to 12 weeks, then disappear for months or years.

Cluster headaches are five times more common in men. Many men who get them are heavy smokers and drinkers. Avoid alcohol and cigarettes during an attack.

See your doctor if you think you have cluster headaches or if you have persistent, severe headaches with no apparent cause.

Also see "Headache Emergencies" on page 125.

The head may feel like it is in a vise. Some people feel a dull, pressing, burning sensation above the eyes.

The pain may also affect the jaw, neck, and shoulder muscles. You can rarely pinpoint the center or source of pain.

Prevention

- Reduce emotional stress. The next time you do something that causes a headache, take time to relax before and afterwards. See page 252 for good ways to cope with stress.

- Reduce physical stress. Change positions often during desk work and stretch for 30 seconds each hour. Make a conscious effort to relax your jaw, neck, and shoulder muscles.

- Evaluate your neck and shoulder posture at work and make adjustments if needed. See page 66.

- Daily exercise helps relieve tension.

- Cut down on caffeine. People who drink a lot of caffeinated beverages often develop a headache several hours after they have their last beverage, or may wake with a headache that is relieved by drinking caffeine.

Home Treatment

- Stop whatever you are doing and sit quietly for a moment. Close your eyes and inhale and exhale slowly. Try to relax your head and neck muscles.

- Take a stretching break or try a relaxation exercise. See page 252 or Resources 40 and 79 on pages 309 and 311.

Tension Headaches – cont.

- Massage the neck muscles. Rub gently and firmly toward the heart. See page 68 for neck exercises.

- Treat yourself to a massage. Some people find regular massages very helpful in relieving tension.

- Apply heat with a heating pad, hot water bottle, or a warm shower.

- Lie down in a dark room with a cool cloth on your forehead.

- Aspirin, acetaminophen, or ibuprofen often helps relieve a tension headache. However, using over-the-counter or prescription headache medications too often may make headaches more frequent or severe. If this occurs, call your doctor for advice.

- See page 252 for helpful ways to deal with stress.

When to Call Kaiser Permanente

- If a headache is very severe and cannot be relieved with home treatment.

- If a headache occurs with fever of 103° or higher and no other symptoms.

- If unexplained headaches continue to occur more than three times a week.

- If headaches become more frequent and severe.

- If headaches awaken you out of a sound sleep or are worse first thing in the morning.

- If you need help discovering or eliminating the source of your tension headaches. Talking it over with a health professional may be helpful.

- Also see "Headache Emergencies" on page 125.

Tracking Your Headaches

If you have recurring headaches, keep a record of your symptoms. This record will help your doctor if medical evaluation is needed.

1. The date and time each headache started and stopped.

2. Any factors that seem to trigger the headache: food, smoke, bright light, stress, activity.

3. The location and nature of the pain: throbbing, aching, stabbing, dull.

4. The severity of the pain.

5. Other physical symptoms: nausea, vomiting, visual disturbance, sensitivity to light or noise.

6. If you are a woman, note any association between headaches and your menstrual cycle or use of birth control pills or hormone replacement therapy.

Chapter 10

Skin Problems

Skin problems are rarely life-threatening, but they can be a nuisance. Diagnosing skin problems may require a doctor's help, especially the first time you have a particular ailment. Use the chart on the next page and the index to find the skin problem you're interested in. Also see "Childhood Rashes" on page 157.

Acne

Acne is the term for pimples or blackheads that form on the face, chest, upper back, or shoulders. A pimple forms when an oil gland in the skin is blocked and secretions and bacteria build up under the skin. Acne occurs most often in adolescence, but often persists into adulthood.

Many women get a few pimples just before their menstrual period. Stress and some oral contraceptives may make acne worse. Fatty foods such as chocolate and nuts are generally no longer considered a cause of acne.

Most cases of acne will respond to home treatment. For severe or persistent cases, your doctor can prescribe stronger topical medication, antibiotics, or other drugs.

Prevention

- Wash your face with a mild soap, such as Dove, or one that contains benzoyl peroxide, such as Oxy-5. Wash as often as necessary to keep it clean, but do not scrub.

- While foods are no longer considered a significant cause of acne, avoid any food that seems to cause pimples.

Skin Problems

Skin Symptoms	Possible Causes
Raised, red, itchy welt after an insect bite or taking a drug	See Hives, p. 140; Insect Bites and Stings, p. 142.
Red, painful, swollen bump under the skin	See Boils, p. 134.
Red, flaky, itchy skin	See Dry Skin, p. 136; Eczema, p. 137; Fungal Infections, p. 138; Rashes, p. 145.
Crusty, honey-colored rash	See Impetigo, p. 140.
Rash that develops after wearing new jewelry or clothing; exposure to poisonous plants; eating a new food; taking a new drug	See Rashes, p. 145.
Painful blisters in a band around one side of the body	See Shingles, p. 139.
Change in shape, size, or color of a mole, or persistently irritated mole	See Skin Cancer, p. 146.
Cracked, blistered, itchy, peeling skin between the toes	See Fungal Infections (athlete's foot), p. 138.
Red, itchy, weeping rash on the groin or thighs	See Fungal Infections (jock itch), p. 138; Impetigo, p. 140.
Scaly, itchy, bald spots on scalp	See Fungal Infections (ringworm), p. 138.
Flaky, silvery patches of skin, especially on knees, elbows, or scalp	See Psoriasis, p. 137.
Sandpapery skin rash with sore throat; "raspberry" tongue	Scarlet fever. See p. 108.

Acne – continued

Home Treatment

- Cleanliness is essential. Wash your face, shoulders, chest, and back with soapy water. Use a very gentle soap such as Aveeno, Neutrogena, or Basis. Avoid drying soaps such as Ivory. Always rinse very well.

- Keep long hair off the face and shoulders, and wash it daily.

- Don't pop pimples and blackheads. This can cause infection and scarring.

- Benzoyl peroxide gel or cream, an over-the-counter medication, is one of the best treatments for acne. Start with the lowest strength and apply once a day one-half hour after washing. You may experience mild redness and dryness as a side effect. It may take several weeks to work. Never use more than 5 percent strength benzoyl peroxide except on the advice of a doctor.

- Use only non-comedogenic, water-based lotions and cosmetics, and only if they don't aggravate the acne.

When to Call Kaiser Permanente

- If acne cannot be controlled with the above home treatment.

- If there are severe red or purple inflammation, cysts, or nodules under the skin.

Blisters

Blisters are usually the result of persistent or repeated rubbing against the skin. Some illnesses, such as shingles, cause blister-like rashes (see page 139). Burns can also blister the skin. See page 213.

Prevention

- Avoid shoes that are too tight or rub on your feet.

- Wear gloves to protect your hands when doing heavy chores.

Home Treatment

- If a blister is small and closed, leave it alone. Protect it from further rubbing with a loose bandage, and avoid the activity or shoes that caused it.

- If a small blister is in a weight-bearing area, protect it with a donut-shaped moleskin pad. Leave the area over the blister open.

- If a blister is larger than one inch across, it is usually best to drain it. The following is a safe method:

  - Sterilize a needle with rubbing alcohol.

  - Gently puncture the blister at the edge.

  - Press the fluid in the blister toward the hole you have made to drain it.

- Once you have opened a blister, or if it has torn open, wash the area with soap and water.

Blisters – continued

- Do not remove the flap of skin covering the blister unless it is very dirty or torn, or if pus is forming under the blister. Gently smooth it flat over the tender skin underneath.

- Apply an antibiotic ointment and a sterile bandage. Do not use alcohol or iodine. They will delay healing.

- Change the bandage once a day to reduce the chance of infection.

- Remove the bandage at night to let the area dry.

When to Call Kaiser Permanente

- If blisters recur often and you do not know the cause.

- If signs of infection develop:
  - Increased pain, swelling, redness or tenderness
  - Heat or red streaks extending from the blister
  - Discharge of pus
  - Fever of 100° or higher with no other cause

- If you have diabetes or peripheral vascular disease.

Boils

A boil is a red, swollen, painful bump under the skin, similar to an overgrown pimple. Boils are often caused by an infected hair follicle. Bacteria from the infection will form an abscess or pocket of pus. The abscess can become larger than a ping-pong ball and be extremely painful.

Boils occur most often in areas where there is hair and chafing. The face, neck, armpits, breasts, groin, and buttocks are common boil sites.

Prevention

- Wash boil-prone areas often with soapy water. An antibacterial soap may help. Dry thoroughly.

- Avoid clothing that is too tight.

Home Treatment

- Do not squeeze, scratch, drain, or lance the boil. Squeezing can push the infection deeper into the skin. Scratching can spread the bacteria and form new boils.

- Wash yourself well with an anti-bacterial soap to prevent the boil from spreading.

- Use moist heat often. Apply hot, wet washcloths to the boil for 20 to 30 minutes, three to four times a day. Do this as soon as you notice a boil. The heat and moisture can help bring the boil to a head, but it may take five to seven days. A hot water bottle or heating pad applied over a damp towel may also help.

- Continue using warm compresses for three days after the boil opens. Apply a bandage to keep draining material from spreading, and change it daily.

Birthmarks

Birthmarks are common in babies and small children and most will fade as the child grows. Report any changes in birthmarks to your health professional.

Salmon patches ("stork bites") are light pink birthmarks that may appear on the upper lip, eyelids, forehead, and back of the neck. They will fade within a few months.

Strawberry birthmarks are soft, red lumps formed by clusters of blood vessels. They may be present at birth or appear during the first few months. They may grow for up to six months, are stable for a short time, and then usually begin to recede and fade. Sixty percent are gone by age five; nearly all have disappeared by age nine. No treatment is necessary unless they continue to grow.

Port-wine stains are light pink or wine-colored birthmarks that appear most often on the head and face. They are permanent, and become darker as the child grows.

Birthmarks need to be removed only if they interfere with breathing or vision, or if they disfigure the face. If surgery is desired for cosmetic reasons, it is best to wait until the child is older.

When to Call Kaiser Permanente

If needed, your medical provider can drain the boil and treat the infection. Call if:

- The boil is on your face, near your spine, or in the anal area.
- Worsening signs of infection develop:
  - Increased pain, swelling, heat, redness, or tenderness
  - Red streaks extending from the boil
  - Continued discharge of pus
  - Fever of 100° or higher with no other cause
- The pain limits your normal activities.
- You have diabetes.
- Any other lumps, particularly painful ones, develop near the infected area.
- The boil is as large as a ping-pong ball.
- The boil is not improving after five to seven days of home treatment.
- Many boils develop and persist over several months.

Dandruff

Dandruff occurs when the skin cells of the scalp flake off. This flaking is natural and occurs all over your body. On the scalp, however, flakes can mix with oil and dust to form dandruff. Dandruff cannot be cured, but it can be controlled.

Dandruff – continued

Home Treatment

- Try frequent and energetic shampooing with any shampoo. Wash hair daily if it controls dandruff.

- If the dandruff is excessive and itchy, try a dandruff shampoo (Selsun Blue, Sebulex, Tegrin) three times a week. Experiment to find the one that works best for you. Alternate with your regular shampoo.

When to Call Kaiser Permanente

- If frequent shampooing, or shampooing with a dandruff shampoo, doesn't control dandruff. Your doctor may prescribe a stronger dandruff shampoo.

Dry Skin

Dry, itchy, flaky skin is a common problem. It results when the skin loses water (not oil) to the air. Dry indoor air is a common cause, as is excessive bathing with strong soaps and hot water. Dry skin is often worse in the winter due to lower humidity and indoor heat.

Prevention

- Humidify your home, especially the bedroom.

- Avoid hot showers and baths. They strip the skin's natural oil, which helps hold in moisture.

Relief from Itching

- Keep the itchy area cool and wet. Try a compress soaked in ice water.

- An oatmeal bath may help relieve itching. Wrap one cup of oatmeal in a cotton cloth and boil as you would to cook it. Use this as a sponge and bathe in tepid water without soap. Or try an Aveeno Colloidal Oatmeal bath.

- Calamine lotion is helpful for poison ivy or oak rashes.

- Try an over-the-counter 1 percent hydrocortisone cream for small itchy areas. Use very sparingly on the face or genitals. If itching is severe, your doctor may prescribe a stronger cream.

- Try an over-the-counter oral antihistamine (Chlor-Trimeton, Benadryl).

- Cut nails short or wear gloves at night to prevent scratching.

- Wear cotton clothing. Avoid wool and acrylic fabrics next to the skin.

- Avoid strong detergents and deodorant soaps. Avoid Ivory as it is very drying. Limit use of perfumes and perfumed products.

- Avoid overexposure to the sun. See page 147.

Home Treatment

- Follow the prevention guidelines above.

- Bathe every other day instead of every day. Use warm or cool water and a gentle soap (Dove, Tone,

Basis). Use little or no soap on dry skin areas. Pat dry with a towel; don't rub skin.

- Apply a moisturizer (Vaseline, Moisturel, Nutraderm) while skin is still damp to seal in moisture. A light layer of petroleum jelly is also an effective and inexpensive moisturizer. Reapply lotion often.

- For very dry hands, try this for a night: Apply a thin layer of petroleum jelly, and wear thin cotton gloves to bed. (May also help dry feet.)

- Avoid scratching, which damages the skin. If itching is a problem, see "Relief from Itching" on page 136.

When to Call Kaiser Permanente

- If you itch all over your body without obvious cause or rash.

- If itching is so bad that you cannot sleep and home treatment methods are not helping.

- If the skin is badly broken due to scratching.

Eczema

Eczema (atopic dermatitis) is a chronic skin disorder common in people with asthma, hay fever, and other allergies. It causes a very itchy, red, scaly rash that may weep or ooze a clear fluid. The rash may also be thick, skin colored, and slightly silvery. The rash may first develop as tiny blisters, which break and crust over. It is prone to infection, especially if scratching is not controlled.

In children, eczema appears most often on the face, scalp, buttocks, thighs, and torso. In adults, it usually affects the neck, inside the elbows, and backs of the knees.

Eczema is often worse during infancy and greatly improves by early adulthood. Many children improve by age two.

Psoriasis

Psoriasis is a chronic skin condition that causes flaky, silvery patches on the knees, elbows, or scalp. The fingernails, palms, and soles of the feet may also be affected. It is not contagious.

The patches, called plaques, are made up of dead skin cells that accumulate in thick layers. Normal skin cells are replaced every 30 days. In psoriasis, skin cells are replaced every three to four days.

Small patches of psoriasis can often be treated with regular use of hydrocortisone cream.

Tar products (lotions, gels, shampoos) may also be useful, although they may increase sensitivity to the sun. Limited exposure to the sun may also help (protect unaffected skin with sunscreen). If psoriasis affects the scalp, try a dandruff shampoo.

Stress may contribute to psoriasis. Stress reduction may help in some cases. See page 252.

Call your doctor if psoriasis covers much of your body or is very red. More extensive cases often need professional care.

Eczema – continued

Home Treatment

Helping the skin retain moisture is important to successful treatment.

- Take brief daily baths or showers with lukewarm (not hot) water. Use a gentle soap (Dove, Basis, Aveeno, Neutrogena) or non-soap cleanser (Cetaphil or Aveeno). If possible, bathe without soap.

- After bathing, pat skin dry and apply a lubricating cream (Vaseline, Nutraderm, DML, Moisturel). The cream may help keep your skin from drying out. Reapply cream often.

- An oral antihistamine (Benadryl) may help relieve itching and relax you enough to allow sleep. Avoid antihistamine and antiseptic creams and sprays, as they irritate the skin.

- Use a humidifier in the bedroom.

- Avoid contact with any irritants or allergens that cause problems.

- Wash clothes and bedding in mild detergent and rinse at least twice. Do not use fabric softener if it is irritating.

- For more tips on relieving itching, see page 136.

When to Call Kaiser Permanente

- If crusting or weeping sores appear. A bacterial infection may be present.

- If a red patchy rash appears on the face accompanied by joint pain and fever.

- If itching interferes with sleep and home treatment is not working.

Fungal Infections

Fungal infections of the skin may affect the feet, groin, scalp, or nails. Fungi grow best in warm, moist areas of the skin, such as between the toes, in the groin, and the area beneath the breasts.

Athlete's foot (tinea pedis) is the most common fungal skin infection. Symptoms include cracked, blistered, and peeling areas between the toes, redness and scaling on the soles, and intense itching. It rarely affects children before puberty; if it does, it may resemble eczema. Athlete's foot often recurs and must be treated again each time.

Jock itch (tinea cruris) causes severe itching and moistness on the skin of the groin and upper thighs. There may be red, scaly, raised areas on the skin that weep or ooze pus or clear fluid.

Ringworm is a contagious fungal infection of the scalp or body. It is *not* caused by worms. Its symptoms include round spots that may be scaly and itchy. It may appear on the torso as a small, red, scaly spot that itches and grows until it is about an inch across. It is more common in children than in adults.

Fungal infections of the fingernails and toenails cause discoloration, thickening, and often softening of the nails. They are difficult to treat and often cause permanent damage to the nails.

Thrush is a yeast infection that occurs in the mouth, especially in babies. It causes a white coating inside the mouth, often on the cheeks, that may look like milk but is hard to remove.

Prevention

- Keep the feet clean and dry. Dry well between the toes after swimming or bathing.

- Wear leather shoes or sandals that allow your feet to "breathe," and wear cotton socks to absorb sweat. Use powder on your feet and in your shoes. Give shoes 24 hours to dry between wearings.

- Wear thongs or shower sandals in public pools and showers.

- Keep the groin clean and dry. Wash and dry well, especially after exercise, and apply talcum powder to absorb moisture. Wear cotton underclothes and avoid tight pants and pantyhose.

- Teach children not to play with dogs or cats that have bald or mangy spots on their coats.

- Don't share hats, combs, or brushes.

Home Treatment

- Follow the prevention guidelines above.

- For athlete's foot and jock itch, use an over-the-counter antifungal powder or lotion, such as Micatin or Lotrimin AF. Use the medication for a week or two after the symptoms clear up to prevent recurrence. Do not use hydrocortisone on a fungal infection.

- Consider wearing cotton socks, and change them twice a day to keep your feet dry. If possible, wear open sandals with cotton socks. When indoors, go in stocking feet.

- Ringworm on the body can be treated with one of the antifungals listed above.

When to Call Kaiser Permanente

- If signs of infection are present: increased swelling and redness or signs of pus.

- If you have diabetes and develop athlete's foot. People with diabetes are at increased risk of infection and may need professional care.

- If home treatment fails to clear up athlete's foot or jock itch after two weeks.

Shingles

Shingles (herpes zoster) is caused by the reactivation of the chicken pox virus in the body years after the initial illness. The virus usually affects one of the large nerves that spread outward from the spine, causing pain and a rash in a band around one side of the chest, abdomen, or face. The rash will blister and scab, then clear up over the course of a few weeks.

No one knows what makes the virus active again. Shingles is more common in older adults and people who have weakened immune systems, but can affect anyone who has had chicken pox.

Shingles itself is not contagious, but exposure to the rash can cause chicken pox in a person who has not had it before.

If you suspect shingles, call your doctor or advice nurse, within a day after the rash starts if possible, to discuss drugs that can limit the pain and rash.

Fungal Infections – continued

- If there is a sudden loss of hair associated with flaking, broken hairs, and inflammation of the scalp, or if there are several household members with hair loss.

- If ringworm is severe and spreading. Prescription medicine may be needed.

- If ringworm is present on the scalp.

Hives

Hives (urticaria) are an allergic reaction of the skin. Hives are raised, red, itchy patches of skin (wheals or welts) that may appear and disappear at random. They range in size from less than a quarter-inch to an inch or more, and they may last a few minutes or a few days.

Multiple hives often occur in response to a drug, food, or infection. A single hive commonly develops after an insect sting. Other possible causes include plants, inhaled allergens, stress, cosmetics, and exposure to heat, cold, or sunlight. Often a cause cannot be found.

Prevention

- Avoid foods, medications, and insects that have previously caused hives.

Home Treatment

- Continue to avoid the substance that causes hives.

- Cool water compresses will help relieve itching. Also see page 136.

- An oral antihistamine (Benadryl, Chlor-Trimeton) may help treat the hives and relieve itching. Once the hives have disappeared, decrease the dose of the medication slowly over five to seven days.

When to Call Kaiser Permanente

- Call *immediately* if hives occur with dizziness, wheezing, difficulty breathing, tightness in the chest, or swelling of the tongue, lips, or face.

- If hives develop soon after taking a new drug.

- If hives persist for several days despite home treatment and avoiding the suspected irritants.

Impetigo

Impetigo is a bacterial infection that is much more common in children than in adults. It often starts when a small cut or scratch becomes infected. Symptoms are oozing, scabbed, honey-colored, crusty sores. These sores often appear on the face between the upper lip and nose, especially after a cold. Scratching the sores may spread impetigo to other parts of the body.

Prevention

- Wash all scratches and sores with soap and water.

- If your child has a runny nose, keep the area between the upper lip and nose clean to prevent infection.

- Keep fingernails short and clean.

Home Treatment

Small areas of impetigo may respond well to prompt home treatment.

- Remove crusts by soaking the area in warm water (use a warm washcloth for the face) for 15 to 20 minutes, then scrub gently with a washcloth and antibacterial soap such as Betadine or Hibiclens. Pat dry gently; do not rub. Repeat several times a day.

- Apply an antibiotic ointment (see page 295). Cover the area with gauze taped well away from the area. This will help keep the infection from spreading and prevent scratching.

- To prevent spreading the infection, do not share towels, washcloths, or bath water. Men should shave around the sores, not over them, and use a clean blade daily. Do not use a shaving brush.

When to Call Kaiser Permanente

- If impetigo covers an area larger than two inches in diameter.

- If, after three to four days, you have not progressed in controlling impetigo or any new infected areas appear. Your doctor may prescribe an antibiotic.

- If the area around the nostrils, lips, or face swells and becomes tender.

- If signs of infection develop after two to three days:

  ○ Pain, swelling, or tenderness

  ○ Heat and redness, or red streaks extending from the area

  ○ Discharge of pus

  ○ Fever of 100° or higher with no other cause

Ingrown Toenails

Ingrown toenails are caused when an improperly trimmed toenail cuts into the skin at the edge of the nail. Shoes that are too tight can also cause ingrown toenails. Because the cut can easily become infected, prompt care is needed.

Prevention

- Cut toenails straight across so the edges cannot cut into the skin. Leave the nails a little longer at the corners so that the sharp ends don't cut into the skin.

- Wear roomy shoes and keep your feet clean and dry.

Home Treatment

- Soak your foot in warm water.

- Wedge a small piece of wet cotton under the corner of the nail to cushion the nail and keep it from cutting the skin.

- Repeat daily until the nail has grown out and can be trimmed.

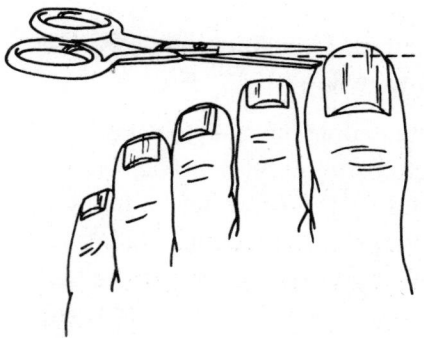

Cutting toenails

Ingrown Toenails – continued

When to Call Kaiser Permanente

- If signs of infection develop:

  ○ Increased pain, swelling, or tenderness

  ○ Red streaks extending from the area

  ○ Discharge of pus

  ○ Fever of 100° or higher with no other cause

- If you have diabetes or circulatory problems.

Insect Bites and Stings

Insect and spider bites and bee, yellow jacket, and wasp stings usually cause a localized reaction with swelling, redness, and itching. In some people, especially children, the redness and swelling may be worse, and the local reaction may last up to a day. In most cases, bites and stings do not cause reactions all over the body. (In a few areas, mosquitos may spread illnesses, including encephalitis and malaria.)

Some people have severe skin reactions to insect or spider bites or stings, and a few have allergic (anaphylactic) reactions that affect the whole body. Symptoms may include hives all over the body, shortness of breath and tightness in the chest, dizziness, wheezing, or swelling of the tongue and face. If these symptoms develop, *immediate* medical attention is needed.

Few spiders cause serious bites, although any bite may be serious if the person has an allergic reaction.

Black widow spiders can be up to two inches across (although they are generally much smaller) and are shiny black with a red hourglass mark on their undersides. Their bites may cause chills, fever, nausea, and severe stomach pain. Infants and children will be more affected by a bite than adults.

Brown recluse (fiddler) spiders are smaller with long legs, and brown with a white violin-shaped mark on their back. Their bites cause intense pain and may result in a blister that turns into a larger sore.

Jellyfish are common on some ocean beaches. If touched, their tentacles release a stinging poison that causes a painful reaction.

Prevention

- To avoid bee stings, wear white or light-colored solid fabrics. Bees are attracted to dark colors and flowered prints.

- Avoid wearing perfumes and colognes when you are outside.

- Apply an insect repellent containing DEET every few hours when in insect- and spider-infested areas. Use a lower-concentration DEET product for small children and pregnant women. Wash DEET off when you come inside. Alpha-Keri and Skin-So-Soft bath oils also seem to repel insects.

- Wear gloves and tuck pants into socks when working in woodpiles, sheds, and basements where spiders are found.

Home Treatment

- Remove a bee stinger by scraping or flicking it out (if the stinger isn't visible, assume there isn't one). Don't squeeze the stinger; you may release more venom into the skin.

- If the bite is from a black widow or brown recluse spider, apply ice to the bite and call your doctor.

- Apply a cold pack or ice cube to the bite or sting. Some people also find that a paste of baking soda, meat tenderizer, or activated charcoal mixed with a little water helps relieve pain and decrease the reaction.

- An oral antihistamine (Benadryl, Chlor-Trimeton) may help relieve pain and swelling, and relieve itching if there are many bites. Calamine lotion, hydrocortisone cream, or a local anesthetic containing benzocaine (Solarcaine) may also help.

- Anyone who has had a severe systemic allergic reaction to insect venom should carry an emergency kit containing a syringe and adrenalin (epinephrine). Ask your doctor or pharmacist how to use the kit.

- Trim fingernails to prevent scratching, which can lead to infection.

For jellyfish stings:

- Rinse the area immediately with saltwater. Do not use fresh water and do not rub; it will release more poison.

- Splash vinegar, alcohol, or meat tenderizer dissolved in saltwater on the area to neutralize the poison.

- Remove any attached tentacles carefully. Protect your hand with a towel and apply a paste of sand or baking soda and saltwater to the area. Scrape the tentacles off with the cloth or the edge of a credit card.

- Apply calamine lotion to relieve pain and itching.

- If you are stung by a Portuguese man-of-war jellyfish, scrape the stinging tentacles off with sand and seek medical care immediately.

When to Call Kaiser Permanente

- Call *immediately* if signs of a severe allergic reaction develop soon after being stung by an insect:

  ○ Wheezing, difficulty breathing

  ○ Swelling around the lips, tongue, or face, or significant swelling around the site of the insect sting (e.g., entire arm or leg is swollen)

  ○ Skin rash, itching, feeling of warmth, or hives

- If a blister appears at the site of a spider bite, or if the surrounding skin becomes discolored.

- To talk with your doctor about adrenalin kits or allergy shots (immunotherapy) for insect venom. See page 92.

Lice and Scabies

Lice are tiny, white, wingless insects that may live on the skin, hair, or clothing. They feed by biting the skin and sucking blood. The bites itch. Lice lay tiny eggs, called nits, which can often be seen on the hair. Head lice live in the hair on the head; body lice live on clothing; and pubic lice (also called crabs) live in the groin, underarms, and eyelashes. Lice are spread by close physical contact or contact with the clothing, bedding, brushes, or combs of an infected person. Pubic lice can be spread by sexual contact.

Scabies are tiny mites that burrow under the skin and lay eggs. This burrowing causes an allergic reaction with a rash that itches intensely. They are often found between folds of skin on the fingers and toes, wrists, underarms, and groin. They are usually treated with a prescription medication that is applied over the entire body and left on overnight. Itching may last for several weeks after treatment. Over-the-counter lotions for lice may not be strong enough to treat scabies.

Prevention

- Be alert for signs of lice: itching and signs of lice or nits along the hair shafts of the head. Prompt treatment can help prevent spreading them to others.

Bald Spots

Bald spots are not the same as baldness. Men often have a natural tendency toward baldness. This natural hair loss is largely hereditary. It poses no major health risks other than sunburn (wear a hat and use sunscreen).

Bald spots may be caused by repeated pulling of the hair, such as tight braids or habitual tugging or twisting. Ringworm is a fungal infection that causes scaly bald spots. See page 138.

Bald spots that appear on a normal scalp may indicate a more significant problem. If hair loss is sudden, or if it develops after beginning a new medication, call your doctor.

Home Treatment

- Nix and RID are over-the-counter medications for lice. Follow the manufacturer's directions for use. Treat the entire family. For head lice, comb the hair well with a fine-toothed comb after treatment to remove all nits.

- On the day you start treatment, wash all clothing worn in the last week, bedding, and towels in hot water to help get rid of lice, nits, and mites. Iron things that cannot be washed.

- Contact your pharmacist or health department for more information on treatment and preventing reinfestation.

When to Call Kaiser Permanente

- If treatment with over-the-counter medication is not successful. Stronger prescription drugs are available.

- If you suspect scabies. (Prescription medications are needed to treat scabies.)

Rashes

A rash (dermatitis) is any irritation or inflammation of the skin. Rashes can be caused by illness, allergy, or heat, and may sometimes be caused by emotional stress. When you first get a rash, ask yourself these questions to help determine the cause:

- Did the rash follow contact with anything new that could have irritated your skin: poison ivy, oak, or sumac; soaps, detergents, shampoos, perfumes, cosmetics, or lotions; jewelry or fabrics?

- Have you eaten anything new that you may be allergic to?

- Are you taking any medications, either prescription or over-the-counter?

- Have you been unusually stressed or upset recently?

- Is there joint pain or fever with the rash?

- Is the rash spreading?

- Does the rash itch?

Also see page 157.

Prevention

- If you are exposed to poison ivy, oak, or sumac, wash the skin with dish soap and water within 30 minutes to get the irritating oil off the skin. This may help prevent or reduce the rash. Also wash your dog, your clothes, and anything that may have come in contact with the plant.

- Use fragrance- and preservative-free or hypoallergenic detergents, lotions, and cosmetics if you have frequent rashes.

Home Treatment

- Wash affected areas with water. Soap can be irritating. Pat dry thoroughly.

- Apply cold, wet compresses to reduce itching. Repeat frequently. Also see page 136.

- Leave the rash exposed to the air. Baby powder can help keep it dry. Avoid lotions and ointments until the rash heals. However, calamine lotion is helpful for plant rashes. Use it three to four times a day.

- Hydrocortisone cream can provide temporary relief of itching. Use very sparingly on facial rashes.

- Avoid products that cause the rash: detergents, cosmetics, lotions, clothing, jewelry, etc.

- Rashes on the feet or groin may be due to fungal infections. See page 138.

Rashes – continued

When to Call Kaiser Permanente

- If signs of infection develop after two to three days:

  ○ Pain, swelling, or tenderness

  ○ Heat and redness, or red streaks extending from the area

  ○ Discharge of pus

  ○ Fever of 100° or higher with no other cause

- If you suspect a medication reaction caused the rash.

- If rash occurs with fever and joint pain.

- If rash occurs with sore throat. See page 108.

- If a rash appears and you aren't sure what is causing it.

- If rash continues after two to three weeks of home treatment.

Skin Cancer

Skin cancer is the most common type of cancer. Fortunately, many types of skin cancer are easy to cure.

Most skin cancer is caused by sun damage. Ninety percent of skin problems occur on the face, neck, and arms, where sun exposure is greatest. Light-skinned, blue-eyed people are more likely to develop skin cancer. Dark-skinned people have less risk.

Most skin cancers are generally slow growing, easy to recognize, and easy to treat in a doctor's office. A small percentage of skin cancers are more serious.

Skin cancers of the non-melanoma type (**basal cell** and **squamous cell cancers**) tend to develop in sun-exposed areas. They differ from non-cancerous growths in several important ways. Skin cancers:

- Tend to bleed more and are often open sores that do not heal.

- Tend to be slow growing.

Most moles are harmless. However, **malignant melanomas** (cancerous moles) can be fatal and should be promptly treated.

Prevention

Most skin cancers can be prevented by avoiding excessive exposure to the sun. Much damaging sun exposure has occured by age 20, so keep your children protected (see page 147). Cumulative exposure to sun is a major factor in some types of skin cancers.

Home Treatment

Examine your skin with a mirror or another person's help. Look for unusual moles, spots, or bumps. Pay special attention to areas that receive a lot of sun exposure: hands, arms, chest, and neck (especially the back of the neck), face, ears, etc. Note any changes and report them to your doctor.

When to Call Kaiser Permanente

Monitor your moles. If they do not change over time, there is little cause for concern. Call your health professional if you observe any of the following changes:

- Asymmetrical shape: One half does not match the other half.

- Border irregularity: The edges are ragged, notched, or blurred.

- Color: The color is not uniform. Watch for shades of red and black, or a red, white, and blue mottled appearance.

- Diameter: Larger than a pencil eraser (harmless moles are usually smaller than this.)

- Scaliness, oozing, bleeding, or spreading of pigment into surrounding skin.

- Appearance of a bump or nodule on the mole, or any change in appearance of the mole.

- Itching, tenderness, or pain.

- Unusual skin changes or growths, especially if they bleed and keep growing.

- If you have a family history of malignant melanoma, let your doctor know. You may be at higher risk.

Sunburn

A sunburn is usually a first-degree burn that involves just the outer surface of the skin. Sunburns are uncomfortable, but are usually not dangerous unless they are extensive. Severe sunburns can be serious in infants and small children.

Prevention

If you are going to be in the sun for more than 15 minutes, take the following precautions:

- Use a sunscreen with a sun protection factor (SPF) of at least 15.

- Apply the sunscreen 15 minutes before exposure. Reapply every two hours or as directed.

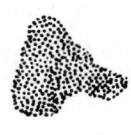

Asymmetrical shape

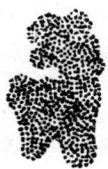

Border irregular

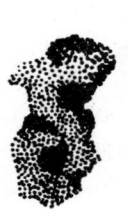

Color varied

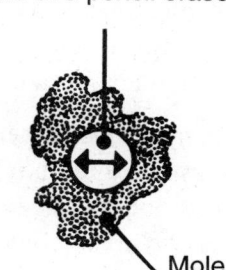

Size of a pencil eraser

Mole

Diameter larger than a pencil eraser

Mole changes to watch for

Sunburn – continued

- If you are allergic to PABA, the active ingredient in many sun-screens, use non-PABA alternatives. Ask your pharmacist.

- Wear light-colored, loose-fitting, long-sleeved clothes and a broad-brimmed hat to shade your face.

- Drink lots of water. Sweating helps cool the skin.

- Avoid the sun between 10 a.m. and 2 p.m., when the burning rays are strongest.

- Don't forget the kids. Early sun exposure may be very hard on their tender skin. Teach your young children healthy sun habits—hats and sunscreen—early.

Home Treatment

- Watch sunburned infants or children for signs of dehydration. See page 43. Also watch for signs of heat exhaustion. See page 225. Drink lots of water.

- Cool baths or compresses can be very soothing. Take acetaminophen or aspirin for pain. Don't give aspirin to children.

- A mild fever and headache can accompany a sunburn. Lie down in a cool, quiet room to relieve headache.

- There is nothing you can do to prevent peeling; it is part of the healing process. Lotion can help relieve itching.

When to Call Kaiser Permanente

- If signs of heat stroke develop. See page 225.

- If there is severe blistering accompanied by fever or you feel very ill.

- If there is fever of 102° or higher.

- If dizziness or vision problems persist after the person has cooled off.

Tick Bites

A tick is a small insect that fastens itself to the body. A tick should be removed as soon as you discover it.

Lyme disease (which is relatively uncommon in Colorado) is a bacterial infection spread by deer ticks. Deer ticks are tiny, about the size of the period at the end of this sentence. Therefore, if the tick is large enough that it can be seen easily, it is probably not a deer tick.

Early symptoms of Lyme disease include a red "bulls-eye" rash with a white center around the bite. The rash develops four days to three weeks after the bite. Flu-like symptoms such as fever, fatigue, headache, muscle aches, and joint pain may also occur. Lyme disease can be treated with antibiotics to prevent later symptoms, such as arthritis and heart problems.

Prevention

- Wear light-colored clothing and tuck pant legs into socks.

- Apply an insect repellent containing DEET to exposed areas of skin or to clothing when in tick-infested areas.

  ◦ Use a lower-concentration product on children and pregnant women.

  ◦ Use caution around eyes and mouth. Don't put repellent on small children's hands, as they often put their hands in their mouths.

  ◦ After returning indoors, wash the repellent off with soap and water.

Home Treatment

- Check regularly for ticks when you are out in the woods and thoroughly examine your skin and scalp when you return home. Check your pets, too. The sooner ticks are removed, the less likely they are to spread bacteria.

- Remove a tick by gently pulling with tweezers, as close to the skin as possible. Pull straight out and try not to crush the body. Save the tick in a jar for tests if symptoms of Lyme disease develop.

- Wash the area and apply an antiseptic.

When to Call Kaiser Permanente

- If you are unable to remove the entire tick.

- In areas where Lyme disease is common, see a doctor if a tick has been attached for more than 24 hours.

- If a red "bulls-eye" rash, fever, fatigue, or flu-like symptoms develop up to three weeks after a tick bite.

Warts

Warts are skin growths that are caused by a virus. They can appear anywhere on the body. Warts are not dangerous, but can be bothersome.

Little is known about warts. Most types are only slightly contagious. They can spread to other areas on the same person but rarely to other people. Genital and anal warts are an exception; they are easily transmitted through sexual contact and may increase the risk of cervical cancer. See page 199.

Plantar warts appear on the soles of the feet. Most of the wart lies under the skin surface, and may make you feel like you are walking on a pebble.

Because warts seem to come and go for little reason, it's possible they are sensitive to slight changes in the immune system. In some cases, you can "think" them away.

When necessary, your doctor can remove warts. Unfortunately, they often come back.

Home Treatment

- Warts appear and disappear spontaneously. They can last a week, a month, or even years. To get rid of your warts, it helps to believe in the treatment. If something works for you, stick with it.

- If the wart bleeds a little, cover it with a bandage and apply light pressure to stop the bleeding.

Warts – continued

- If the wart is in the way, use a pumice stone or salicylic acid ointment. This drug can be irritating in high concentrations; you may need to use a milder form for a longer period of time. These are over-the-counter products.

- If you use a pumice stone, both the debris from the wart and the area of the pumice stone that touched the wart can be infectious. Do not handle this material. Discard both the wart debris and pumice stone promptly.

- For plantar warts, apply a donut-shaped pad to cushion the wart and relieve pain. Apply salicylic acid solution to the wart at night, and rub the whitened skin off in the morning. Do not use salicylic acid if you have diabetes or peripheral vascular disease.

- Try the least expensive method of treating warts. You may save a trip to your doctor.

- Don't cut or burn off a wart.

When to Call Kaiser Permanente

- If a wart looks infected after being irritated or knocked off.

- If a plantar wart is painful when you walk and foam pads do not help.

- If you have warts in the anal or genital area. See page 199.

- If the wart causes continual discomfort.

- If a wart develops on the face and is a cosmetic concern.

Calluses and Corns

Calluses are hard, thickened skin on parts of the foot exposed to friction. Corns are caused by pressure on the skin from the inside, such as a bone.

Soak your feet in warm water and rub the callus or corn with a pumice stone. You may need to repeat for several days before the thickened skin is gone.

Do not try to cut or burn off corns or calluses. If you have diabetes or peripheral vascular disease, talk with your doctor about removing troublesome corns or calluses.

Chapter 11

Infant and Child Health

When your child gets sick or hurt, you are usually the first person around to provide care. Your calmness, confidence, and competence in caring for your children's health problems will help them enjoy healthy childhoods and learn the importance of self-care for their own use as they mature.

Virtually every health problem in this book may affect children. However, a few are almost exclusively childhood concerns. For convenience, we have grouped these problems into this chapter. If the problem you are looking for is not in this chapter, please look for it in the index.

Facts About Infants and Young Children

The following brief notes are of particular concern to parents. This information may help dispel some unnecessary fears and give you some guidance.

For more information on child health, see Resources 23 to 31 on page 308.

Umbilical Cords and Belly Buttons

The umbilical cord will drop off and the navel will usually heal in one to three weeks. After the cord comes off, there may be a moist or bloody oozing for a few days, less than the size of a quarter, between diaper changes. This does not need special treatment.

Clean the navel three or four times a day with a bit of cotton wet with rubbing alcohol. Pull the cord up gently but firmly to clean the base (try to avoid getting alcohol on the skin around the navel). Vigorous cleaning will reduce the risk of infection. Keep the navel dry and do not give a tub or pan bath until it is healed. Fold diapers below and shirts above the cord to promote drying.

Call your doctor if there is redness or swelling around the navel, or a large

Facts About Infants – cont.

amount of foul-smelling discharge from the navel.

The appearance of the navel is not affected by the way the cord is tied off. A small nodule of tissue some-times remains after the cord falls off. If it is small, no treatment is usu-ally needed. If it is larger or persists longer than two weeks, call your doctor.

Breast-feeding

Breast milk is the ideal food for babies younger than four to six months. The American Academy of Pediatrics recommends that babies be breast-fed for the first year of life. Up until age four to six months, infants should be fed only breast milk or for-mula. Discuss with your child's provider when you may start giving cow's milk.

Breast-feeding has many advantages both for baby and mother. Breast milk contains antibodies and other disease-preventing substances. Breast-fed babies have fewer colds, ear infec-tions, diarrhea, and vomiting. Breast milk protects against allergies and asthma, and also is easier to digest than formula.

Breast-feeding helps build strong bonds between baby and mother, helps reduce post-delivery bleeding, and often helps the mother lose weight after the baby is born.

Child Car Seats

Infant and child car seats save lives. Many states require them for all children under age four and those weighing less than 40 pounds. Children who are not in car seats can be seriously injured or killed during crashes or even abrupt stops at low speeds. For maximum safety, follow the manu-facturer's recommendations for car seat use.

Infants under 20 pounds: Use an infant car seat that reclines and faces the rear. If your car has a passenger-side air bag, you may need to put the car seat in the back seat. Check the manufacturer's instructions.

Infants and children over 20 pounds: Use a toddler seat that faces the front and has a shield or harness. Some infant seats can be converted into toddler seats.

Children over age four and over 40 pounds: Use a booster seat that elevates the child so he can see out of the window. Use regular lap and shoulder belts. Adjust the shoulder belt to fit across the shoulder, not the neck.

Set a good example for your chil-dren by always wearing your own seat belt, and always insist that they buckle up.

Some instruction in the art of breast-feeding helps ensure that you will have a positive breast-feeding experience. Childbirth preparation classes offered through Kaiser Permanente provide such instruction, or call for advice. Also see Resources 86 and 87 on page 311. The La Leche League and the Nursing Mother's Council are other good sources of breast-feeding information, advice, and support.

Nursing mothers need an extra 500 calories per day above their pre-pregnancy intake. Although you don't need to drink milk to make milk, extra calcium and protein are important, and your doctor may prescribe a vitamin supplement. Anything you consume will cross over into your breast milk. For this reason, avoid smoking, drinking alcohol, and limit caffeine to one or two beverages per day. Do not take any medication while breast-feeding unless it was prescribed by a health professional.

Although breast-feeding is best for your baby, babies can also get good nutrition from formula. If, because of your job or for other reasons, you are unable to breast-feed, add an extra amount of cuddling at feeding time.

Circumcision

Circumcision is surgery to remove the foreskin of a newborn boy's penis. About 60 percent of boys in the U.S. are circumcised, down from over 80 percent in the late 1970s.

There are both benefits and risks associated with circumcision. It reduces the risk of cancer of the penis, which affects about 1 in 600 uncircumcised men in the U.S. Penile cancer is rare in circumcised boys and men. For uncircumcised males, the risk of penile cancer can be greatly reduced by regular washing of the penis after pulling back the foreskin. Circumcision may also reduce the risk of urinary tract infections in young boys.

The risks of circumcision are slight. Complications of local infection or bleeding occur in about one in every 250 cases. Local anesthetic will reduce the pain of circumcision. Generally, circumcision is not recommended for a sick infant. Discuss the risks and benefits of circumcision with your doctor. The decision is entirely up to you.

After circumcision, apply petroleum jelly liberally to the head of the penis at each diaper change to prevent the scab from sticking to the diaper. Wash the penis by dripping warm water over it (do not use alcohol or baby wipes). Pat dry with a soft towel.

If the circumcision site is red, apply an antibiotic ointment (Bacitracin or Polysporin). Call your doctor if the redness extends down the shaft of the penis.

If you choose not to have your son circumcised, clean the exposed foreskin gently during the first four years. Starting around age four, gently begin to retract the foreskin. Do not forcibly retract the foreskin; it may not be fully retractable until puberty. Teach your son to wash the penis well at every bath, and to gently retract the foreskin and clean beneath it.

Facts About Infants – cont.

Uniqueness

No two children are exactly alike. Each child has his own special way of approaching the world. Study your child's behavior and temperament. What is "normal" for him may be far different from the "normal" behavior of a sibling, neighbor, or friend of the same age.

Discipline

Discipline is a way to help children develop self-control and responsible behavior. Children best accept discipline that is fair, firm, consistent, and loving. Focus on the child's behavior, not the child's personality. Set limits and offer the child choices within those limits. For older children and teens, be specific and firm in setting rules and expectations.

Use reflective listening to improve communication with your child. When she expresses her feelings, paraphrase them back to her. This lets her know you are listening and helps her clarify what she is feeling.

Look for and praise good behavior, and ignore bad behavior. If bad behavior doesn't get attention, a child will usually stop doing it.

When your child misbehaves:

• If you are angry, take a few minutes to calm down before disciplining him. Make it clear that you like the child, but you don't like the behavior.

• Use "time-outs" to interrupt problem behaviors and help the child build self-control.

• Discipline older children with loss of privileges or allowances.

• Do not use physical punishment to discipline your children.

Temper Tantrums

Children often have temper tantrums when they are frustrated, want attention, or to get their own way. Children tend to have more temper tantrums when they are tired, hungry, or sick.

• Be supportive if the tantrum is due to frustration, fatigue, or hunger. Offer encouragement, suggest a nap, or provide a snack.

• Stay calm. Getting angry will prolong the tantrum. Avoid spanking, because it tells the child that you have lost control.

• Use time-outs to help the child calm down.

• Don't let tantrums change your behavior as a parent. Children will learn quickly that a tantrum is not the way to get their own way.

Toilet Training

Every child has a unique timetable for becoming toilet trained. Most children are ready to begin toilet training between age 18 and 36 months. Look for these other signs of readiness in your child:

• Understands words referring to bowel movements and urination.

• Knows what the toilet is for and has watched others use it.

- Prefers clean, dry diapers to soiled ones.

- Understands that using the potty means having a dry diaper.

- Recognizes the sensation of a full bladder and the urge to have a bowel movement.

If you think your child is ready to begin toilet training, the following tips may make it go more smoothly:

- Get the child a potty chair. Make sure the child's feet can rest on the floor or on a footrest. Encourage the child to sit on the chair at least once a day at about the same time each day. Let the child use the chair for looking at books or watching TV.

- After he has had a bowel movement in a diaper, sit the child on the chair, and put the contents of the diaper in the pot.

- Once the child is interested, let her play for short periods without a diaper and with the chair nearby. Encourage her to use the chair if she needs to "go potty."

- Reward every success with hugs and words of praise. Relapses are common in the first few weeks, but don't criticize for mistakes. Keep a casual attitude.

- Bladder control may take longer than bowel control. If the child is aware of a full bladder, try putting him on the potty every 30 to 60 minutes. Praise the child for success and give gentle encouragement when he wets his pants.

Sleep Habits

Babies have both deep and light sleep cycles. In each four-hour sleep period, there is an hour of light sleep, 60 to 90 minutes of deep sleep, and another half hour of light sleep. At the end of this cycle, the baby is semi-alert and can be wakened easily.

Parents can help the baby sleep through the night by helping him learn to soothe himself back to sleep during the light sleep cycles.

For infants (birth to 2 months):

- Put the baby in the crib when she is drowsy but awake.

- Make middle-of-the night feedings short and boring.

- Don't wake the baby for diaper changes unless they are soiled or the baby has a bad diaper rash.

- Set a late bedtime and give the last feeding then.

- As the baby gets older, delay the middle-of-the-night feeding, and discontinue it sometime after age four months.

Bed-Wetting

Bed-wetting (enuresis) is common among young children. Most will outgrow the problem by age six to eight as their bladders grow larger and bladder control improves. Bed-wetting is rarely caused by urinary tract infection or emotional problems.

Bed-Wetting – continued

Prevention

- Limit what the child drinks during the two hours before bedtime (but don't argue over a few sips of water).

- Remind the child to get up during the night to urinate. Providing a bedside potty chair and night light may help.

Home Treatment

- Do not punish or embarrass the child. Praise your child's dry nights, and do not overreact to wet ones.

- Let children over age four help solve the problem. Reward them for dry nights and have them help clean up after wet nights.

- Do not force a child to wear diapers at night. Waterproof, extra-absorbent underwear may help avoid daily bed changes. Wash them with one-half cup of vinegar to eliminate odor.

When to Call Kaiser Permanente

- If bed-wetting occurs with painful or burning urination.

- If prevention and home treatment are not successful after four to six weeks, or if bed-wetting becomes more frequent or severe. Your doctor can rule out or treat any physical causes of bed-wetting.

- If bed-wetting continues past age six, or occurs in a child who had previously been dry for several months.

- If bed-wetting occurs with soiling of the underwear with bowel movements after age three.

- If a child over age three has daytime bladder control problems.

Chickenpox

Chickenpox (varicella) is a relatively minor illness. Almost all children will get it. The first couple of days, your child will be in generally ill health, with a cold, cough, fever, and abdominal pain. Then a rash of red, pimple-like spots appears. A child may have just one or two spots or the rash may cover the entire body, including the throat, mouth, ears, groin, and scalp.

The spots turn into clear blisters that become cloudy, break open, and crust over. This rash itches a lot. Spots continue to appear for one to five days, and subside over a week or two.

Chickenpox is very contagious. After exposure, symptoms occur in two to three weeks. Chickenpox is contagious for one to two days before the spots appear, and for up to five days after the spots appear. Children can generally return to school or day care when all the spots have scabbed. Encephalitis (see page 102) is a rare complication of chickenpox.

Prevention

A new vaccine is available for the prevention of chickenpox. The vaccine, given as a single shot at age one, is safe and effective. However, it is unknown at this time whether or not booster shots will be necessary to protect children as they grow up.

Because the disease is less serious in children than in adolescents and adults, parents may choose instead to allow their children to catch the natural disease, which provides lifelong immunity.

Children who have not had chickenpox by age 11 to 12 should be immunized. Adults who have never had chickenpox should also be immunized, but need a blood test to confirm that they need the vaccine. For adults, two shots are needed for immunity.

Pregnant women cannot receive the vaccine. If a pregnant woman has never had chickenpox and has not been vaccinated, she should be especially careful to avoid people with chickenpox, since the virus can harm the developing fetus.

Home Treatment

• No aspirin! Do *not* give aspirin to children and teens under age 20 who may have chickenpox because aspirin use is related to Reye's Syndrome. Use acetaminophen to relieve fever.

• Control the itching (see page 136). Oral Benadryl and warm baths with

---

Childhood Rashes

Rashes that come with childhood illnesses are hard to tell apart. Review all symptoms before deciding what to do.

Description	Possible Illness
Red, pimple-like spots that turn to blisters; fever	Chickenpox, p. 156
Rash in diaper area only	Diaper Rash, p. 161
Red rash on face that looks like slapped cheeks; pink rash on torso that comes and goes; possible fever	Fifth Disease, p. 168
Red or pink dots on head, neck, shoulders; more common in infants	Prickly Heat, p. 167
Sudden high fever for 2–3 days followed by rose-pink rash on torso, arms, neck after fever goes down	Roseola, p. 168
Fine pink rash; starts on face and covers whole body; swollen glands behind ears	Rubella (rare), p. 166
Fever, runny nose, hacking cough; red eyes 2–3 days before spotty red rash covers whole body	Rubeola (measles) (rare), p. 166
High fever, sore throat, sandpapery rash, and raspberry-textured tongue	Scarlet fever, p. 108

Chickenpox – continued

some baking soda, or Aveeno Colloidal oatmeal added to the water will help.

- Cut the child's fingernails to prevent scratching. If scabs are scratched off too early, they may become infected.

When to Call Kaiser Permanente

- If your child is at risk of complications from chickenpox (is taking steroid medications or cancer chemotherapy, or has immuno-deficiency problems).

- If a child age three months to three years has a fever of 103° or higher for 24 hours. See Fever on page 163.

- If severe itching cannot be controlled by Benadryl and warm baths.

- If bruising appears without injury.

- If sores appear in the eyes.

- If you notice signs of encephalitis (see page 102). These signs are:

  ○ Severe headache

  ○ Unusual sleepiness

  ○ Continued vomiting

Colic

Parents of young babies are often painfully aware of colic, which often occurs in the late afternoon, evening, and at night. Colic is not really a disease; it is the name for an assortment of problems that cause babies to draw up their legs, tighten their abdomens, and cry.

Doctors aren't sure what causes colic. With some babies, it seems unavoidable. However, colic is generally not caused by a feeding problem or intolerance to cow's milk.

Fortunately, colic goes away as the baby matures, almost always by the end of the third month. It is over sooner for many babies and may never appear in many others. Although no one method always works to relieve colicky babies, there are a number of possible remedies you can try. Unfortunately, what works one time may not work the next. Be creative and persistent.

Home Treatment

- Most important: stay calm and try to relax. If you start to lose control, take a minute to collect your thoughts. *Never* shake a baby; it can cause permanent brain damage.

- Make sure the baby is getting enough to eat and not too much. The problem may be hunger, not colic.

- Make sure the baby isn't swallowing too much air while eating. Feed the baby slowly, holding him almost upright. Burp the baby periodically. Prop the baby up for 15 minutes after feeding.

- If the baby is bottle-fed, use nipples with holes large enough to drip cold formula at least one drop per second. Babies will swallow more air from around the nipple if the hole is too small.

- Heat formula to body temperature. Don't overheat.

- Keep a regular routine for meals, naps, and playtime. Mealtime should be quiet and undisturbed by bright lights and loud noise.

- Make sure the baby's diaper is clean, that the baby isn't too hot or cold, and isn't bored.

- Use a pacifier, and try rocking or walking the baby. Putting the baby stomach-down over your knee or forearm may be helpful.

- Calm the baby with a car ride or a walk outside. Placing the baby near a clothes dryer, dishwasher, or bubbling aquarium may help soothe him.

- Don't worry about spoiling a baby during the first three months; comforting a baby makes both of you feel better.

- Ask a friend or neighbor to babysit some evening while you go to dinner and a movie!

- Don't feel guilty about shutting the bedroom door and turning up the stereo once in a while; if it will help you to relax, it will help the baby. However, don't let your baby cry alone for more than 5 to 10 minutes during the first three months. After 10 minutes, try the above suggestions again.

When to Call Kaiser Permanente

Colic generally does not require professional treatment unless it is accompanied by vomiting and/or diarrhea or other signs of more serious illness. If the baby looks healthy and acts normally between episodes, and if your emotions can stand the noise for the first three months, you have little cause for worry.

However, if colic lasts more than three hours a day, or if you feel like you are losing self-control, contact your doctor for advice.

In rare cases, colic may be so severe that you and your doctor may consider a medication. Ask about side effects.

Cradle Cap

Cradle cap is an oily yellow scaling or crusting on the scalp of infants. It is caused by a build up of normal oils on the skin. Cradle cap is common in babies and is easily treated.

Home Treatment

- Wash the baby's head with baby shampoo once a day. Gently scrub the scalp with a soft-bristled brush (a soft toothbrush works well) for a few minutes to remove the scales. Don't worry about hurting the baby's skull; it is sturdier than you think. Rinse well.

- You can also rub mineral oil on the scalp one hour before shampooing to loosen the scales.

- If scrubbing with regular shampoo doesn't work, try using a dandruff shampoo, such as Ionil-T, Sebulex, or Selsun Blue. Use these carefully as they will irritate your baby's eyes.

- If the rash is irritated and red, a mild hydrocortisone cream (Cortaid) will probably help.

Croup

Croup is a respiratory problem most common in children age two to four years. It may accompany a viral infection, such as a cold. The main symptom is a harsh cough that sounds like a seal's bark. A fever of 100° to 101° is common. The child may become very frightened. Croup usually gets worse at night and may last one to seven days.

Home Treatment

- Stay calm. The child is already frightened and needs you to be calm.

- Bundle up and take the child outside for a walk in the cool fresh air. Cool moist air is best.

- Get moisture into the air to make it easier for the child to breathe. Take the child into the bathroom, turn on all hot-water faucets, then sit on the floor in the steamy room and read a story together.

- Set up a vaporizer in the child's bedroom. With a cold-mist vaporizer, the air will be quite cold. Dress the child in warm pajamas, cover with the usual covers, and place a light sheet over the blankets to catch moisture. Don't worry about your child getting chilled. The cool, moist air is the important part.

- If the child starts crying, the worst is usually over. A child who can cry can breathe.

When to Call Kaiser Permanente

- If the child stops breathing or begins to turn blue, call 861-3434, 911, or emergency services. If the child stops breathing, give rescue breathing (see page 206) until help arrives.

- Medical care is needed immediately if these signs of respiratory distress appear and persist despite home treatment:

  ○ Squeaky or raspy sound as child inhales (stridor)

  ○ Sucking in or retraction between ribs as child inhales

  ○ Flaring nostrils

- If the child is so short of breath that she can't walk or talk.

- If the child drools or is breathing with the chin jutting out and the mouth open.

- If 20 minutes of steam inhalation or cold outdoor air do not relax the child enough to allow sleep.

- If the child has a fever of 102° or higher.

- If you or your child get hysterical and cannot calm down.

- If it is the first case of croup in your family and you need reassurance.

- If croup lasts longer than three nights.

Diaper Rash

Diaper rash is a reaction to the moisture and bacteria in babies' urine and stools, or to the soap used to wash diapers. While it is uncomfortable, diaper rash is usually not dangerous.

Symptoms of the rash are a red bottom and thighs. It will be easier for you to recognize after you have seen it the first time.

Prevention

- Change diapers as soon as possible after they have been soiled or wet.

- Leave the skin open to the air as often as possible.

- Wash diapers with mild detergent and rinse twice. Do not use bleach.

- Avoid using plastic pants for a while if your baby has frequent problems. These items trap moisture against the baby's skin.

Home Treatment

- Change diapers frequently. Rinse and dry the skin in the diaper area at every diaper change. Use a washcloth with water. Wash with a mild soap once a day.

- Try protecting the skin with Desitin, Diaparene, A & D Ointment, or zinc oxide. Apply cream only to dry skin. Discontinue creams if a rash develops as they slow healing.

- Baby powder on the diaper area may increase comfort. Sprinkle it in your hand first, then pat it onto the baby (you and your baby will inhale less powder).

- Try another brand or type of diaper. Some babies tolerate one kind better than another.

- Avoid excessively bulky or multilayered diapers.

- Stop using plastic pants when the rash appears.

- Try changing detergents if the rash does not clear.

When to Call Kaiser Permanente

- If the diaper rash becomes very red, raw, or sore looking.

- If the rash has blisters, pus, or crusty patches.

- If the rash is mainly in the skin creases. This may indicate a yeast infection.

- If a significant rash lasts longer than five days.

- If the problem is caused by frequent diarrhea, see Diarrhea below and Dehydration on page 43.

Diarrhea and Vomiting

Diarrhea and vomiting may be caused by viral stomach flu, or by eating unusual foods or unusual amounts of foods. An infant's developing digestive system sometimes will not tolerate large amounts of juice, fruit, or even milk. Breast-fed babies are less likely to develop diarrhea.

Diarrhea and Vomiting – cont.

Stomach flu often starts with vomiting that is followed in a few hours (sometimes eight to 12 hours or longer) by diarrhea. Sometimes there is no diarrhea.

Infants and children under age four, and especially under six months, need special attention when they have diarrhea or are vomiting. They can quickly become dehydrated. Careful observation of the child's appearance and fluid intake can help prevent problems. For children age four and older, see Diarrhea on page 45 and Vomiting on page 50.

Home Treatment

Infants age 3 months to 2 years:

• If the baby is breast-fed, continue breast-feeding. If the diarrhea gets worse (larger, more frequent stools), or if the child begins vomiting, supplement feedings with an oral rehydration drink (Pedialyte, Ricelyte, or store brand).

• If the baby is formula-fed, switch to an oral rehydration drink. Gradually add back formula feedings within 24 hours. Return to the usual amount of formula within another day.

• For children over age six months, you can improve the taste of the rehydration drink by adding a pinch of NutraSweet or sugar-free Kool-Aid or Jell-O powder.

• Give four to eight ounces of fluid (breast milk or rehydration drink) for each large loose stool.

• Do not use sports drinks, fruit juice, or soda. These drinks contain too much sugar and not enough of the electrolytes that are being lost.

• Do not use rehydration drinks as the sole source of fluid for more than 12 to 24 hours.

• After 12 to 24 hours, offer the child solid foods, if he was eating solids before. Allow the child to eat what he prefers; the particular food is not important. Avoid high-fiber foods (such as beans) and foods with a lot of sugar, such as juice and ice cream.

Children age 2 years and older:

• Give one-half to one cup each hour of an oral rehydration drink. Give smaller amounts more often if the child is vomiting. Add NutraSweet flavorings if needed.

• Gatorade or sports drinks may be used *temporarily* if the diarrhea is mild to moderate, but oral rehydration drinks are better. Do not give fruit juice or soda.

• Offer easily digestible foods in addition to the rehydration drink. Resume a regular diet within a day or so. Do not use a rehydration drink as the sole source of fluids and nutrients for more than 24 hours.

As the child gets better, the stools will get smaller and less frequent. Some types of diarrhea may cause four to six days of watery diarrhea. However, as long as the child is taking in enough fluids and nutrients, is urinating normal amounts, and seems to be improving, you can treat the illness at home.

Watch for signs of dehydration. See page 43.

When to Call Kaiser Permanente

- If the diarrhea is bloody, tarry, or dark red.

- If the urine becomes bloody or cola colored.

- If there is blood in the vomit.

- If vomiting occurs with severe headache, sleepiness, lethargy (child cannot be awakened easily) or a stiff neck (child may cry out when the neck is moved). See page 102.

- If signs of dehydration appear (also see page 43):

  ○ No urine output for 12 hours or less than 3 urinations in 24 hours

  ○ Sunken eyes

  ○ Child cries without tears

  ○ Pale, mottled skin

  ○ Extreme thirst

- If a child with diarrhea or vomiting refuses to drink or cannot take in enough liquid to replace lost fluids.

- If vomiting lasts longer than two to four hours in a child under six months, or one day in a child under age four.

- If severe diarrhea (many watery stools in a child who appears very sick) lasts longer than 12 to 24 hours in an infant under six months, or one to two days in a child under age four. If diarrhea is mild to moderate (a few stools that are looser than usual without other signs of illness), call after four to seven days.

- If the child has a fever of 103° or higher, or a lower fever with diarrhea for more than two days.

- If the child has severe stomach pain.

- If stomach pain is persistent and there is frequent vomiting for more than 12 hours with little or no diarrhea.

- If stomach pain starts several hours before the vomiting and seems like more than stomach cramps.

- If stomach pain is not located near the bellybutton, especially if it seems to be in the lower right abdomen. This can be difficult to determine in small children.

Fever

Fever is usually defined as a rectal temperature greater than 100.4° or an oral temperature above 99.8°. Body temperature can also rise above normal when an infant is overdressed or in a room that is too warm.

In most, but not all, cases, fever indicates that an illness is present. By itself, a fever is not harmful; in fact, it may help the body fight infections more effectively.

In children, viral infections, such as colds, flu, or chickenpox can cause high fevers. Bacterial infections, such as strep throat, also cause fevers. Teething may cause a low-grade fever up to 100°.

Children tend to run higher fevers than adults. Although high fevers are uncomfortable, they do not often cause medical problems. Convulsions from fever (febrile convulsions) occur only occasionally. See page 165.

Fever – continued

For information on taking accurate temperatures in infants and children, see page 33. All temperatures in this section are rectal.

There is no medical evidence that prolonged high fevers can cause brain damage. The body limits a temperature from going above 106°. However, when heat from external sources (like a car parked in the sun) raises the body temperature above 107°, brain damage can occur.

Home Treatment

It can be hard to know when to call your doctor when your child has a fever, especially during an influenza or other viral illness outbreak. Flu (see page 103) can cause a high fever for five days or longer, along with body aches, headache, and cold-like symptoms.

The degree of the fever is not always related to the severity of the infection. How your child looks and acts is a better guide than the thermometer.

Most children will be less active when they have a fever. However, if there are periods during the day when your child is more active, cheerful and playing, and is taking fluids well, it is a good sign.

Generally, if a child over three is comfortable, leave the fever alone. It will do more good than harm. If the child is eating well and playing as usual, there is usually no cause for concern.

- Dress the child lightly, and do not wrap him in blankets.

- Encourage the child to drink extra liquids or suck on ice chips or popsicles.

- If the fever is over 102° and the child is uncomfortable:

  ○ Give acetaminophen or ibuprofen. See page 300 for dose information. Do *not* give aspirin to children or teens under age 20.

  ○ Sponge the child with lukewarm water for 20 minutes. Do not use cold water, ice, or rubbing alcohol.

When to Call Kaiser Permanente

- Call a health professional *immediately* if fever is accompanied by these symptoms:

  ○ Stiff neck, headache or confusion, or bulging soft spot on an infant's head

  ○ Headache, nausea, vomiting, and excessive sleepiness or lethargy

  ○ Rapid, difficult breathing

  ○ Drooling or inability to swallow

  ○ Purple rash that does not lighten when you press on it

- If an infant under three months has a fever of 101° or higher.

- If a child age three months to three years has a fever of 103° or higher for 24 hours.

- If a child has a fever of 104° or higher that does not come down after four to six hours of home treatment.

- If a child with a fever seems sicker than you would expect with a viral illness such as a cold or flu.

- If fever occurs with pain that isn't relieved by home treatment.

- If a fever has lasted more than three days.

- If a child becomes delirious or has hallucinations.

- Call a health professional within 24 hours if fever is accompanied by:

  ○ Vomiting, diarrhea, and stomach pain

  ○ Signs of dehydration (see page 43)

  ○ Unexplained skin rash (see page 157 for common childhood illnesses that cause rash)

  ○ Ear pain (babies often pull at painful ears)

  ○ Painful urination

  ○ Joint pain

  ○ Any unusual or significant pain

Fever Convulsions

Fever (febrile) convulsions or "fits" are involuntary spasms of muscles that sometimes occur in children who have had a rapid increase in temperature.

Convulsions usually occur when the temperature has risen quickly (often before you have noticed that your child has a fever). Once a high fever has developed, the risk of a convulsion is probably gone.

The child having a convulsion stiffens up, clenching arms, legs, and teeth. The eyes may roll back, and the child may also stop breathing for a few seconds, vomit, urinate, or pass stools. Convulsions usually last one to five minutes.

Although frightening, fever convulsions in children age six months to four years are seldom serious and do not cause any harm. Only one percent of children at this age are prone to fever convulsions. About 30 percent of children who have a fever convulsion will have another one, usually within two years.

Home Treatment

During a convulsion:

- Protect the child from injury. Ease the child to the floor, or hold a very small child face down on your lap. Do not restrain the child.

- Turn the head to the side to clear the mouth of any vomit or saliva so the child can breathe.

- Do not put anything in the child's mouth to prevent tongue biting. This may injure the child.

- Try to stay calm, which will help calm the child.

- Time the length of the convulsion, if possible.

After a convulsion:

- Check for injuries.

- Reduce fever with acetaminophen or ibuprofen and lukewarm sponge baths. See page 164.

- Put the child in a cool room to sleep. Drowsiness is common following a convulsion.

Fever Convulsions – continued

When to Call Kaiser Permanente

- Call 861-3434, 911, or emergency services:

  ° If the child stops breathing for longer than 30 to 60 seconds. Begin rescue breathing. See page 206.

  ° If a convulsion lasts longer than five minutes, or a second convulsion occurs.

- If a convulsion occurs without fever.

- If it is the child's first convulsion, or if you haven't discussed with your doctor what to do if there is another one.

- If the child is under six months old, is five years or older, or if an adult has a convulsion.

- If you are unable to reduce fever to 102° after a convulsion.

- If a high fever occurs with severe headache, vomiting, stiff neck, or bulging soft spot on an infant's head. See "Encephalitis and Meningitis" on page 102.

Pinworms

Pinworms are tiny, thread-like worms that infect the digestive tracts of young children. Pinworms are most common in four- to six-year-olds, although anyone may be infected. The worms live in the upper end of the large intestine, near the appendix, and travel to the outside of the anus to lay their eggs.

Measles, Mumps, and Rubella

Measles (rubeola), mumps, and rubella (German measles) were once common childhood illnesses. Today, they are quite rare, thanks to the measles, mumps, and rubella (MMR) vaccine. Two shots, one given at age 12 months and a second at age 11 to 12 years, provide lifelong protection. Adults who have not been immunized may also need both shots.

Local outbreaks of measles, mumps, or rubella can occur where immunization rates are not high enough.

Measles symptoms:
- Fever, runny nose, hacking cough
- Reddened eyes
- Spotty red rash on entire body

Mumps symptoms:
- Swelling along the jawline
- Fever and vomiting

Rubella symptom:
- Fine pink rash starting on face and covering entire body

Call Kaiser Permanente for information about the MMR vaccine, or if you suspect your child has measles, mumps, or rubella.

The egg-laying almost always occurs at night and usually causes the child to scratch the anal area.

When the child later sucks a thumb or licks a finger, the eggs are ingested and the cycle begins again. The eggs are very sticky, and can survive on clothing and bedding for days, where they can be picked up by other family members.

Rectal itching, especially at night, is the most common symptom of pinworm infection. If the infection is very severe, there may also be abdominal pain and loss of appetite.

Pinworms are common and affect many families. If you suspect pinworms, it's easy to find out for sure in your own home and at no cost. Go into your child's darkened bedroom several hours after bedtime and shine a flashlight on the child's anus. The light will make the worms move back into the anus. If you don't see the worms after checking for two or three nights, it is unlikely that the child is infected.

Prevention

Teach children to wash their hands after using the toilet and before meals.

Home Treatment

- Call the advice nurse to get a medication for pinworms.

- Treat every family member in the household over age two who has symptoms. If infection recurs, consider treating everyone in the family over age two.

- On the first day of treatment, wash all underwear, nightclothes, bedding, and towels in hot water to get rid of any eggs and prevent reinfection. Sanitize toilet and sleeping areas with a strong disinfectant cleaner.

- Trim and keep all fingernails short.

- Require frequent hand washing, morning showers, and daily changes of pajamas and underwear.

When to Call Kaiser Permanente

- If any drug produces reactions such as vomiting or pain.

- If you suspect pinworms but the nighttime checks reveal nothing.

- If you continue to see worms at night three days after treatment. Stronger prescription drugs are available.

Prickly Heat (Sweat Rash)

Prickly heat, also called heat rash, sweat rash, or miliaria, is a rash of red or pink dots that appears over an infant's head, neck, and shoulders. The dots look like tiny pimples.

Prickly heat is often caused by well-meaning parents who dress their baby too warmly, but it can happen to any baby in really hot weather. An infant should be dressed just as lightly as an adult and will be comfortable at the same temperature. Babies' hands and feet feel cold to your touch because most of their blood is near the stomach helping digestion.

Prevention

Do not overdress your baby. Place your hand between the baby's shoulder blades. If the skin is hot or moist, the baby is too warm.

Home Treatment

- Dress the baby in as few clothes as possible during hot weather.

- Keep the skin cool and dry.

Prickly Heat – continued

- Keep the baby's sleeping area cool.
- Hydrocortisone cream (0.5 percent) can be helpful.

When to Call Kaiser Permanente

- If the rash looks infected or persists over three to four days.
- If the infant looks sick.
- If sweat rash is accompanied by a fever of 101° that doesn't come down after you remove extra clothing.

Roseola

Roseola (roseola infantum) is a mild viral illness that often starts with a sudden high fever (103° to 105°) and irritability. The fever lasts two to three days. As the fever drops, a rosy-pink rash appears on the torso, neck, and arms. It may last one to two days. Since the fever is quite high and may come on quickly, fever convulsions may occur (see page 165). Roseola is most common in children six months to two years of age. It is rare after age four.

Home Treatment

- If the child is uncomfortable, reduce the fever. See page 164.
- Give lots of liquids.
- If a convulsion occurs, see page 165.

Fifth Disease

Another common childhood illness that causes rash is erythema infectiosum, or "fifth disease." The main symptom is a red rash on the face that looks like slapped cheeks, and a lacy pink rash on the backs of the arms and legs, torso, and buttocks. There may be a low fever. The rash may come and go for several weeks in response to changes in temperature and sunlight.

This illness is most contagious the week before the rash appears. Once the rash has developed, the child is no longer contagious. Fifth disease is harmless in children, but it poses a slight risk to developing fetuses. Pregnant women should avoid exposure if possible.

If you are pregnant and are exposed to a child with fifth disease, or if you develop a fifth disease-like rash, contact your obstetrician.

Home treatment for fifth disease is simply to keep the child comfortable and watch for signs that a more serious illness is present (fever over 102°; child seems very sick).

When to Call Kaiser Permanente

- See When to Call Kaiser Permanente under Fever on page 164.

Chapter 12

Women's Health

Women have always been health experts. Throughout history, women have been the chief providers of health and healing to others. Even now, when hospitals, clinics, and a vast array of health professionals are available to treat illness and injury, a full 80 percent of all health problems are still treated in the home, often by moms and grandmoms.

Women need to be health experts for themselves, too. From puberty to menopause, women must cope with unique health care problems. This chapter covers health issues of special concern to women. By becoming knowledgeable about the female body and how to take care of it, women can take greater control of their health, and with it, their lives.

Breast Health

Breast cancer is the leading cause of cancer deaths in women age 40 to 55. However, breast cancer is highly treatable if detected early. There are three methods of early detection: breast self-exam, clinical breast exam, and mammogram.

Breast Self-Exam

Many women examine their breasts for lumps once a month. Although breast self-exams have not been proven to save lives, we still suggest that women begin to practice monthly breast self-exams as soon as their breasts develop. (Mammography after age 50 does save lives and is strongly recommended. See page 172.)

Most breast lumps are discovered by women themselves, often quite by accident. The breast self-exam is a simple technique to help you learn what is normal for you and become aware of any changes.

Establish a regular time each month to examine your breasts, such as a few days after your period when your breasts are not swollen or tender. Women who do not menstruate (after menopause and women who have had

Breast Health – continued

hysterectomies) can examine their breasts the first day of each month.

Most women's breast tissue has some lumps or thickening. When in doubt about a particular lump, check the other breast. If you find a similar lump in the same area on the other breast, both breasts are probably normal. Be on the lookout for a lump that feels much harder than the rest of the breast.

Have any areas of concern checked by your health professional. The important thing is to learn what is normal for you and to report changes to your doctor.

The breast self-exam takes place in two stages.

Stage 1: In front of the mirror

Examine your breasts visually in a mirror. Few women have breasts that match exactly. It is normal for one breast to be slightly larger than the other. Learn what is normal for you.

Look at your breasts in four positions:

• Stand with your arms at your sides

• With your hands on your hips

• With your arms raised overhead

• While bending forward

 In each position, look for changes in the contour and shape of your breasts, the color and texture of the skin and nipple, and any discharge from the nipples.

Squeeze the nipple of each breast gently between thumb and index finger. Look for a discharge.

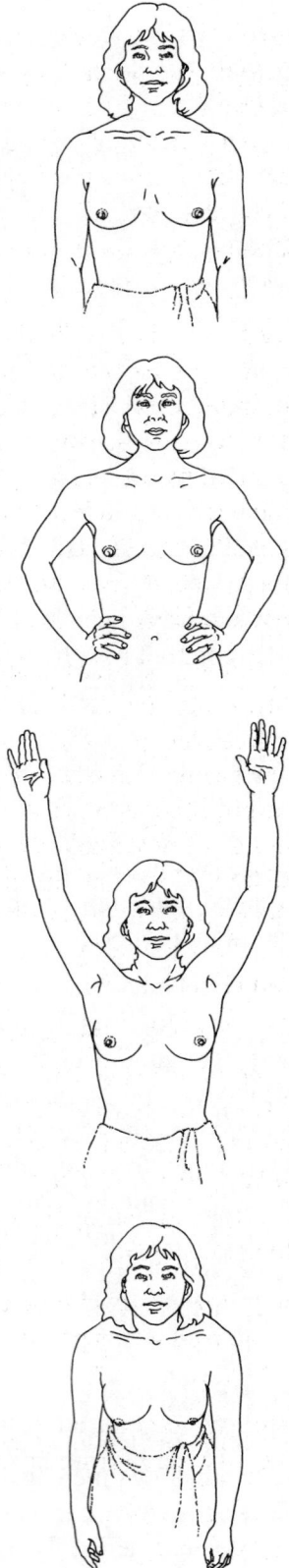

Stage 1

Stage 2: Lying down

To examine your left breast, place a pillow or folded towel under your left shoulder. Use your right hand to examine your left breast. If your breasts are large, lie on your right side and turn your left shoulder back flat to spread the breast tissue more evenly over your chest wall.

Use the pads of your middle three fingers to examine your breast. Move the fingers in small, dime-sized circles. Don't lift your fingers away from the skin. Use light, medium, and deep pressure in each spot to feel the full thickness of the breast tissue. You are feeling for lumps, thickening, or changes of any kind.

Examine your entire breast using a vertical strip pattern (see illustration). Examine all tissue from the collarbone to the armpit and from the bra line to the breastbone. Start in the armpit and work down to the bottom of the bra line. Move one finger width toward the middle and work up to the collarbone. Repeat until you have covered all the breast tissue.

Another way of doing this is to imagine that your breast is a clock. Start on the outside of the breast at 12:00, move slowly to 1:00 and then around the clock back to 12:00. Then move one inch in toward the nipple and go around the clock again.

Move the pillow or towel to the other shoulder and repeat this procedure for the other breast.

If you discover any unusual lumps, thickening, discharge from the nipple, or changes of any kind, report them to your doctor immediately. Remember, most lumps are not malignant, but you will need your doctor to make a diagnosis.

If you examine your breasts monthly, you will learn what is normal for you and quickly recognize if something changes. The breast self-exam takes some practice. You can learn more about breast self-exams at your Kaiser Permanente Health Education Department.

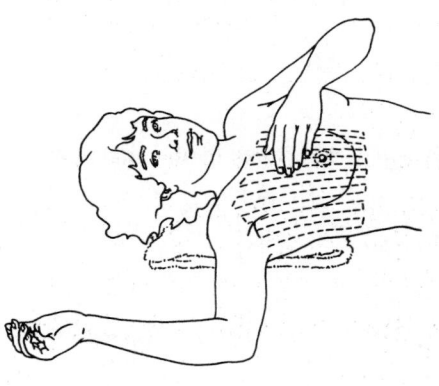

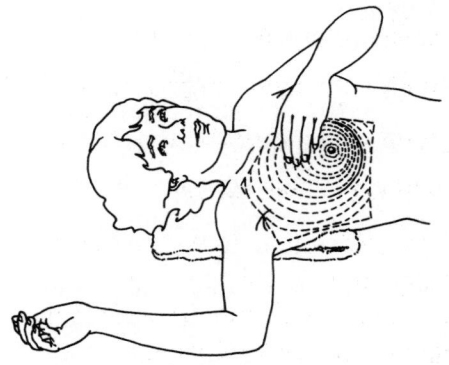

Stage 2

Breast Health – continued

Clinical Breast Exam

The second component for early detection of breast problems is your health professional's physical exam. This exam is very similar to the self-exam. A clinical breast exam is recommended with regular physical examinations, at least every 2 years starting at age 35.

Mammogram

A mammogram is a breast X-ray. It helps to find breast tumors too small to be detected by breast self-exam.

Mammograms have been shown to save lives in women over 50, reducing breast cancer death rates by up to one-third. Research has found that mammography in women under age 50 is of uncertain benefit. This may be due to differences in younger women's breast tissue, or in the types of tumors that develop before menopause.

Abnormal mammograms that require biopsies are quite common, so given the absence of benefit, many experts, including the U.S. Preventive Services Task Force, no longer recommend mammograms before age 50. On the other hand, the American Cancer Society recommends mammograms every two years starting at age 40. If you are interested in mammography before age 50, discuss the potential risks and benefits with your health care provider. A shared decision-making document is available to help you with this decision. After age 50 (more specifically, after menopause), mammograms are recommended every one to two years.

Mammograms are recommended before age 50 if:

- Your mother, sister, or daughter has had breast cancer.

- You have had a breast biopsy that showed abnormal changes (atypical hyperplasia).

- You have been diagnosed with breast cancer.

Scheduling an Exam

- When possible, schedule your mammogram 7 to 14 days after your period, for comfort.

- Do not wear deodorant, perfume, powder, or lotion, which can affect the quality of the X-ray.

- Wear clothing that allows you to remove only your top.

Breast Health Tips

- Do your breast self-exam every month. Most breast lumps are discovered by women themselves. If detected early, breast cancer usually can be successfully treated.

- Have a clinical breast exam with your regular physical exams.

- Have a periodic mammogram. See Tests for Early Detection on page 31 for frequency.

Gynecological Health

Pap smears are a vital component of women's health. These exams can give you early indications of any abnormalities in your cervix. It is better to catch any disease in its early stages, when it is much easier to treat.

Self-Exam

A female's genitals include two sets of lips: the inner (labia minora) and the outer (labia majora). These lips form around the urinary opening, the vaginal opening, and the clitoris.

Periodically examine your entire genital area for any sores, warts, red swollen areas, or unusual discharge. A normal discharge may be white to yellowish-white and smell slightly like vinegar. It can be either thick or thin and present in large or small amounts; every woman is different. During ovulation (the midpoint between periods) there is often a large amount of clear, slippery mucus. If your discharge seems unusual in amount, smell, or texture, see Vaginitis on page 186.

There should be no pain or straining on urination, and the urine should come out in a fairly steady stream. The urine should be pale yellow and it should not have a strong ammonia smell. If you experience pain or burning on urination, see Urinary Tract Infections on page 184.

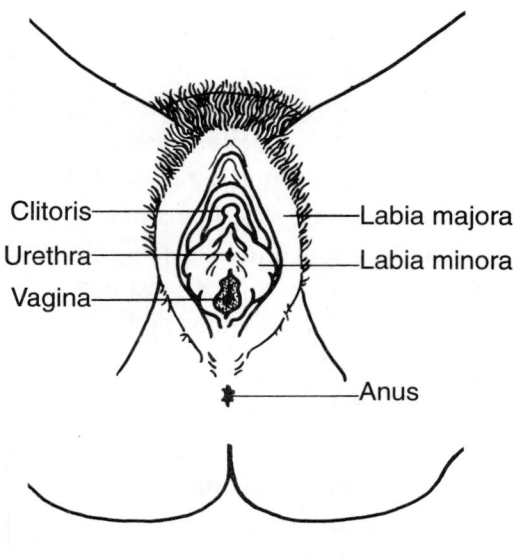

Clitoris—————Labia majora
Urethra—————Labia minora
Vagina—

—Anus

Female genitals

Self-exams will help you better understand your own body and what is normal for you.

The Pelvic Exam

A pelvic exam given by a health care professional will generally consist of an external genital exam, a Pap test, and a manual exam.

The Pap test is the screening exam for cancer of the cervix. Pap smears detect 90 to 95 percent of cervical cancers, making it a reliable and important test. The clinician will insert a speculum into your vagina and gather some cells from your cervix and vagina.

The cells are put on a slide and sent to a lab for classification. If abnormal cells are found, your doctor will ask you to return for more testing. In any case, you will be notified of the results of your Pap test. Ask for an explanation of your results.

For a manual exam, the clinician inserts two gloved and lubricated fingers into your vagina and presses on your lower abdomen with the other hand to feel the ovaries and uterus.

Scheduling an Exam

The first Pap test is recommended when a girl or woman becomes sexually active. Therefore, a 16-year-old girl who is sexually active should have an exam.

Pap smears are recommended every two years. There is a long precancerous stage before cervical cancer develops. Women with a single sexual partner and several normal Pap smears need less frequent exams.

Gynecological Health – cont.

Women with multiple sexual partners or a history of abnormal exams need yearly exams. Discuss this with your health care provider.

Schedule the exam one to two weeks after your period. Do not douche, have intercourse, or use feminine hygiene products for 24 hours before the exam as they can alter the results.

For more information on women's health, see Resources 83 to 85 on page 311.

Pregnancy: How to Make a Healthy Baby

You can increase the chances that your baby will be healthy. The following guidelines will help.

Before Conception

The mother's health, before and during the first weeks after conception, is particularly important for the baby's health. Start helping your baby even before you become pregnant.

- If you have diabetes, high blood pressure, seizure disorders, or any inherited diseases, talk with your doctor before getting pregnant. Your doctor may want to modify your treatment and may be able to prescribe medicine that is safer for the developing baby.

- Before you start trying to get pregnant, have a blood test to check your rubella immunity. If you test negative, you will want to receive your immunization and then use some form of birth control for at least three months.

- If you have any symptoms of sexually transmitted diseases or you are unsure of the sexual history of your partner, read pages 199 to 203 and arrange for an examination and testing with your doctor.

- Eat well. Make sure your diet includes plenty of green leafy vegetables and legumes, and take a folic acid supplement containing 0.4 mg of folate or a prenatal vitamin that contains 0.4 mg of folic acid. Folic acid helps prevent certain birth defects, such as spina bifida. Other good sources of folic acid include fortified cereal and whole-wheat bread.

- Stop smoking. See page 112.

- Stop drinking.

- Stop all illegal drug use and eliminate any medications that are not absolutely essential.

- If you are anxious or depressed, get help. See pages 278 to 280.

- Buy a good book on pregnancy and begin reading. See Resources 71 to 73 on page 311.

Home Pregnancy Tests

If you become pregnant, it is important that you know right away. The quickest way is with a home pregnancy test. Home pregnancy tests are inexpensive and very reliable when done correctly. Some tests can show positive results within a few days of the missed period. Select a test that has simple instructions and follow them *exactly*. Mistakes can lead to false results.

If the test is positive, schedule an appointment with your doctor to confirm the test and to begin pregnancy counseling and/or prenatal care.

Morning Sickness

For many women, the first few months of pregnancy bring morning sickness, which can happen at any time of the day. This is a normal result of the body's adjustment to pregnancy. The following home treatment can help:

- Eat five or six small meals a day to avoid an empty stomach. Include some protein in each of these meals.

- Eat crackers or dry toast before getting up in the morning.

- Increase your intake of vitamin B_6 by eating more whole grains and cereals, wheat germ, nuts, seeds, and legumes.

- Keep a positive attitude. Morning sickness usually passes in three to four months.

Early Pregnancy (First Trimester)

- Continue to avoid smoking, alcohol, and drugs.

- Get regular prenatal care from your family doctor or obstetrician.

- Continue to improve your nutrition. Call your health department to learn if you are eligible for food supplements through the WIC program (Women, Infants, and Children). WIC gives vouchers for nutritious food to pregnant women at high risk for pregnancy problems.

- Continue taking 0.4 mg of folic acid or your prenatal vitamin with 0.4 mg of folic acid daily. For some women, prenatal vitamin supplements may cause more morning sickness early in the pregnancy. If this happens, call your health care provider for advice.

- Avoid touching cat feces and litter boxes. Also, cook all meats well before eating. Cat feces and under-cooked or raw meat can carry toxoplasmosis, an infection that can cause brain damage in the fetus or miscarriage.

- Avoid all chemical vapors, paint fumes, and poisons.

- If you drink coffee or soda with caffeine, cut back to two cups per day.

Middle Pregnancy (Second Trimester)

- Continue with the safeguards described above.

- Reduce the risk of trauma and falls:

  ○ Always wear your seat belt.

  ○ Wear sensible shoes.

  ○ Continue moderate levels of your regular exercises so you don't become exhausted or short of breath.

  ○ Avoid sports with a high risk of falls or impact.

- Increase your calcium intake by drinking more milk (a quart of skim or low-fat milk a day) or through other sources of calcium. See page 264.

- Control your weight as advised by your health care provider.

Pregnancy – continued

Late Pregnancy (Third Trimester)

- Maintain all of the other guidelines listed above.

- Get plenty of rest.

- Take childbirth classes with your partner or designated coach, and take a tour through the Labor and Delivery area of the hospital.

- If appropriate, have your other children take a class to help them adjust to the new baby.

- Practice the relaxation exercises on page 252. They will be helpful during labor.

- Develop a written birth plan with your doctor that outlines your wishes and expectations throughout the labor and delivery.

- Maintain a good sense of humor.

Cesarean Deliveries

Most babies are delivered vaginally, just as nature intended. However, when the health of the baby or mother is at risk, doctors can also deliver the baby through an incision in the abdomen. This is called a cesarean delivery or a C-section.

There are three main concerns with cesarean deliveries:

- More risk. Some mothers who have C-sections develop infections or bleeding that require additional medications or treatment. Although the maternal death rate for C-sections is four times higher than the rate for vaginal deliveries, the rate for both types of delivery is very low.

- Longer recovery. You can usually go home within one day after a vaginal delivery. Hospital stays after cesarean deliveries may be two to three days. After a cesarean, you must limit your activity over the next four to six weeks to allow the incision to heal.

- Less involvement. The mother and other family members can be more involved with a vaginal delivery. Cesarean delivery is a surgery, which limits family involvement.

C-sections are a good idea when either the baby or the mother is in danger. A cesarean should not be done just because it is easier to schedule or because you have previously had a C-section delivery. Ask your doctor what you can do to help avoid the need for a cesarean delivery.

Breast-feeding

Breast milk is the ideal food for your new baby. See page 152.

Bleeding Between Periods

Many women experience bleeding or spotting between periods. It does not necessarily mean a serious condition is present. Use of an intrauterine device (IUD) may increase your chances of spotting. Some minor bleeding is common during ovulation and during the first three months of using birth control pills. It is also common to spot or bleed irregularly while breast-feeding.

If the bleeding is not heavy and occurs only occasionally, it is probably not a cause for concern.

Use tampons or pads, and avoid aspirin, which may prolong the bleeding.

When to Call Kaiser Permanente

- If bleeding is accompanied by unusual pain, cramping, or fever.

- If the bleeding is heavy (changing a maxi pad or super tampon every hour for more than six hours).

- If bleeding between periods lasts more than 10 days in a row or occurs three months in a row.

- If bleeding occurs after intercourse.

- If you are over age 35 and have any bleeding between periods or prolonged bleeding with periods.

Birth Control During Menopause

Some women may continue to ovulate during menopause, which means there is a slight chance that they could become pregnant, even though they are no longer menstruating regularly.

Women who have their last period *before* age 50 and who do not want to become pregnant should continue using contraceptives. They should discuss contraception options with their health care provider.

Menopause

Menopause occurs for most women between the ages of 45 and 55, when the production of female hormones (estrogen and progesterone) begins to decline. These hormonal changes will cause irregular menstrual periods before they stop altogether. You may also experience hot flashes, vaginal dryness, and mood changes. Osteoporosis is also directly linked to the decrease in estrogen that comes with menopause. See page 79.

Irregular periods may mean lighter or heavier menstrual flows, either shorter or longer intervals between flows, or spotting. Some women have irregular periods for years during menopause. Others have regular periods until they suddenly stop. Each woman is unique and will experience menopause differently.

Hot flashes are sudden periods of intense heat, sweating, and flushing. A hot flash usually begins in the chest and spreads out to the neck, face, and arms. They are experienced by 75 to 80 percent of women going through menopause. They may occur as frequently as once an hour and last as long as three to four minutes. If they occur at night, they may disrupt your sleep. Most hot flashes cease within one or two years, but may persist for several years.

Vaginal dryness, the loss of lubrication and moisture in the vagina, may lead to soreness during and after intercourse. These vaginal changes may also increase the risk of infections. See Vaginitis on page 186.

Menopause – continued

Mood changes are caused by the hormonal and physical changes of menopause. Symptoms such as nervousness, lethargy, insomnia, moodiness, or depression are common.

With menopause, many women fear emotional upheaval and the loss of sexuality. On the other hand, many women look forward to the freedom that menopause brings, particularly freedom from menstrual cycle discomfort and freedom from contraception.

Understanding what is happening to you and using home care techniques to relieve any discomfort will help you through menopause.

Home Treatment

Irregular Periods:
• Keep a written record of your periods in case you need to discuss them with a health professional.

Hot Flashes:
• Keep your home and work place cool.

• Wear layers of loose clothing that can be easily removed.

• Drink lots of water and juices. Avoid caffeine and alcohol if they bring on hot flashes.

• Exercise regularly. This will help to stabilize hormones and prevent insomnia.

Vaginal Dryness:
• Use a water-soluble vaginal lubricant such as K-Y Jelly, Surgilube, or Today Personal Lubricant. Do not use a petroleum-based product such as Vaseline.

Mood Changes:
• The best thing you can do for yourself is to realize you are not alone. Discuss your symptoms with other women. Give yourself, and ask from others, abundant amounts of love, caring, and understanding.

When to Call Kaiser Permanente

• If you have prolonged irregular bleeding, particularly if you are overweight.

• If you are considering hormone replacement therapy.

Hormone Therapy

Hormone therapy helps relieve the short-term symptoms of menopause and reduces some long-term risks associated with lower estrogen levels. There are two types of hormone therapy. Estrogen replacement therapy (ERT) is estrogen alone. Hormone replacement therapy (HRT) combines estrogen with progestin, another hormone.

ERT is usually prescribed only for women who have had a hysterectomy, since it increases the risk of endometrial cancer. HRT is usually prescribed only for women who have a uterus. Women with a uterus who take ERT need regular checkups for uterine lining changes.

Hormone therapy reduces some health risks and increases others. Consider the following factors in your decision.

Osteoporosis

Both ERT and HRT reduce the risk of osteoporosis and slow the rate of bone loss that occurs after menopause, which helps reduce the risk of fractures. See page 79 for information on preventing osteoporosis.

Heart Disease

ERT reduces a woman's risk of heart disease by increasing high-density lipoprotein (HDL or "good") cholesterol. Studies of HRT suggest it also has a significant "heart-protective" effect.

Because the risk of heart disease is much greater than other health risks for postmenopausal women, the "heart-protective" effect of ERT may make it a wise choice for many women.

Colon Cancer

Recently, a reduction in the risk of colon cancer has been noted among women taking estrogen therapy.

Breast Cancer

It is not clear whether hormone therapy increases the risk of breast cancer. Some studies find that it may increase the risk slightly; others find no increase in risk. However, women who currently have breast cancer should not take ERT or HRT. Some women who have had breast cancer in the past but have been cancer-free for at least two to three years may be able to take HRT. Discuss this with your health care provider.

Endometrial Cancer

Estrogen alone (ERT) increases the risk of endometrial (uterine) cancer. Estrogen combined with progestin (HRT) protects against this increased risk.

Gallbladder Disease

Both ERT and HRT increase the risk of gallbladder disease.

Considerations

Hormone therapy reduces the discomfort caused by menopausal symptoms. However, HRT also has side effects that may be unacceptable to some women. They include periodic vaginal bleeding, bloating, cramping, nausea, and breast tenderness. Your doctor may be able to ease these side effects by adjusting the dose.

To gain the long-term benefits of hormone therapy, the medications must be taken for many years. Women on long-term hormone therapy need regular visits to a health professional.

Should You Take Hormones?

Hormone therapy is usually not recommended for women who have had breast cancer, trouble with blood clots, liver disease, or undiagnosed vaginal bleeding.

On the other hand, hormone therapy can be beneficial for most women. Discuss the potential risks and benefits with your health care provider.

Menstrual Cramps

Many women suffer from painful menstrual cramps (dysmenorrhea). Symptoms include mild to severe cramping in the lower abdomen, back, or thighs, headaches, diarrhea, constipation, nausea, dizziness, and fainting.

During the menstrual cycle, the lining of the uterus produces a hormone called prostaglandin. This hormone causes the uterus to contract, often painfully. Women with severe cramps may produce higher than normal amounts of prostaglandin, or may be more sensitive to its effects.

Home Treatment

- Exercise. Regular workouts decrease the severity of cramps. See Chapter 17.

- Ibuprofen and naproxen (Aleve) inhibit the production of prostaglandins, and generally help ease cramps better than aspirin or acetaminophen. Take it the day before your period starts, or at the first sign of pain. Take ibuprofen or naproxen with milk or food, as they can upset your stomach.

- Use heat (hot water bottles, heating pads, or hot baths) to relax tense muscles and relieve cramping.

- Herbal teas, such as chamomile, mint, raspberry, and blackberry are good for soothing tense muscles and anxious moods.

- Try using sanitary napkins instead of tampons.

- If you have symptoms other than cramping, such as weight gain, headache, and tension, see Premenstrual Syndrome on page 182.

When to Call Kaiser Permanente

- If menstrual bleeding is very heavy (changing more than one maxi pad or super tampon an hour for more than six hours) or lasts longer than 10 days.

- If periods come closer than 21 days apart.

- If you suspect that your intrauterine device (IUD) is causing the cramping.

- If cramps fail to respond to home treatment.

- If your period is accompanied by sudden high fever, diarrhea, or skin rash.

- If painful cramping suddenly occurs after years of less painful periods.

- If cramps begin five to seven days before your period begins, or if cramps do not cease when menstrual flow stops.

- If pelvic pain seems unrelated to your menstrual cycle.

Missed or Irregular Periods

Missed or irregular periods have a variety of causes. Pregnancy is usually the first cause to be considered, but others include:

- Stress, weight loss or gain, increased exercise (missed periods are common in endurance athletes), and travel.

- Use of birth control pills, which may cause lighter, less frequent, or skipped periods.

- Menopause or menarche (starting of menstrual periods). For the first few years of menstruation, periods may be irregular.

- Hormone imbalance or problems in the reproductive system.

- Medications, including steroids, tranquilizers, and diet pills.

Prevention

- Avoid fad diets that greatly restrict calories and food variety. Avoid rapid weight loss.

- Learn and practice relaxation exercises to cope with stress. See page 252.

- Increase exercise gradually.

Home Treatment

- If you had intercourse during the previous month, do a home pregnancy test. See page 174.

- Follow the prevention guidelines above.

- Work on ways to reduce and cope with stress. See Chapter 17.

- If you are an endurance athlete, cut back on training or talk with a doctor about estrogen/progesterone/calcium supplements to protect against bone loss.

- If dieting, include more variety and calories in your diet.

- If age 45 or older, you may be starting menopause. See page 177.

- Try to relax. Restoring your life to emotional and physical balance will help. Many women miss periods now and then. Chances are, unless you are pregnant, your cycle will return to normal next month.

When to Call Kaiser Permanente

- If pregnancy is possible, to confirm your home pregnancy test and begin pregnancy counseling and/or prenatal care.

- If you have missed two regular periods, are not pregnant, are not approaching menopause, and are not dieting, exercising a lot, or under psychological stress.

- If you are an endurance athlete who is unable to cut back on training. You may need hormones or calcium supplements.

- If you miss two periods while taking birth control pills, and you have not skipped any pills.

Premenstrual Syndrome

Premenstrual syndrome (PMS) occurs 7 to 10 days before the menstrual period begins. It is estimated that 90 percent of women have had some of the symptoms associated with PMS. Only about 10 percent of women have severe problems with PMS.

Over 150 physical and psychological symptoms are associated with PMS. Physical symptoms include: headaches, backaches, weight gain, breast tenderness, water retention and bloating, food cravings and increased appetite, diarrhea or constipation, dizziness or fainting, and clumsiness.

Emotional symptoms include: irritability and anger, mood swings, anxiety, sudden bouts of crying, sadness, fatigue, poor concentration, diminished sex drive, and aggression. Symptoms generally improve with the onset of bleeding.

A self-test to determine if you have PMS:

- Do the same symptoms occur each month?

- Do symptoms improve or disappear when bleeding begins?

- Do you have at least one symptom-free week per month?

Keep a diary charting your menstrual symptoms, their timing, and severity. If symptoms appear fairly consistent over several months, chances are you have PMS.

Home Treatment

- Eat smaller meals every three to four hours with plenty of whole grains, fruit, and vegetables. Limit fats and sweets, and reduce salt to help limit bloating.

- Eliminating tobacco, alcohol, and caffeine may help relieve some symptoms.

- Get some exercise. Regular exercise will help minimize PMS symptoms. See Chapter 17.

- Try an over-the-counter PMS medication, such as Midol or Pamprin. Many products contain a combination of drugs to help relieve symptoms of cramps, bloating, and headache.

- Taking 50 mg of vitamin B_6 twice a day is often helpful. Do not take more than 100 mg per day.

- Be good to yourself. Reduce your stress level as much as possible. Try relaxation techniques such as yoga and deep breathing. See Chapter 17.

- Talk with others. Your PMS also affects those with whom you live and work.

When to Call Kaiser Permanente

- If physical or emotional symptoms are severe and you feel out of control.

- If symptoms do not stop when menstrual bleeding starts.

Urinary Incontinence

If you suffer from urinary incontinence (loss of bladder control), you are not alone. Many people are coping with this problem.

Many cases of incontinence can be controlled, if not cured outright. Temporary incontinence can be caused by water pills (diuretics) and many other common medications. Urinary infections, stones in the urinary tract, or extended bed rest are other causes. If the underlying problem is corrected, the incontinence can be cured.

There are three types of persistent or chronic loss of bladder control:

Stress incontinence refers to small amounts of urine leaking out during exercise, coughing, laughing, sneezing, or other movements that squeeze the bladder. It is most often seen in women, although men may experience it after prostate surgery.

This kind of incontinence is often helped by Kegel exercises (right).

Urge incontinence happens when the need to urinate comes on so quickly there is not enough time to get to the toilet. Stroke, Parkinson's disease, kidney or bladder stones, and bladder infection are some of the causes of urge incontinence.

Overflow incontinence occurs when the bladder cannot empty itself completely. Diabetes or an enlarged prostate may be the underlying cause.

Kegel Exercises

Kegel exercises can help cure or improve stress incontinence. They strengthen the muscles that control the flow of urine.

- Locate the muscles by stopping your urine in midstream and starting again. The muscles that you feel squeezing around your urethra and anus are the ones to focus on.

- Practice squeezing these muscles while you are not urinating. If your stomach or buttocks move, you are not using the right muscles.

- Hold the squeeze for three seconds, then relax for three seconds.

- Repeat the exercise 10 to 15 times per session.

- Do at least 10 Kegel exercise sessions per day.

Kegel exercises are simple and effective. You can do them anywhere and anytime. No one will know you are doing them except you.

Home Treatment

- Don't let incontinence embarrass you. Take charge and work with your doctor to treat any underlying conditions that may be causing the problem.

- Don't let incontinence keep you from doing the things you like to do. Absorbent pads or briefs, such as Attends and Depend, are available in pharmacies and supermarkets. No one will know you are wearing one.

Incontinence – continued

- Avoid coffee, tea, and other drinks that contain caffeine, which overstimulates the bladder. Do not cut down on over-all fluids; you need these to keep the rest of your body healthy.

- Practice "double-voiding." Empty your bladder as much as possible, relax for a minute, and then try to empty your bladder again.

- Urinate on a schedule, perhaps every three to four hours during the day, whether the urge is there or not. This may help you to restore control.

- Wear clothing that can be easily removed, such as pants with elastic waistbands. If you have difficulty with buttons and zippers, consider replacing them with velcro closures.

- Keep skin in the genital area dry to prevent rashes. Vaseline or Desitin ointment will help.

- Pay special attention to any medications you are taking, including over-the-counter drugs, since some affect bladder control.

- Incontinence is sometimes caused by a urinary tract infection. If you feel pain or burning when you urinate, see the home treatment for urinary tract infections (right).

- For stress incontinence, practice Kegel exercises daily. See page 183.

When to Call Kaiser Permanente

- If you haven't been able to adequately control your symptoms by these home measures.

Urinary Tract Infections

Urinary tract infection (UTI), also called bladder infection or cystitis, is a common health problem for women, young girls, and some infant boys. It may also occur in men.

Early symptoms may include burning or pain during urination and itching or pain in the urethra (the tube that carries urine from the bladder). There may also be discomfort in the lower abdomen and a frequent urge to urinate without being able to pass much urine. Men with these symptoms may have an infection of the prostate gland. See page 193.

Urinary infections are generally caused by *E. coli* bacteria, which are normally present in the digestive system. Because women have shorter urethras, they are much more susceptible to the infection than men.

Other causes of irritation to the genital area that may be associated with bladder infection include intercourse, diaphragms, wearing tight jeans or pants, bike riding, infrequent urination, perfumed soaps and powders, even spicy food.

Apply home treatment at the very first hint of irritation or painful urination. Because the organs of the urinary tract are connected, infection can easily spread from one organ to the next. Untreated infections may spread to the kidneys and cause more serious problems.

Prevention

- Drink more fluids; water is best.

- Urinate frequently.

- Women should wipe from front to back after going to the toilet to reduce the spread of bacteria from the anus to the urethra. Teach young girls this habit during toilet training.

- Avoid frequent douching, and do not use vaginal deodorants or perfumed feminine hygiene products.

- Wash the genital area once a day with plain water or mild soap. Rinse well and dry thoroughly.

- Women susceptible to urinary infections should urinate promptly after intercourse. Drinking extra water after intercourse may also help prevent infection.

- Wear cotton underwear, cotton-lined pantyhose, and loose clothing.

- Drinking cranberry juice may protect against infection, especially in women after menopause.

Blood in the Urine

A blow to the kidneys, excessive running, or a urinary tract infection can cause blood in the urine. Blood in the urine can be a sign of a serious illness in both women and men and should always be discussed with a health professional.

Eating foods such as beets, blackberries, and those containing red dyes can temporarily color the urine. Urine may also appear pink or red due to blood or natural or artificial food colorings.

Home Treatment

- Drink as much water (think in terms of gallons) as you can in the first 24 hours after symptoms appear. This will help flush bacteria out of the bladder.

- Avoid alcohol and caffeine.

- A hot bath may help relieve pain and itching.

- Examine the genital area and check temperature twice daily. Fever may indicate a more serious infection is present.

- Avoid intercourse until symptoms improve.

- If abdominal pain or vaginal burning and redness occur in a young girl, consider the possibility of an allergy to bubble bath or soap.

When to Call Kaiser Permanente

- If painful urination occurs with any of the following symptoms:

  ○ Chills and/or fever over 101°

  ○ Inability to urinate when you feel the urge

  ○ Lower back pain just below rib cage

  ○ Blood or pus in the urine

  ○ Unusual vaginal discharge

  ○ Nausea or vomiting

- If symptoms do not improve after 24 hours of home treatment.

- If you are pregnant or have diabetes, and have symptoms of a urinary tract infection.

Vaginitis

Vaginitis is any vaginal infection, inflammation, or irritation that causes a change in normal vaginal discharge. General symptoms include a change in the amount, color, odor, or consistency of the discharge, itching, painful urination, and pain during intercourse. Common types of vaginitis include yeast infection and nonspecific infection (bacterial vaginosis). Some types of sexually transmitted diseases can also cause an unusual vaginal discharge. See page 199.

Vaginitis is usually caused by an upset to the normal balance of the vagina. Causes may include:

• A recent change in sexual partners or sexual practices.

• Irritation caused by excessive douching, strong soaps or perfumed feminine hygiene products, wearing tight pants or jeans, intercourse, or bicycling.

• Antibiotics, which kill protective bacteria.

• Stress, pregnancy, diabetes, and birth control pills. The hormonal changes of menopause may also cause a type of vaginitis. See page 177.

Vaginitis is common and not necessarily a symptom of a sexually transmitted disease. Some women seem more susceptible than others. An aggravating fact about vaginitis is that it tends to recur.

Prevention

• Wear cotton underpants. The organisms that cause vaginitis grow best in warm, moist places. Nylon underwear and pantyhose tend to trap heat and perspiration. Avoid pants that are tight in the crotch and thighs.

• Wipe from front to back after using the toilet to avoid spreading bacteria from the anus to the vagina.

• Wash the genital area once a day with plain water or a mild, non-perfumed soap. Rinse well and dry thoroughly.

• Avoid douching. A healthy vagina will clean itself.

• Avoid using feminine deodorant sprays and other perfumed products. They irritate tender skin.

• Change tampons at least three times a day or alternate tampons with pads. Be sure to remove the last tampon used during the period.

• Eat a cup of yogurt containing active acidophilus cultures each day. Some women find this helps prevent yeast infections. It may be especially helpful if you are taking antibiotics.

• Some women find that applying yogurt containing active acidophilus cultures to the vagina may be helpful. This may be done with a spoon or douche apparatus.

Home Treatment

- Bacterial vaginosis or a nonspecific vaginitis may go away by itself in three to four days.

- Avoid intercourse for two weeks to give irritated vaginal tissues time to heal.

- Avoid scratching. Relieve itching with a cold water compress or over-the-counter hydrocortisone cream applied thinly to vaginal tissues three times daily.

- Make sure that the cause of the vaginitis is not a forgotten tampon or other foreign object.

- Over-the-counter antifungal creams (Gyne-Lotrimin, Monistat) are available to treat yeast infections.

- If you have burning and pain on urination and feel the need to urinate often, see Urinary Tract Infections on page 184.

When to Call Kaiser Permanente

- If the discharge is accompanied by discomfort or pelvic pain and fever.

- If the discharge and other symptoms are very uncomfortable.

- If you think you've been exposed to a sexually transmitted disease (see page 199). Your partner may need to be treated as well.

- If home treatment with an over-the-counter product fails to clear up a yeast infection within three to four days. A different organism may be causing the infection.

- If you are using over-the-counter antifungal creams repeatedly.

- If you have pain with intercourse that is not eased by use of a vaginal lubricant, such as K-Y Jelly.

- If any unusual discharge lasts more than two weeks.

- If you plan to see a health professional, do not douche, use vaginal creams, or have intercourse for 48 hours before your appointment, since they may make diagnosis difficult.

Medication can be prescribed to clear up the infection. See page 302, which describes appropriate use of antibiotics. If vaginitis returns after treatment, your partner may need to be treated as well. (The infection usually does not cause symptoms in men.)

Man who say it cannot be done should not interrupt man doing it.
Old Chinese Proverb

Chapter 13

Men's Health

The average man lives seven years less than the average woman. A good part of this seven-year gap is because more women than men have developed healthy habits. To start living longer, men need to start living smarter.

Risky Lifestyles

Poor health habits contribute to the gender gap in each of the seven most common causes of death for men ages 25 to 44. (These risks apply to other ages and women, too.)

1. Injuries (21 percent of deaths)

• Men are twice as likely to drive after drinking as women.

• Men are nine percent less likely to wear their seatbelts than women.

2. HIV Infection (16.5 percent of deaths)

• Closely related to unprotected male-male and male-female sex practices, as well as intravenous drug use.

3. Heart Disease (11 percent of deaths)

• Men consume 45 percent more dietary cholesterol than women.

• Men are six percent more likely to smoke than women.

• Men are four percent more likely to be overweight than women.

4. Cancer (10 percent of deaths)

• Men are 12 percent more likely to be heavy smokers than women.

5. Suicide (10 percent of deaths)

• Men are half as likely to seek help for emotional problems as women.

6. Homicide (10 percent of deaths)

• Men are nearly 70 percent more likely to own guns than women.

7. Liver Disease (three percent of deaths)

• Men are five times more likely to drink alcohol daily than women.

Risky Lifestyles – continued

If you want to live longer and feel better, start living smarter, one small step at a time.

While this chapter is entitled Men's Health, its purpose is not to address the primary areas of nutrition, stress management, and safety that men must deal with if they are to close the longevity gap. This chapter focuses on specific health problems that are of particular interest to men. For more information, see Chapters 17 and 18, and Resource 61 on page 310.

Genital Health

Daily cleaning of the penis, particularly under the foreskin of an uncircumcised penis, can prevent bacterial infection. Daily washing also reduces the already low risk of penile cancer. Boys should be taught by age three or four how to retract the foreskin, wash the penis, and replace the foreskin over the head of the penis after cleaning. The foreskin may not be fully retractable until age three or older. Do not forcibly retract a child's foreskin if it is painful or difficult to do so.

Testicular Self-Exam

Teen males and young men who are at increased risk of testicular cancer (due to family history of testicular cancer or personal history of undescended testicles) are encouraged to examine their testes once a month. Testicular cancer is very rare and highly curable when detected early.

The best time to do the exam is after a warm bath or shower when the scrotal skin is relaxed.

• Stand and place your right leg on an elevated surface. A tub side or toilet seat works fine.

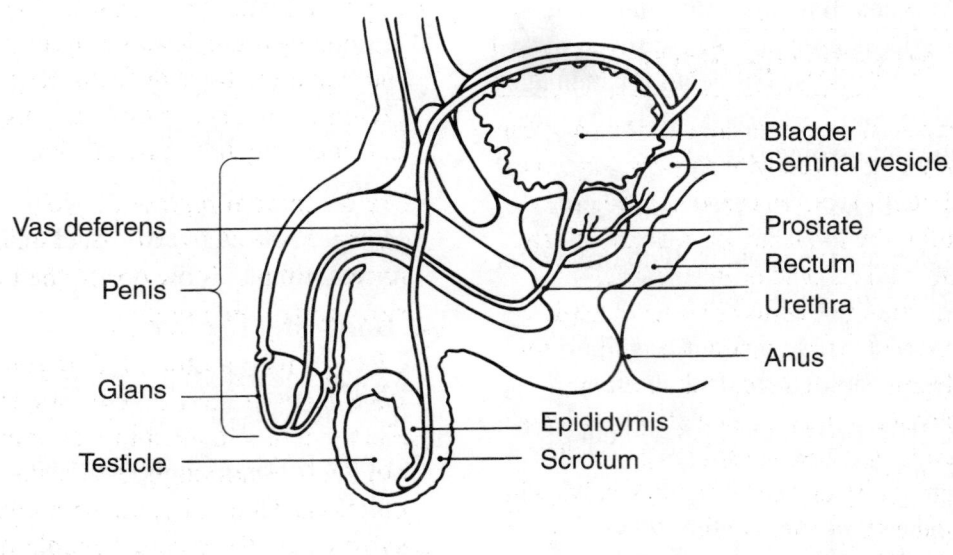

Male genitals

• Explore the surface of the right testicle by gently rolling it between the thumb and fingers of both hands. Feel for any hard lumps or nodules. The testicle should feel round and smooth.

• Notice any enlargement of the testicle or a change in its consistency. It is normal for one testicle to be slightly larger than the other. Any major size differences should be reported to a health professional.

• Repeat, lifting the left leg and examining your left testicle.

Call your health professional for an immediate appointment if you notice any of the following:

• Unusual lumps or nodules in the testes

• Unexplained pain or swelling in the testes or scrotum

• If you notice any penile discharge, or sores on your penis, see page 199 and discuss it with your doctor.

Erection Problems

Erection problems are common and can often be solved with self-care remedies. By definition, an erection problem is difficulty in raising or maintaining an erection capable of intercourse. Erection problems are often due to stress at work, tension in relationships, depression, fatigue, lack of privacy, physical injury, or side effects of medications. These causes are generally temporary and will usually resolve with home treatment. Additional less reversible causes include a long history of smoking or vascular disease.

Prevention

Most erection problems can be prevented by taking a more relaxed approach to lovemaking and watching for possible side effects from medications or illnesses. While the ease of gaining and sustaining erections generally decreases with age, with the right foreplay and environment, there is no age limit to the ability of healthy men to have erections.

Home Treatment

• Rule out medications first. Scores of drugs can cause erection problem side effects. Many blood pressure medicines, diuretics, and mood-altering drugs are particularly troublesome. Ask your doctor or pharmacist to check your medications for possible side effects on sexual function, or look it up yourself. See Resource 2 on page 307.

• Avoid alcohol and smoking, which make erection problems worse.

• Cope with stress (see Chapter 17). Tension in your life can distract you and make erections difficult. Regular exercise and other stress-relieving activities may help ease tension.

• Try for more foreplay. Let your partner know that you would enjoy some stroking. Slow down, then slow down some more.

• Give yourself a little time. If you have experienced a recent loss or change in a relationship, you may not yet be emotionally ready for erections. Generally, the stress will subside and the erection problem will disappear after a few weeks. Do what you can to relax.

Erection Problems – continued

- Find out if you can have erections at other times. If you can have an erection during masturbation or on awakening, the problem is probably stress-related or due to an emotional problem.

When to Call Kaiser Permanente

- If you think that a medication may be causing the problem. Substitutes may be available.

- If you are unable to have an erection at all, or think that your problem may be a physical one.

- If you are still having problems after a few months of self-care, consider talking with a psychological therapist.

- After all other options have been tried for several months without success, you may wish to talk with your doctor about erection-producing injections, a vacuum device, or penile implant.

Hernia

A hernia occurs when part of the intestine bulges out through a weak spot in the abdominal wall. Hernias are more common in men than in women. They commonly occur in the groin and may bulge into the scrotum. An inguinal hernia is one that occurs in the inguinal canal, which leads from the abdomen to the scrotum.

Hernias are often caused by increased abdominal pressure resulting from lifting heavy weights, coughing, or straining during a bowel movement. Sometimes, a weak spot in the abdominal wall is present at birth.

The symptoms of a hernia may come on gradually or suddenly. There may be a feeling that something has given way and varying degrees of pain.

Symptoms may include:

- Feeling of weakness, pressure, burning, or pain in the groin or scrotum.

- A bulge or lump in the groin or scrotum. These bulges may be easier to see when the person coughs, and may disappear when the person lies down.

- Pain in the groin when straining, lifting, or coughing.

A hernia is called reducible if it can be pushed back into place in the abdomen; irreducible if it cannot.

A hernia becomes incarcerated when the intestine becomes trapped outside the abdominal wall. If the blood supply is cut off, the hernia is said to be strangulated. When this occurs, the tissue swells and dies. The dead tissue quickly becomes infected, requiring immediate medical attention. Rapidly increasing pain in the groin or scrotum is a sign that the hernia has become strangulated.

Prevention

- Avoid activities that strain your abdominal area.

- Use proper lifting techniques (see page 59), and avoid lifting weights that are too heavy for you.

- Strengthen your abdominal muscles. See curl-ups on page 60.

- Avoid straining during bowel movements.

When to Call Kaiser Permanente

- If you suspect a hernia, see your doctor for a full diagnosis and evaluation of the risk. Most hernias do not require surgery unless they interfere with your daily life, cause a lot of pain, or if the risk of strangulation is high.

- If you experience increasing pain in the abdomen, scrotum, or groin.

- If mild groin pain or an unexplained groin bump or swelling continues for more than one week.

Prostate Problems

The prostate is a doughnut-shaped cluster of glands located at the bottom of the bladder about halfway between the rectum and the base of the penis. It encircles the urethra, the tube that carries urine from the bladder out through the penis. The walnut-sized gland produces most of the fluid in semen.

The three most common prostate problems are: infection (prostatitis), prostate enlargement (benign prostatic hypertrophy), and prostate cancer.

Prostate Infection (Prostatitis)

There are two types of prostate infection, acute and chronic. Acute infections come on suddenly and have some or all of the following symptoms:

- Fever and chills

- Pain and burning on urination and ejaculation

- Strong and frequent urge to urinate while passing only small amounts of urine

- Lower back or abdominal pain

- Blood in the urine (occasionally)

Symptoms of chronic prostatitis are usually milder than those of an acute infection, and fever and chills are usually not present. Either infection may occur with a urinary tract infection. See page 184.

Sometimes, men will have painful urinary symptoms without infection. This condition may be called prostatodynia, and is often related to stress or anxiety.

Prostate infections usually respond well to home care and antibiotic treatment. If the infection recurs, long-term antibiotic treatment may be needed.

Prevention

- Increase your fluid intake to as much as 8 to 12 glasses per day. You are drinking enough when you are urinating more often than usual. Extra fluids help flush the urinary tract clean.

Prostatitis – continued

- Avoid alcohol and caffeine. Caffeine can cause a strong and frequent urge to urinate. Remember that colas contain caffeine as well as coffee and tea.

- Keep stress under control. A high level of stress is closely associated with prostatodynia.

Home Treatment

- Drink as much water as you can tolerate.

- Eliminate all alcohol and caffeine from your diet.

- Hot baths help soothe pain and reduce stress.

- Aspirin or ibuprofen may help ease painful urinary symptoms.

When to Call Kaiser Permanente

- If urinary symptoms occur with fever, chills, vomiting, or pain in the back or abdomen.

- If urine is red or pink with no dietary reason. See page 185. Always call Kaiser Permanente if you have blood in your urine.

- If symptoms continue for five days despite home care.

- If there is a sudden change or worsening of symptoms.

- If you have pain on urination or ejaculation and a discharge from the penis. See page 199.

Prostate Enlargement (Benign Prostatic Hypertrophy)

As men age, the prostate may enlarge. This seems to be a natural process and is not really a disease. However, as the gland gets bigger, it tends to squeeze the urethra and cause urinary problems, such as:

- Difficulty getting urine started and completely stopped (dribbling)

- Urge to urinate frequently, or being wakened by the need to urinate

- Painful urination

- Decreased force of the urine stream

- Incomplete bladder emptying

An enlarged prostate gland is not a serious problem unless urination becomes extremely difficult, or backed-up urine causes bladder infections or kidney damage. Some dribbling is very common and not necessarily a sign of prostate problems.

Surgery is usually not necessary for an enlarged prostate. Although surgery used to be a common treatment, recent research shows that most cases of prostate enlargement do not get worse over time as previously thought. Many men find that their symptoms are stable and some even clear up on their own. In these cases, the best treatment may be no treatment at all. Drugs are available that may help improve symptoms in some men. Your doctor can advise you on the various treatment options.

Prevention

Since the prostate produces seminal fluid, there is a long-standing belief that regular ejaculations (two to three times per week) will help prevent an enlarged prostate. There is no scientific proof of this, but it is risk-free.

Home Treatment

- Avoid antihistamines and decongestants, which can make urinary problems worse.

- If you are bothered by a frequent urge to urinate at night, cut down on beverages, especially alcohol and caffeine, before bedtime.

- Don't postpone urinating, and take plenty of time. Try sitting on the toilet instead of standing.

- If dribbling after urination is a problem, wash your penis once a day to prevent infection.

- Also see Incontinence on page 183.

When to Call Kaiser Permanente

- If fever, chills, or back or abdominal pain develop.

- Diuretics, tranquilizers, antihistamines, decongestants, and antidepressants can aggravate urinary problems. If you take these drugs, ask your health professional if there are other medications without these side effects.

- If the symptoms of an enlarged prostate last longer than two weeks. Early examination enables you to confirm the diagnosis and consider treatment options.

Prostate Cancer

Prostate cancer is the most common cancer and the second leading cause of cancer deaths in men. It becomes more common with age, and most cases are in men over 65. It is usually a small and slow-growing cancer. Since it is most often present in older men, it usually does not shorten life. However, when it is large, advanced, or appears at a younger age, it can be very serious. When detected early, before it has spread to other organs, the cancer may be curable.

There are no specific symptoms of prostate cancer. Most men have no symptoms at all. In some cases, it can cause urinary symptoms very similar to those of prostate enlargement. In advanced cases, other symptoms may be caused by spread of the cancer to other organs such as bone.

Prostate cancer sometimes runs in families, is more common in African-American men, and tends to be more common in men who eat a high-fat diet.

Prevention

Besides maintaining a low-fat diet, there is no known way to reduce the risk of prostate cancer.

Home Treatment

Prostate cancer treatment is very individual. Work together with your doctor to be sure that you will receive a long-term benefit from treatment. Your age, overall health, other medical conditions, and the characteristics of the cancer are all important factors to consider in making treatment decisions.

Prostate Cancer – continued

Learn all you can about the available treatment options, which may include watchful waiting, so that you can work with your doctor to select the one best suited for you.

When to Call Kaiser Permanente

There is a great deal of controversy about the value of screening men who do not have any symptoms using rectal exams and the prostate-specific antigen (PSA) blood test. Using these tests to detect prostate cancer earlier has not been shown to improve the man's quality of life or to prolong life. Therefore, most experts do not recommend routine rectal exams or PSA tests.

Talk with your doctor or visit a Kaiser Permanente Health Education Department for more information.

I wasn't kissing her, I was whispering in her mouth.
Groucho Marx

Chapter 14

Sexual Health

Sexuality is an important aspect of health. How we love, how we show affection, how we value ourselves, and how we bond with and befriend each other are all influenced by our sexuality. Sexuality is also based on deep personal values we learn from our parents, our culture, our religion, and who we are.

Sexuality can be confusing; myths and misunderstandings abound. Parents have a special obligation to help guide their children as their sexual values develop. Talk with your children about their sexuality and give them good information. Help them learn to make responsible and safe decisions about sex and sexuality.

This chapter covers specific health issues of concern to people who are sexually active—birth control and sexually transmitted diseases, including AIDS.

Birth Control

Birth control can help you prevent unplanned pregnancies. However, no birth control method (except abstinence) is 100 percent effective and without risks. The chart on page 198 briefly describes the most common birth control methods. Review each method with your partner before deciding which one meets your needs. Your health professional can help you better understand the risks and effectiveness of each method.

Condoms are a birth control method that also protect against sexually transmitted disease, although they are not 100 percent effective. A condom used with spermicide containing non-oxynol-9 provides the most reliable, but not total, protection. Other barrier methods (diaphragm, cervical cap, sponge) provide very minimal protection against STDs.

Birth Control

Method	Pregnancies*	Comments
Sterilization Tubal ligation (women) Vasectomy (men)	Less than 1	Consider it permanent.
Hormonal Methods Oral contraceptives (the Pill)	3 (less than 1 with proper use)	Increased risk of circula- tory disorders and high blood pressure in smokers.
Norplant (implant) Depo-Provera (shot)	Less than 1 Less than 1	May cause irregular menstrual bleeding.
Intrauterine Device (IUD)	3	May cause bleeding and cramping. May be expelled without being noticed. Increased risk of pelvic infection.
Barrier Methods Condom alone	12	Use properly for best protection.
Condom + spermicide	5	Provides the most reliable protection against STDs.
Sponge Diaphragm Cervical cap	18 – 28 18 18	
Spermicides Jelly, cream, foam, suppositories	21	Use properly for best protection.
Used with condom	5	
Periodic Abstinence (natural family planning: basal body temperature, mucous, or rhythm/calendar method)	20	
Withdrawal	18	
No method (chance)	85	

*Typical number of accidental pregnancies per 100 women in one year.
Source: R. Hatcher, et al., *Contraceptive Technology, 1990-1992.*

Sexually Transmitted Diseases

Sexually transmitted diseases (STDs) or venereal diseases (VD) are infections passed from person to person through sexual intercourse or genital contact. Chlamydia, genital herpes, genital warts, gonorrhea, hepatitis B, and syphilis are among the most common STDs. AIDS (acquired immune deficiency syndrome), the most virulent and deadly of all STDs, is discussed on page 201.

Chlamydia (kla-mid-ee-uh) is a bacterial infection that affects millions of men and women. It may be difficult to detect chlamydia; about 80 percent of women and 10 percent of men with the disease have no symptoms. If symptoms do show up, they occur two to four weeks after exposure. In women, symptoms may include vaginal discharge or irregular menstrual bleeding, painful urination, genital itching, or lower abdominal pain. In men, there may be a penile discharge and painful urination.

Chlamydia is easily treated with antibiotics. If undetected and untreated, chlamydia can cause pelvic inflammatory disease in women, which may lead to sterility.

Genital herpes is caused by the herpes simplex virus, which also causes cold sores and fever blisters (see page 238). Genital herpes is easily spread through sexual and other direct skin contact. Symptoms occur 2 to 30 days after contact with an infected person.

The first case of genital herpes may be quite severe, with many painful sores or blisters. Fever, swollen glands, and headache or muscle aches may also occur with the first outbreak. If the sores develop inside the urethra or vagina, there may be pain on urination or a vaginal discharge. The sores will crust and disappear in one to three weeks' time. Sometimes, the first episode is so mild it is unnoticed. It is also possible to be infected with herpes and have no symptoms.

There is no known cure for herpes. Once infected, you may have recurrent outbreaks, which are usually shorter and less severe than the first one. Itching, burning, or tingling may occur at the place where the sores will later appear. Medication is available that helps reduce the frequency and severity of recurrent outbreaks. It is generally useful only for people who have frequent and severe outbreaks.

Genital warts are caused by the human papillomavirus (HPV), which is spread by sexual contact. They generally appear as small fleshy bumps or flat white patches on the labia (the lips around the vagina), inside the vagina, on the penis or scrotum, or around the anus. Of most concern to women is the link between HPV and cervical cancer. The virus can be detected by a Pap smear. If warts are bothersome or develop on the cervix, they may be removed by a health professional. In some cases, the warts may recur.

Gonorrhea, also known as clap, drip, or GC, is a bacterial infection spread through sexual contact.

STDs – continued

Symptoms include painful urination, vaginal discharge, irregular menstrual bleeding, or a thick discharge from the penis. Many people who have the bacteria have no symptoms. If untreated, gonorrhea in women may lead to pelvic inflammatory disease and sterility. It can sometimes spread to the joints and cause arthritis.

Hepatitis B is a viral infection spread through sexual contact or contact with infected blood. An infected pregnant woman can also transmit the virus to her baby. Symptoms appear two to five months after exposure, and include vomiting, abdominal pain, loss of appetite, and yellow tint to the eyes and skin (jaundice). About one-third of infected people have no symptoms. Long-term effects of the disease include life-threatening liver damage. A vaccine against hepatitis B is recommended for all infants, adolescents who were not previously immunized, and people in certain high-risk groups. See page 28.

Syphilis is a bacterial infection spread through sexual contact or sharing of contaminated needles. Symptoms appear two weeks to one month after contact. The first symptom is a chancre, a small red blister, ulcer, or sore that appears on the genitals, rectal area, or mouth. This sore is painless and may go unnoticed. The lymph nodes in the groin may also swell.

If syphilis is not treated early, it can proceed to a second phase in two to eight weeks. Symptoms of the second phase include skin rash, patchy hair loss, fever, swollen lymph glands, and flu-like symptoms, which are easily confused with other illnesses.

Syphilis can be treated with antibiotics. If untreated, syphilis will cause serious problems and premature death.

Prevention

Preventing a sexually transmitted disease is easier than treating an infection once it occurs. Only monogamy between uninfected partners or sexual abstinence completely *eliminates* the risk.

• Avoid sexual contact while you or your partner is being treated for a sexually transmitted disease.

• If you or your partner have herpes, avoid sexual contact when a blister or any open ulcer or sore is present, and use condoms at all other times.

• The same behaviors that reduce your risk of HIV also reduce your risk of getting other STDs. See page 202 for additional prevention guidelines.

When to Call Kaiser Permanente

If you notice any unusual discharge, sores, redness, or growths on the genitals, or if you suspect that you have been exposed to a STD, make an appointment as soon as possible.

STDs need to be diagnosed and treated by a health professional. Your doctor or a health department can provide STD diagnosis and treatment. Your sexual partner must also be treated, even if he or she has no symptoms. He or she may reinfect you or develop serious complications.

HIV Infection and AIDS

AIDS (acquired immune deficiency syndrome) is caused by the human immunodeficiency virus (HIV). HIV destroys the immune system, which makes it impossible for the body to fight off disease or even minor illnesses. AIDS is the last phase in HIV disease, when the body is unable to fight a disease or infection.

A person is said to be HIV-positive if antibodies to the virus are detected in his or her blood. It may take up to six months after infection for the antibodies to appear. Someone who is HIV-positive may appear to be healthy for 10 years or longer before the symptoms of AIDS develop.

HIV is *not* spread by mosquitoes, toilet seats, being coughed on by an infected person, casual contact with someone who is HIV-positive or who has AIDS, or by donating blood.

Because all blood has been tested for HIV since 1985, the risk of getting the virus from blood or blood products is extremely low.

HIV is spread only when blood, semen, or vaginal fluids from an infected person enters someone else's body. The specific behaviors that spread HIV include:

1. Sharing injection needles and syringes with someone who is HIV-positive.

2. Unprotected (without a condom) rectal entry intercourse (anal sex) with someone who is HIV-positive. Anal sex often tears the rectal blood vessels, allowing the virus to enter the body.

3. Unprotected vaginal or oral sexual activity with someone who is HIV-positive.

Babies born to or breast-fed by women who are HIV-positive are also at high risk of contracting the virus.

Being touched, hugged, or lightly kissed by someone who is HIV-positive will not transfer the virus to you. As long as you practice the prevention behaviors below, you have virtually no risk of contracting the virus.

If your behavior puts you at risk for HIV infection, a blood test should be done six months after the risky behavior. Early diagnosis and treatment of HIV is important even before symptoms develop.

A simple, confidential blood test, available at Kaiser Permanente or a health department, can determine if you are HIV-positive. Remember that it can take up to six months after infection for HIV antibodies to develop. The virus can be transmitted even before antibodies have developed. Researchers believe that all people who are HIV-positive will eventually develop AIDS. Although there are treatments for some of the symptoms of AIDS, there is currently no cure, and it is apparently always fatal.

HIV Infection and AIDS – cont.

Symptoms of HIV Infection and AIDS

The early symptoms of HIV infection are like flu symptoms that won't go away. Common symptoms are:

- Rapid unexplained weight loss

- Persistent unexplained fever and night sweats

- Persistent severe fatigue

- Persistent diarrhea

- Swelling of glands in neck, armpits, or groin

As the immune system deteriorates, a variety of other symptoms may appear, including:

- Unusual sores on the skin or in the mouth; white patches in the mouth

- Increased outbreaks of cold sores

- Unexplained shortness of breath and dry cough

- Severe numbness or pain in the hands and feet

- Personality change or mental deterioration

- Unusual cancers and infections

These symptoms are usually caused by many illnesses other than HIV infection or AIDS. However, if any symptom develops or persists without a good explanation, especially if your behavior puts you at risk of HIV infection, call your doctor.

Prevention

Only monogamy between uninfected partners or sexual abstinence completely eliminates the risk of HIV and other sexually transmitted diseases. The following actions will *reduce* your risk:

- If you are beginning a sexual relationship, take time before having sex to talk about HIV and other STDs. Find out if your partner has ever been exposed or infected or if your partner's behavior puts him or her at risk of HIV infection. Remember that it is possible to be infected without knowing it.

- Use condoms with any new partner until you are certain that person does not have any sexually transmitted diseases and you are certain that neither of you will have unprotected sexual contact with anyone else while your relationship lasts.

- Remember that it can take up to six months before HIV can be detected in the blood. If you plan to use HIV testing to decide whether condoms are needed, wait six months after any unprotected sexual contact or other high-risk behavior. During this time, both you and your partner need to avoid unprotected sexual contact and use condoms every time you have sexual contact.

- Avoid unprotected sexual contact with anyone who has symptoms of or who has been exposed to an STD. Keep in mind that a person may have no symptoms but still be able to transmit the diseases.

- Avoid unprotected vaginal and anal intercourse and oral sex with anyone whose sexual history may not be risk-free. Use latex condoms from the beginning to the end of sexual contact. "Natural" or lambskin condoms do not protect against HIV infection. For even greater protection, use a spermicide containing nonoxynol-9 in addition to condoms. Apply the spermicide directly into the vagina, not into the condom.

- Do not rely on spermicides, the sponge, or the diaphragm to protect against STDs. They add some protection to condoms, but do not provide adequate protection when used alone. They do not protect against AIDS.

In addition to the guidelines above, the following will reduce your risk of getting HIV:

- Avoid the activities on page 201 that spread HIV. Safer activities include closed-mouth kissing, hugging, massage, and other pleasurable touching.

- Never share needles, syringes, or other personal items that could be contaminated with blood. Even needles that have been boiled can remain contaminated.

For more information, call the National AIDS Hotline at 800-342-AIDS. Also see Resource 6 on page 307.

It is by the presence of mind in untried emergencies
that the native metal of a man (or woman) *is tested.*
James Russell Lowell

Chapter 15

First Aid and Emergencies

This chapter covers both serious medical emergencies and minor first aid situations. Review this chapter before you need it. Then, when you are faced with an emergency or injury, you will know where to turn. Your confidence in dealing with both major and minor emergencies will be reassuring to an injured person. Also see Resource 38 on page 309.

Medical emergencies covered in this chapter include:

- Bleeding, page 219.

- Cardiopulmonary Resuscitation (CPR), page 206.

- Chest Pain, page 216.

- Head Injuries, page 224.

- Poisoning, page 230.

- Shock, page 234.

- Unconsciousness, page 235.

Dealing with Emergencies

Take a deep breath. Count to 10. Tell yourself you can handle this situation.

Assess the danger. Protect yourself and the injured person from fire, explosions, or other hazards. If you suspect a spinal injury, do not move the person unless the danger is great.

If the person is unconscious or unresponsive, check the ABCs: Airway, Breathing, Circulation. If the person is not breathing, see Rescue Breathing and CPR on page 206.

Identify and prioritize the injuries. Treat the most life-threatening problems (bleeding, shock) first. Check for broken bones and other injuries. If you need emergency assistance, call 861-3434 or 911.

Emergencies – continued

Legal Protection

If you are needed in an emergency, give what help you can. Most states have a Good Samaritan law to protect people who help in an emergency. You cannot be sued for giving first aid unless it can be shown that you are guilty of gross negligence.

Rescue Breathing and CPR

Warning: Improper CPR or CPR performed on a person whose heart is still beating can cause *serious* injury. *Never* perform CPR unless:

1. Breathing has stopped.

2. There is no heartbeat.

3. No one with more training in CPR is present.

Be prepared: Take a CPR course from the American Red Cross or the American Heart Association.

For basic life support, think **ABC:** **A**irway, **B**reathing, and **C**irculation, in this order. You must establish an open airway to start breathing, and you must give rescue breathing before you can begin the chest compressions needed if the victim's heart has stopped.

Step 1: Check for consciousness.

Grasp the victim by the shoulders and shout, "Are you okay?" If he does not respond, roll him onto his back, *unless* there is a possible spinal injury. If he may have suffered a spinal injury, gently roll the head, neck, and shoulders together as a unit until he is on his back.

If the victim does not respond, call for help.

- **Children age 8 and under:** Give one full minute of rescue breathing (and CPR if there is no pulse), then call 911 or emergency services.

- **Adults and children age 9 and over:** Call 861-3434, 911, or emergency services immediately. Then give rescue breathing (and CPR if there is no pulse).

Step 2: Open the airway.

Check for breathing. Look to see if the victim's chest and abdomen are moving. Listen and feel for air moving out of the mouth. If the victim is not breathing, open the airway:

- Turn the head to one side and clear any foreign material from the mouth with your fingers.

- Place one hand on the victim's forehead and tilt the head back gently.

- Place the fingers of your other hand under the chin and lift to pull it forward. See Illustration A. **For an infant:** Use care not to tilt the head back too far.

- Sometimes, just opening the airway will allow the victim to breathe. Keep the airway open and look, listen, and feel for signs of breathing. If the victim does not start breathing, begin rescue breathing immediately.

Step 3: Begin rescue breathing.

- Pinch the victim's nostrils shut with your thumb and forefinger. With your other hand, continue tilting the chin forward to keep the airway open.

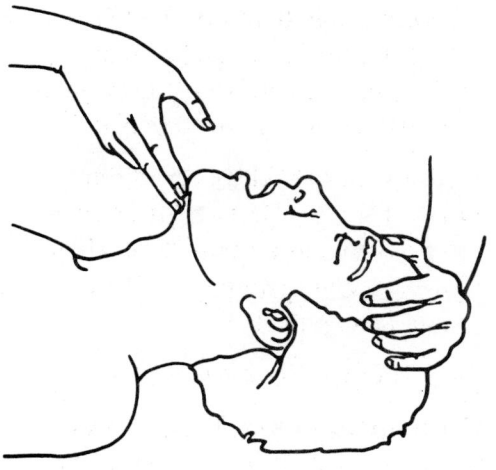

A. Head tilt, chin lift

• Take a deep breath and place your mouth over the victim's, making a tight seal. See Illustration B.

For an infant: Place your mouth over the mouth and nose.

• Slowly blow air in until the victim's chest rises. Take 1½ to 2 seconds to give each breath. Remove your mouth from the victim's and take a deep breath between rescue breaths. Allow the victim's chest to fall and feel the air escape.

• Give 2 full breaths, then check for circulation.

Step 4: Check for circulation.

Locate the carotid artery in the neck:

• Find the voice box or Adam's apple. Slide the tips of your index and middle fingers into the groove beside it.

• Feel for a pulse for 5 to 10 seconds.

If there is no pulse: Begin chest compressions. See Step 5.

If there is a pulse: Continue rescue breathing only until help arrives or the victim starts to breathe on his own. If he begins breathing again, he still needs to be seen by a health professional.

Give rescue breaths:

• Adult (age 9 and older): 1 breath every 5 seconds

• Children age 1 to 8: 1 breath every 4 seconds

• Infant under 1 year: 1 breath every 3 seconds

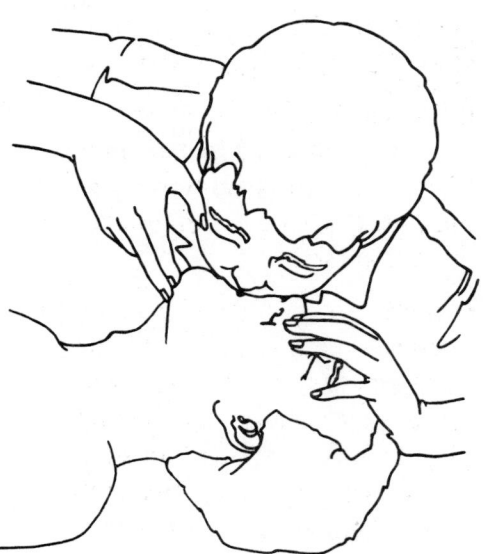

B. Blow air in slowly

Rescue Breathing, CPR – cont.

Step 5: Begin chest compressions.

• **For adults:** Kneel next to the victim. Use your fingers to locate the end of the breastbone (sternum), where the ribs come together. Place 2 fingers at the tip of the breastbone. Place the heel of one hand directly above your fingers. See Illustration C.

• Place your other hand on top of the one that is in position. Do not allow your fingers to touch the chest as that may damage the ribs. See Illustration D.

• Straighten your arms, lock your elbows, and center your shoulders directly over your hands. See Illustration E.

• Press down in a steady rhythm, using your body weight and keeping your arms locked. The force from each thrust should go straight down onto the sternum, compressing it 1½ to 2 inches. It may help to count "one and two and three and four...," up to 15 compressions. Give one downward thrust each time you say a number. Lift your weight, but not your hands, from the victim's chest on the upstroke.

• After 15 compressions, quickly do the head tilt/chin lift, and give 2 full, slow breaths, taking one breath in between.

• Repeat the 15-compressions, 2-breaths cycle 4 times. Check the pulse again. If there is still no pulse, continue the rescue breathing and chest compressions until help arrives, or the victim's pulse and breathing return.

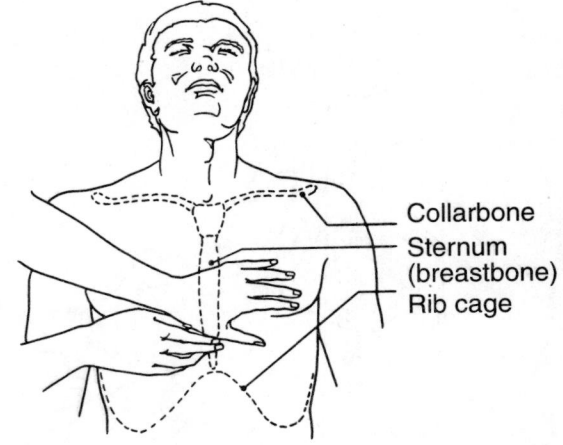

Collarbone
Sternum (breastbone)
Rib cage

C. Location of sternum

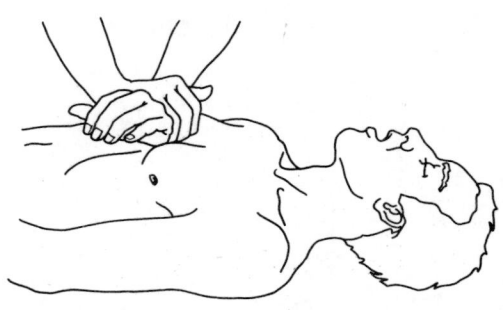

D. Hand position to avoid rib damage

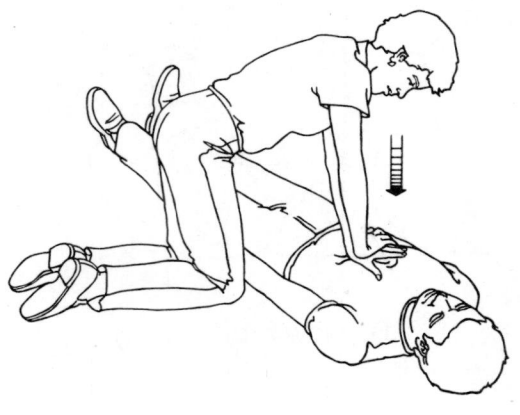

E. Shoulders over sternum

- **For a child:** Using the heel of one hand, press with less force, compressing the sternum 1 to 1½ inches.

- **For an infant:** Place 2 fingers on the sternum, about one finger width below an imaginary line connecting the nipples. Press with gentle force, compressing the sternum about ½ inch.

- **For infants and children:** Give 5 chest compressions, then 1 breath. Repeat 4 times and check the pulse again. If there is still no pulse, continue rescue breathing and chest compressions until help arrives, or until the victim's pulse and breathing are restored.

Accidental Tooth Loss

If a permanent tooth is knocked out, a dentist may be able to reimplant it in the mouth. Baby teeth need to come out anyway, so are usually not reimplanted.

Home Treatment

- Call your dentist immediately for an emergency visit. Teeth reimplanted within 30 minutes have the best chance of success. After two hours, it is unlikely the procedure will be successful.

CPR Ready Reference

	Adults	Children	Infants
If the victim has a pulse, give one rescue breath every:	5 seconds	4 seconds	3 seconds
If the victim has no pulse, locate the chest compression landmark:	Trace ribs into notch; place 2 fingers on sternum	Same as adult	One finger width below nipple line
Do chest compressions with:	2 hands stacked; heel of 1 hand on sternum	Heel of 1 hand on sternum	2 or 3 fingers on sternum
Rate of compressions per minute:	80 to 100	100	100
Compression depth:	1½ to 2"	1 to 1½"	½ to 1"
Ratio of compressions to breaths:			
1 rescuer	15:2	5:1	5:1
2 rescuers	5:1	5:1	N/A

Guidelines from the American Heart Association

Accidental Tooth Loss – cont.

- Clean the tooth and replace it in the socket, or between the gum and cheek (use care not to swallow the tooth), or in a small container of milk. Do not transport the tooth in tap water.

When to Call a Dentist

- If a permanent tooth is knocked out.

- If a baby tooth is knocked out, schedule an appointment within two weeks to determine if a spacer is needed until permanent teeth come in.

Animal Bites

When bitten by an animal, most people want to know if they need a rabies shot. The main wild animal carriers of rabies are raccoons, skunks, foxes, and bats. Pet dogs and cats that have been vaccinated rarely have rabies. However, stray animals are often not vaccinated. Rabies is quite rare, but is fatal if not treated. The treatment is no more painful than a typical injection. Report all wild animal bites to your doctor or health department.

Bites that break the skin often cause bacterial infections. Cat and human bites are particularly prone to infection. Tetanus can occur if shots are not up to date. See page 26.

Prevention

- Vaccinate all pets against rabies. Do not keep wild animals as pets.

- Do not disturb animals while they are eating, even your family pet.

- Teach children not to approach or play with stray dogs or cats.

- Do not touch wild animals or provoke them to attack. Do not handle sick or injured animals.

Home Treatment

- Scrub the bite immediately with soap and water. Treat it as a puncture wound. See page 231.

- If you are bitten by a pet dog or cat, find out whether it has been vaccinated for rabies.

- A healthy pet that has bitten someone should be confined and watched for 10 days to see if it develops symptoms of rabies. If the owner cannot be located or relied on to watch the animal, contact the local health department.

- If you are bitten by a wild animal, contact the health department. They can tell you whether that animal is a rabies carrier in your area, and whether treatment is needed.

When to Call Kaiser Permanente

- If the bite is from a wild animal.

- If the bite is from a dog or cat that is acting strangely, foaming at the mouth, or if the animal attacked for no apparent reason.

- If the bite is from a pet whose owner cannot confirm that it has been vaccinated for rabies.

- If the bite is severe and may need stitches, or if it is on the hand or face.

- If signs of infection develop:

  ○ Increased pain, swelling, redness, or tenderness

  ○ Heat or red streaks extending from the bite

  ○ Discharge of pus

  ○ Fever of 100° or higher with no other cause

Blood Under a Nail

Fingernails and toenails often get crunched, bashed, or smashed. These injuries usually aren't too serious, but if there is bleeding under the nail, the pressure can be very painful.

The throbbing and pain can be relieved only by making a hole in the nail to drain the blood. This can be done at home. You may feel squeamish about trying this, but it is the same thing a health professional would do.

Draining is helpful only if there is severe, throbbing pain (the person can feel the pulse beating under the nail) that is bad enough to keep the person from sleeping.

Home Treatment

- Apply ice as soon as possible after the injury to minimize swelling and relieve pain.

- To make a hole in the nail and relieve throbbing, follow these steps:

  ○ Straighten a paper clip and heat the tip in a flame until it is red hot.

  ○ Place the tip of the paper clip on the nail and let it melt through. You do not need to push. This will not be painful as the nail has no nerves. A thick nail may take several tries.

  ○ As soon as the hole is complete, blood will escape and the pain will be relieved.

- Soak the finger three times a day in a half-and-half mixture of hydrogen peroxide and warm water.

- If the pressure builds up again in a few days, repeat the procedure, using the same hole.

When to Call Kaiser Permanente

- If the person is uncooperative and won't let you try the procedure.

- If signs of infection appear after two to three days:

  ○ Increased pain, swelling, redness or tenderness

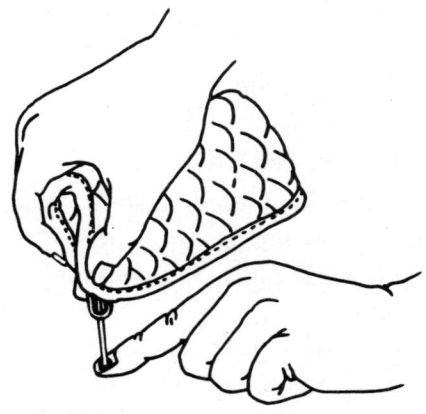

Relieve pressure

Blood Under a Nail – cont.

- Heat or red streaks extending away from the area

- Discharge of pus

- Fever of 100° or higher with no other cause

Blunt Abdominal Wounds

Blunt abdominal wounds caused by a blow to the stomach can cause severe bruising of the abdominal wall and bleeding from the internal organs. Such injuries are often caused by automobile, bicycle, tobogganing, or skiing accidents, where the victim is thrown into something or to the ground.

The symptoms of abdominal injury are similar to those of shock: rapid pulse, low blood pressure, and cold, clammy skin. The abdomen may become rigid or tender. The injured person may become confused and unable to remember or describe the injury.

Home Treatment

- Monitor the injured person's pulse, blood pressure, and breathing. A rapid, weak pulse, falling blood pressure, or very rapid or very slow breathing may indicate internal bleeding. If these signs develop, call 861-3434 or 911, or take the patient to the emergency room.

- Have the injured person lie down with the feet elevated above the heart. Loosen his clothing and cover him with a blanket to keep him warm. Do not give him anything to eat or drink, even though he may be thirsty.

- Watch for signs of shock: faintness, weakness, drowsiness, or confusion; sweating, and cool, clammy skin.

When to Call Kaiser Permanente

Call 861-3434 or 911, or take the patient to the emergency room:

- If signs of shock (see above and page 234) develop up to 48 hours after an abdominal injury.

- If there is bleeding from the rectum, urethra, or vagina following a blow to the abdomen.

- If the injury causes nausea, vomiting, heartburn, or loss of appetite.

- If the abdomen is swollen and hard, or if pressing on the abdomen causes severe pain.

- Call a health professional if you have any concerns about the symptoms you observe.

Bruises

Bruises (contusions) are usually caused by a bump or fall, which ruptures small blood vessels under the skin. Blood seeps into the surrounding tissues, causing the black and blue color of a bruise.

People who take blood thinners (anticoagulants) or aspirin may bruise easily. A bruise may also develop after blood is drawn.

A black eye is a type of bruise. Apply home treatment for a bruise and inspect the eye.

Home Treatment

- Apply ice or cold packs for 15-minute intervals during the first 48 hours to help vessels constrict and to reduce swelling. The sooner you apply ice, the less bleeding will result.

- If possible, elevate the bruised area. Blood will leave the area and there will be less swelling.

- Rest the limb so you don't injure it further.

- If the area is still painful after 48 hours, apply heat with warm towels, a hot water bottle, or a heating pad.

When to Call Kaiser Permanente

- If signs of infection develop:

  ○ Increased pain, swelling, redness, or tenderness

  ○ Heat or red streaks extending away from the area

  ○ Discharge of pus

  ○ Fever of 100° or higher with no other cause

- If a blow to the eye causes:

  ○ Severe bleeding in the white of the eye, or blood in the colored part of the eye

  ○ Impaired or double vision

  ○ Inability to move the eye normally in all directions

  ○ Severe pain in the eyeball rather than in the eye socket

- If you suddenly begin to bruise easily, or if you have unexplained recurrent or multiple bruises.

Burns

Burns are classified as first, second, or third degree depending on their depth, not on the amount of pain or the extent of the burn. A first-degree burn involves only the outer layer of skin. The skin is dry, painful, and sensitive to touch. A mild sunburn is an example.

A second-degree burn involves several layers of skin. The skin becomes swollen, puffy, weepy, or blistered.

A third-degree burn involves all layers of skin and any underlying tissue or organs. The skin is dry, pale white or charred black, swollen, and sometimes breaks open. Nerves are destroyed or damaged, so there may be little pain except on the edge where there is a second-degree burn.

Prevention

- Install smoke detectors on each story of your home. Check and replace batteries regularly.

Burns - continued

- Keep a fire extinguisher near the kitchen. Have it inspected yearly.

- Set your water heater at 120° or lower to avoid burns.

- Don't smoke in bed.

If your clothing catches fire:

- Do not run, as it will fan the flames. Stop, drop, and roll on the ground to smother the flames.

- Smother the flames with a blanket, rug, or coat.

- Use water to douse the fire and cool the skin.

To avoid kitchen burns:

- Use caution when handling hot foods.

- Turn pot handles toward the back of the stove.

- Smother burning food or grease with a lid or pot.

- Supervise children closely.

Home Treatment

- For home treatment of sunburn, see page 147.

- Run cold tap water over the burn for 10 to 15 minutes. Cold water is the best immediate treatment for minor burns. The cold lowers the skin temperature and lessens the severity of the burn. Do not use ice, as it may further damage the injured skin.

- Remove rings, bracelets, watches, or shoes from the burned limb. Swelling may make them difficult to remove later.

For first-degree burns, and second-degree burns with intact blisters:

- Leave the burn alone for 24 hours. Don't cover the burn unless clothing rubs on it. If it rubs, cover it with a gauze pad taped well away from the burn. Do not encircle a hand, arm, or leg with tape. Change the bandage after 24 hours, and then every two days.

- After two to three days of healing, the juice from an aloe leaf can soothe minor burns.

- Do not put salve, butter, grease, oil, or ointment on a burn. They increase the risk of infection and don't help heal the burn.

- For second-degree burns, do not break blisters. If the blisters break, clean the area by running tap water over it. Apply an antibiotic ointment, such as Polysporin or Bacitracin, and cover the burn with a sterile dressing. Don't touch the wound with your hands or any non-sterile objects. Remove the dressing every day, clean the wound and cover it again.

- Aspirin or ibuprofen can help relieve pain from minor burns.

Third-degree burns require immediate medical treatment. Call a health professional and apply home treatment:

- Make sure the source of the burn has been extinguished.

- Have the person lie down to prevent shock.

- Cover the burned area with a clean sheet soaked in cool water.

- Do not apply any salve or medication to the burn.

When to Call Kaiser Permanente

• For all third-degree burns.

• If in doubt as to the extent of burn, or in doubt if it is a second- or third-degree burn.

• If a second-degree burn involves the face, hands, feet, genitals, or a joint.

• If the burn encircles an arm or leg, or covers more than one-quarter of the body part involved.

• Electrical burns are often more extensive than they appear and should be seen by a doctor.

• If the pain lasts longer than 48 hours.

• If signs of infection develop:

  ○ Increased pain, swelling, redness, or tenderness

  ○ Heat or red streaks extending from the area

  ○ Discharge of pus

  ○ Fever of 100° or higher with no other cause

• If an infant, older adult, or person with diabetes is burned.

Chemical Burns to the Eye

Chemical burns to the eye occur when something caustic is splashed into it, such as a cleaning product, gasoline, or turpentine. The vapors or fumes of strong chemicals can also burn or irritate the eyes. The eye becomes red, watery, and may be sensitive to light. If the damage is severe, the eye appears whitish.

Home Treatment

• Immediately flush the eye with water to wash out the chemical. Fill a sink or dishpan with water, immerse the face in the water, and then open and close the eyelids to force the water to all parts of the eye. It may be necessary to move the eyelids with the fingers. Another method is to put the face under a running faucet or shower.

• Continue flushing for 15 to 20 minutes, or until the eye stops hurting, whichever takes longer.

• After flushing the eye with water, cover it with a clean bandage or cloth.

When to Call Kaiser Permanente

• If there is major exposure to a strong acid, such as battery acid, or to a caustic substance, such as lye or Drano, go immediately to an emergency center after flushing the eye.

• Call anytime a chemical is splashed into the eye which required you to flush the eye.

• If the eye still hurts after 20 minutes of home treatment.

• If the eye appears to be damaged. Symptoms include:

  ○ Persistent redness

  ○ Discharge or watering

  ○ Any visual impairment, such as double vision, blurring, or sensitivity to light

  ○ Colored part of the eye (iris) appears white

Chest Pain

CALL 861-3434, 911, OR OTHER EMERGENCY SERVICES IMMEDIATELY if chest pain is crushing or squeezing, increases in intensity, or occurs with any of these symptoms of a heart attack:

- Sweating

- Shortness of breath

- Pain radiating to the shoulder, neck, arm, or jaw

- Nausea or vomiting

- Dizziness

- Rapid and/or irregular pulse

See page 206 for cardiopulmonary resuscitation (CPR).

See page 98 for more information on chest pain.

Choking Rescue Procedure (Heimlich Maneuver)

WARNING: Do *not* begin choking rescue unless the person *cannot breathe* or is turning blue and cannot speak, and you are *certain* they are choking. Also see Choking on page 218. **CALL 861-3434, 911, OR EMERGENCY SERVICES if the person loses consciousness or if you are unable to dislodge the object.**

Adults and Children Over One Year

If victim is standing or sitting:

- Stand behind the victim and wrap your arms around her waist.

- Make a fist with one hand. Place the thumb side of your fist against her abdomen, just above the navel but well below the breastbone. See Illustration A.

- Grasp your fist with the other hand. Give a quick upward thrust into the victim's abdomen. This may cause the object to pop out. Use less force for young children. See Illustration B.

- Repeat until the object pops out or the victim loses consciousness.

- If you choke while alone, do abdominal thrusts on yourself, or lean hard over the back of a chair to pop out the food.

If victim is on the floor:

- Turn the victim face up.

- Straddle him on your knees next to his hips.

- Place the heel of one hand against the victim's abdomen, just above the navel but well below the breastbone. Place your other hand directly over the first. See Illustration C.

- Give a quick upward thrust into the victim's abdomen. Use less force for children. Repeat until the object pops out.

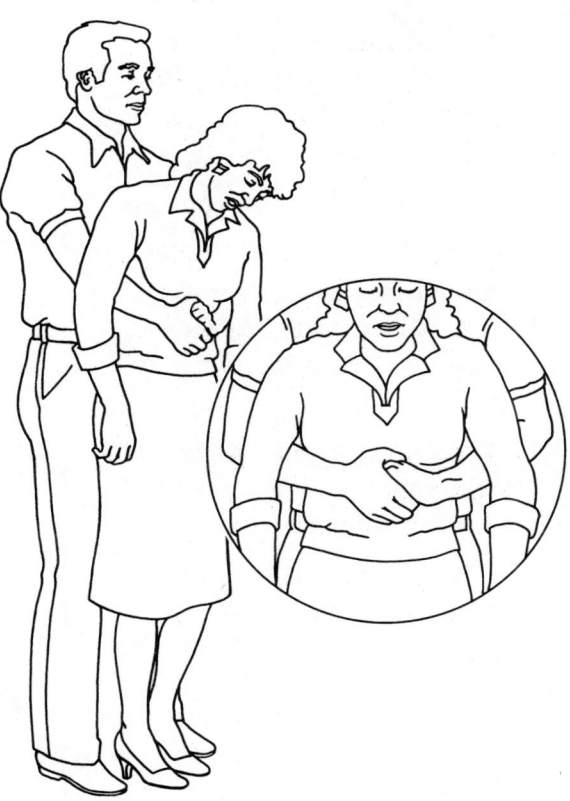

Illustrations A and B

Infant Under One Year

- Hold infant as in Illustration D.

- Use the heel of one hand to jar the child between the shoulder blades in an attempt to dislodge the object. Repeat four times.

- If the airways remains blocked, support the infant's head and turn him over on your thigh with his head down.

- Place two or three fingers just below a line between the nipples, and give up to four upward thrusts until the object pops out.

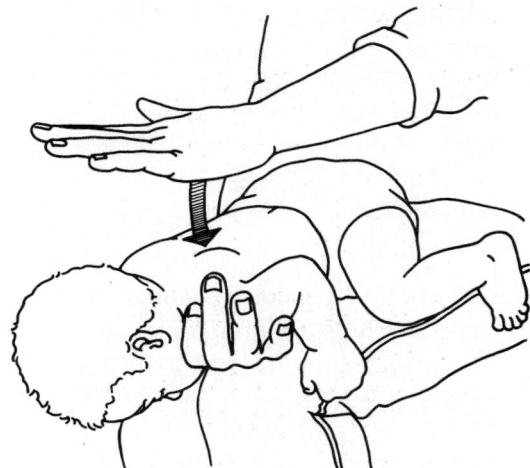

Illustration D

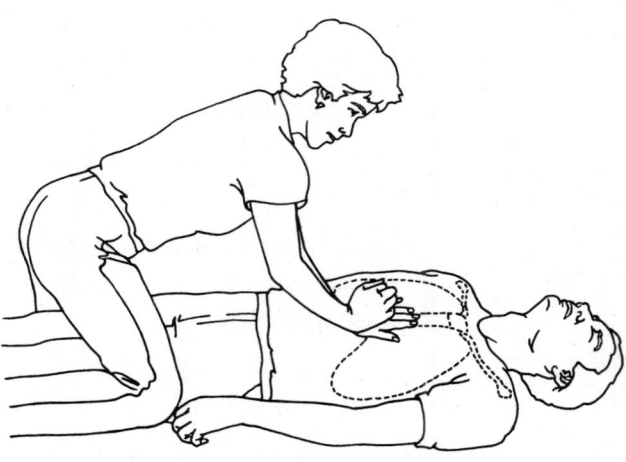

Illustration C

Choking

Choking is usually caused by food or an object stuck in the windpipe. The **Heimlich Maneuver**, described in the Choking Rescue Procedure on page 216, can help pop out the food or object.

A person who is choking cannot cough, talk, or breathe, and may turn blue or dusky.

Prevention

• Don't drink too much alcohol before eating. A person with dulled senses may not chew food properly or may try to swallow too large a portion of food.

• Take small bites. Cut meat into small pieces. Chew your food thoroughly.

• Do not give popcorn, peanuts, or hard candy to children under age three, and supervise older children when they eat these foods.

• Do not allow children under age three to play with toys that have very small parts (smaller than a 50-cent piece) that could be swallowed.

When to Call Kaiser Permanente

• If the person loses consciousness. Call 861-3434 or 911 and attempt rescue breathing. See page 206.

• Call even if the food has been dislodged. The throat could be damaged by the object or there could be abdominal damage from the maneuver.

Disaster Preparation and Response

Prepare for earthquakes, fires, hurricanes, and tornadoes:

• Learn how to shut off your gas, water, and electricity.

• Secure shelves and heavy objects (bookcases, water heaters, etc.) that could cause injury if they fell.

• Keep an emergency kit stocked with supplies for at least 3 days (replace supplies regularly):

  ◦ Two to four quarts of water per person per day

  ◦ First-aid kit

  ◦ Packaged/canned nonperishable food and can opener

  ◦ Blankets/sleeping bags

  ◦ Plastic bags to store waste

  ◦ Small radio with batteries

• Renew prescriptions for essential medications so that you always have a 7- to 10- day supply on hand.

• Have a family plan on what to do if you can't go home.

During a natural disaster:

• Stay calm. Check for and treat injuries.

• Check for gas or water leaks and fires. If you suspect a gas leak, turn off the gas.

• Listen to the Emergency Broadcast System.

Cuts

When you see a cut (laceration), the first steps are to stop the bleeding and determine whether or not stitches are needed.

If the cut is bleeding heavily or spurting blood, see "Stopping Severe Bleeding" at right.

Bleeding from minor cuts will usually stop on its own or with a little direct pressure. To decide whether stitches are needed, see "Are Sutures Necessary?" on page 221. If stitches are needed, apply home treatment and seek medical care as soon as possible, certainly within eight hours.

If stitches are not needed, you can clean and bandage the cut at home.

Home Treatment

- Wash the cut well with soap and water. Treat an animal bite like a puncture wound. See page 231.

- Stop any bleeding by applying direct pressure over the wound for 10 to 15 minutes.

- Leave small cuts unbandaged, unless they will become irritated. They heal best when exposed to the air.

- If a cut needs bandaging, apply antibiotic ointment (Polysporin or Bacitracin). The ointment will keep the cut from sticking to the bandage. Do not use rubbing alcohol, hydrogen peroxide, iodine, or mercurochrome, which can harm tissue and slow healing.

Stopping Severe Bleeding

- Have the person lie down and elevate the site that is bleeding.

- Remove any visible objects. Do not attempt to clean out the wound.

- Press firmly on the wound with clean cloth or the cleanest material available. If the edges of the wound gape, hold them together. If there is an object in the wound, apply pressure around the cut, not directly over it.

- Apply steady pressure for 15 minutes. If blood soaks through the cloth, apply another one without lifting the first. Maintain steady pressure.

- If direct pressure does not slow or stop bleeding after 15 minutes, press firmly on a pressure point between the wound and the heart (see below). Continuous pressure on these points can stop the bleeding with less risk than a tourniquet. Tourniquets should be used *only* as a last resort.

- Watch for shock. See page 234.

- Call 861-3434 or 911 or go to the emergency room if the bleeding has not been controlled after 15 minutes.

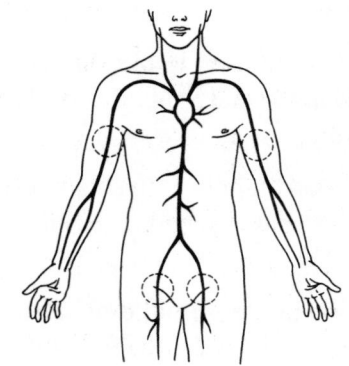

Pressure points

Cuts – continued

- Use an adhesive bandage (Band-Aid) to continue the pressure. Always put an adhesive strip across a cut rather than lengthwise. A butterfly bandage (made at home or purchased) can help hold cut skin edges together:

  ○ Cut a strip from a roll of one-inch adhesive tape and fold it sticky side out. Cut notches into the tape as shown in A.

  ○ Unfold the tape, then fold the notched pieces together sticky side in as in B. The center of the tape will be non-sticky. Keep the part clean that will be over the cut.

  ○ Place one end of the tape on the skin, then pull the other end to close the wound tightly as in C.

  ○ If the cut is long, use more than one bandage.

- Apply a clean bandage at least once a day, or when it gets wet. Leave the bandage off whenever possible.

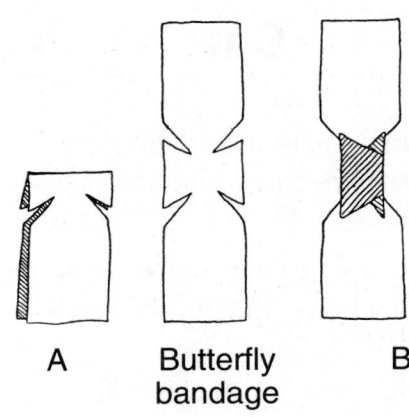

A   Butterfly bandage   B

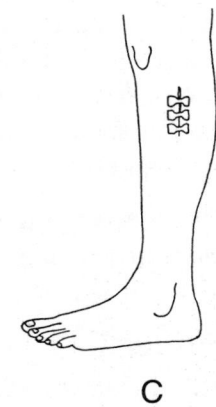

C

When to Call Kaiser Permanente

- If the cut needs stitches. They need to be done within eight hours.

- If a cut continues to bleed through bandages after 15 minutes of direct pressure.

- If the person goes into shock, even if bleeding has stopped. See Shock on page 234.

- If blood or clear fluid drains from the ears or nose following a blow to the head (not due to a cut or direct blow to the nose).

- If there is numbness, tingling, or loss of feeling, or if the person is unable to move a limb below the wound.

- If your tetanus shots are not up to date. See page 26.

- If the cut contains, or might contain, foreign objects such as wood or gravel.

- If signs of infection develop:

  ○ Increased pain, swelling, or tenderness

  ○ Heat and redness or red streaks extending away from the cut

  ○ Discharge of pus

  ○ Fever of 100° or higher with no other cause

Are Sutures Necessary?

For best results, a cut should be sutured within eight hours. Wash the cut well and stop the bleeding, then decide if sutures are needed. Pinch the sides of the cut together. If it looks better, you may want to consider stitches. If stitches are needed, avoid using an antibiotic ointment until after a health professional has examined the cut.

Sutures may be needed for:

- Deep cuts (more than ¼ inch deep) that have jagged edges or gape open.

- Deep cuts on a joint: elbow, knuckle, knee.

- Deep cuts on the palm side of the hand or fingers.

- Cuts on the face, eyelids, or lips.

- Cuts in an area where you are worried about scarring, especially the face.

- Cuts that go down to the muscle or bone.

- Cuts that continue to bleed after 15 minutes of direct pressure.

Cuts like these that are sutured usually heal with less scarring than those that are not.

Sutures may not be needed for:

- Cuts with smooth edges that tend to stay together during normal movement of the affected body part.

- Shallow cuts less than ¼ inch deep that are less than one inch long.

Fishhook Removal

In the excitement of fishing, sometimes fingers are hooked instead of fish. It is useful to know how to remove a fishhook for yourself, or a companion, especially if you are far from medical help.

Home Treatment

Remove the hook as follows:

- Use ice, cold water, or hard pressure to provide temporary numbing.

- **Step A:** Tie a piece of fishing line to the hook near the skin surface.

- **Step B:** Grasp the eye of the hook with one hand and press down about 1/8 inch to disengage the barb.

- **Step C:** While still pressing the hook down (barb disengaged), jerk the line parallel to the skin surface so that the hook shaft leads the barb out of the skin.

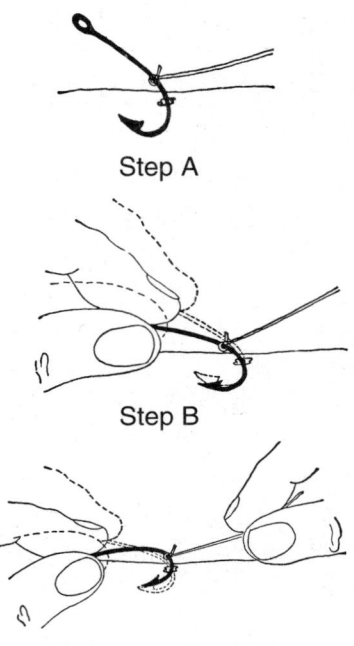

Step A

Step B

Step C

Fishhook Removal – continued

- If the fishhook is deeply embedded, another option is to push the hook the rest of the way through the skin, snip off the barb, and remove the hook.

- Wash the wound thoroughly. Use soap if available. Treat as you would a puncture wound. See page 231.

- Do not try to remove a fishhook from the eye.

When to Call Kaiser Permanente

- If you cannot remove the hook.

- If your tetanus shots are not up to date. See page 26.

- If the hook is in the eye.

- If signs of infection develop:

  ○ Increased pain, swelling, redness, or tenderness

  ○ Heat or red streaks extending from the area

  ○ Discharge of pus

  ○ Fever of 100° or higher with no other cause

Freeing Trapped Limbs

Fingers, arms, or legs sometimes get caught in objects such as bottles, jars, or pipes. Stay calm; panic will only make the situation worse.

Home Treatment

- Don't force the limb. This will only make it swell and become more difficult to remove.

- Try to relax the limb. Relaxation alone will sometimes enable you to free the limb.

- If possible, elevate the limb.

- Apply ice around the exposed limb. This may reduce any swelling and allow it to be released.

- If ice doesn't work, dribble soapy water or cooking oil on the limb. Turn the limb or the object so you "unscrew" it rather than pulling it out directly.

Frostbite

Frostbite is freezing of the skin or underlying tissues that occurs as a result of prolonged exposure to cold.

Frostbitten skin is pale or blue, stiff or rubbery to touch, and feels cold and numb. There may be loss of function in the frozen area. The severity is divided into three degrees:

First degree: Frostnip. Numbness and whitening of the skin with little likelihood of blistering if rewarmed promptly.

Second degree: Superficial frostbite. Outer skin feels hard and frozen but tissue underneath has normal resilience. Blistering is likely.

Third degree: Deep frostbite. Skin is white or blotchy and blue. Skin and tissue underneath is hard and very cold.

Prevention

Stay dry and out of the wind in extreme cold and cover areas of exposed skin. Keep the body's core temperature up:

• Wear layers of clothing. Wool and polypropylene are good insulators. Wear wind- and waterproof outer layers. Wear wool socks and well-fitting, waterproof boots.

• Wear a hat to prevent heat loss from your head. Wear mittens rather than gloves.

• Keep protective clothing and blankets in your car in case of a breakdown in an isolated area.

• Don't drink alcohol or smoke when out in extreme cold.

Home Treatment

• Get inside or take shelter from the wind.

• Check for signs of hypothermia (see page 227) and treat it before treating frostbite.

• Don't rewarm the area if refreezing is possible. Wait until you reach shelter.

• Warm small areas (ears, face, nose, fingers, toes) with warm breath or by tucking hands or feet inside warm clothing next to bare skin. Protect the body part from further exposure. If possible, immerse the frozen part in warm water (104° to 108°) for 15 to 30 minutes.

• Don't rub or massage the frozen area, as it would further damage tissues. Avoid walking on frostbitten feet if possible.

• Keep the frostbitten part warm and elevated. Wrap with blankets or soft material to prevent bruising.

• Blisters may appear as the skin warms. Do not break them. The skin may turn red, burn, tingle, or be very painful. Aspirin or acetaminophen may help.

When to Call Kaiser Permanente

• Immediately if skin is white or blue, hard, and cold (third-degree frostbite). Careful rewarming and antibiotic treatment are needed to prevent infection and permanent tissue damage.

• If blisters develop during rewarming (second- or third-degree frostbite). Do not break blisters. The risk of infection in the blistered area is very high.

• If signs of infection develop:

  ○ Increased pain, swelling, redness, or tenderness

  ○ Heat or red streaks extending from the area

  ○ Discharge of pus

  ○ Fever of 100° or higher with no other cause

Head Injuries

Most bumps on the head are minor and heal as easily as bumps anywhere else. Head injuries that cause cuts often bleed heavily because the blood vessels of the scalp are close to the surface. This bleeding is alarming, but does not always mean the injury is severe.

However, head injuries that do not cause visible external bleeding may have caused life-threatening bleeding and swelling inside the skull. Anyone who has experienced a head injury should be watched carefully for 24 hours for signs of a severe head injury.

Prevention

- Wear your seat belt when in a motor vehicle. Use child car seats.

- Wear a helmet while biking, motor-cycling, and skating.

- Don't dive into shallow or unfamil-iar water.

Home Treatment

- If the victim is unconscious, make sure there is no spinal injury before moving him (see page 234). Check for other injuries.

- If there is bleeding, apply firm pressure directly over the wound with a clean cloth or bandage for 15 minutes. If the blood soaks through, apply additional cloths over the first one. See page 219.

- Apply ice or cold packs to reduce the swelling. A "goose egg" will likely appear anyway, but ice will help ease the pain.

- Watch for the following signs of a severe head injury immediately afterwards and then every two hours for the next 24 hours:

  ○ Confusion. Ask the person his name, address, age, the date, etc.

  ○ Inability to move arms and legs on one side of the body, or slower movement on one side than the other.

  ○ Lethargy, abnormally deep sleep, or difficulty waking up.

  ○ Vomiting that continues after the first two hours.

- Continue observing the person every two hours during the night. Wake him up and check for any unusual symptoms. Call 861-3434 or 911 or go to an emergency room *immediately* if you cannot wake him or if he has any of the above symptoms.

- Check for injuries to other parts of the body, especially if the person has fallen. The alarm that accompanies a head injury may cause you to overlook other injuries that need attention.

When to Call Kaiser Permanente

- If bleeding cannot be stopped or the wound needs stitches. See page 221.

- If the person lost consciousness anytime after the injury.

- If blood or clear fluid drains from the ears or nose following a blow to the head (not due to a cut or direct blow to the nose).

- If the person is confused or has any loss of memory after the first few minutes.

• If double vision or speech difficulty occur after the first minute.

• If a severe headache develops: "The worst headache I've ever had."

• If there are seizures or convulsions.

• If weakness or numbness occur on one side.

• If vomiting occurs after the first two hours or violent vomiting persists after the first 15 minutes. Mild nausea or vomiting at first is usually not serious.

Automobile Seat Restraints

Wearing seat belts saves lives and prevents injuries. No one is strong enough to brace against a sudden impact, even at very low speeds. Seat belts reduce the risk of serious injury and death.

• Wear your seat belt every time you are in a vehicle. Keep the belt snug and close to your body. Always use both the lap and shoulder belts.

• Seat belts are necessary even if your car is equipped with air bags. Air bags inflate from the steering wheel or dashboard of your car in the event of sudden impact. They are very effective in protecting front-seat riders, but must be used with seat belts.

• Use child car seats for infants, children under four, and those weighing under 40 pounds. See page 152.

Heat Exhaustion and Heat Stroke

Heat exhaustion occurs when your body cannot sweat enough to cool you off. It generally happens when you are working or exercising in hot weather. Symptoms include:

• Fatigue, weakness, dizziness, or nausea

• Cool, clammy, pale, red, or flushed skin

Heat exhaustion can sometimes lead to **heat stroke.** Heat stroke requires emergency treatment. It happens when your body stops sweating but the body temperature continues to rise, often to 105° or higher. Symptoms include:

• Confusion, delirium, or unconsciousness

• Hot, dry, red or flushed skin, even under the armpits

Prevention

• Avoid strenuous outdoor physical activity during the hottest part of the day.

• Wear light-colored, loose-fitting clothing to reflect the sun.

• Avoid sudden changes of temperature. Air out a hot car before getting into it.

• If you take diuretics, ask your doctor about taking a lower dose during hot weather.

Heat Exhaustion – continued

- Drink 8 to 10 glasses of water per day. Drink even more if you are working or exercising in hot weather.
- If you exercise strenuously in hot weather, drink more liquid than your thirst seems to require. For example, runners should drink about one cup of water 10 to 15 minutes before running and another cup of water every two miles or so.

Home Treatment

- Get out of the sun to a cool spot and drink lots of cool water, a little at a time. If you are nauseated or dizzy, lie down.
- Sponge the body with cool water.
- If the body temperature reaches 105°, immediate cooling is essential. Use cold, wet cloths all over the body. A cool water bath may be necessary.
- If the temperature is lowered to 102°, use care to avoid over-cooling.

When to Call Kaiser Permanente

- Call 861-3434 or 911 or go to the emergency room if signs of heat stroke develop. Work fast to lower the temperature and seek immediate help if:
  - The skin is dry, even under the armpits, and bright red or flushed.
  - The body temperature reaches 104° and keeps rising.
  - The person is delirious, disoriented, or unconscious.

Hyperventilation

When you breathe fast and deep (hyperventilate), the carbon dioxide (CO_2) level in your blood can drop too low. Symptoms that may occur with hyperventilation include:

- Numbness or tingling in the hands, feet, or around the mouth
- Pounding, racing heartbeat and anxiety
- Feeling you can't get enough air
- Lightheadedness
- Chest pain

In severe cases, the person may lose consciousness.

Prevention

If you have hyperventilated before:

- Ask people to mention it if you start to breathe too fast.
- As soon as you notice fast breathing or other symptoms, slow your breathing to one breath every five seconds, or slow enough that symptoms subside.

Home Treatment

- Sit down and concentrate on slowing your breathing.
- Practice a relaxation technique. See page 252.
- Breathe in and out of a paper bag held over the nose and mouth. This will help bring the amount of CO_2 in the blood back to normal. Continue this treatment intermittently for 5 to 15 minutes.

When to Call Kaiser Permanente

- If hyperventilation occurs in a person who doesn't appear tense or anxious. See page 278 to help determine if a person is anxious.

- If anxiety and hyperventilation are frequent and interfere with your daily activities.

Hypothermia

Hypothermia occurs when the body temperature drops below normal. It occurs when the body loses heat faster than heat can be produced by muscle contraction and shivering.

Early symptoms include:

- Shivering

- Cold, pale skin

- Apathy

- Impaired judgment

Later symptoms include:

- Cold abdomen

- Slow pulse and breathing

- Weakness or drowsiness

- Confusion

Shivering may stop if body temperature drops below 96°.

Hypothermia is an emergency. It can quickly lead to unconsciousness and death if the heat loss continues. Hypothermia can happen at temperatures of 45°, or even higher in wet and windy weather. Frail and inactive people can develop hypothermia indoors if they are not dressed warmly.

Early recognition is very important in the treatment of hypothermia. Often a hiker or skier will lose heat to a critical degree before others notice anything is wrong. If someone begins to shiver violently, stumble, or respond incoherently to questions, suspect hypothermia and warm them quickly.

Prevention

Whenever you plan to be outdoors for several hours in cold weather, take the following precautions:

- Dress warmly and wear wind- and waterproof clothing. Wear fabric that remains warm even when wet, such as wool or polypropylene.

- Wear a warm hat. An unprotected head loses a great deal of the body's total heat production.

- Head for shelter if you get wet or cold.

- Eat well before going out and carry extra food.

- Don't drink alcohol while in the cold. It makes the body lose heat faster.

- Older or less active people can prevent indoor hypothermia by dressing warmly and keeping temperatures above 65°.

Home Treatment

The goal of home or "in-the-field" treatment is to stop additional heat loss and slowly rewarm the person. Warming one degree per hour is best.

Hypothermia – continued

- For mild cases, get the person out of the cold and wind, give him dry or wool clothing, and warm fluids to drink.

- For moderate cases, remove cold, wet clothes first, then warm the person with your own body heat by wrapping a blanket or sleeping bag around both of you.

- Give warm liquids to drink, and high-energy foods, such as candy. Do not give food or drink if the person is disoriented or unconscious.

- Do not give alcoholic beverages.

- Rewarming the victim in warm water can cause shock or heart attack. However, in emergency situations when help is not available and other home treatments are not working, you can use a warm water (100° to 105°) soak as a last resort.

When to Call Kaiser Permanente

- If the person loses consciousness or seems confused.

- If the victim is a child or older adult. It's a good idea to call regardless of the severity of the symptoms.

- If the body temperature does not return to normal after four hours of warming.

Nosebleeds

Nosebleeds are inconvenient and messy, but they can usually be stopped with home treatment. Some common causes of nosebleeds are low humidity, colds and allergies, blows to the nose, medications (especially aspirin), high altitudes, and blowing or picking the nose.

Prevention

- Low humidity is a common cause of nosebleeds. Humidify your home, especially the bedrooms, and keep the heat low (60° to 64°) in sleeping areas.

- If your nose becomes very dry, breathe moist air for awhile (e.g., from a shower) and then put a little petroleum jelly on the inside to help prevent bleeding. A saline nasal spray may also help.

- Limit your use of aspirin, which can contribute to nosebleeds.

Home Treatment

- Sit up straight and tip your head slightly forward. Tilting the head back may cause blood to run down the throat.

- Blow all the clots out of the nose. Pinch the nostrils shut between your thumb and forefinger or apply firm pressure against the bleeding nostril for *10 full minutes*. Resist the urge to peek after a few minutes to see if it has stopped bleeding.

- After 10 minutes, release the nose. If it is still bleeding, hold it for 10 more minutes. Most nosebleeds will stop after 10 to 30 minutes of direct pressure.

- Stay quiet for a few hours and do not blow the nose for at least 12 hours after the bleeding has stopped.

When to Call Kaiser Permanente

- If the bleeding hasn't stopped after 30 minutes of direct pressure.

- If blood runs down the back of your throat even when the nose is pinched.

- If there is a deformity in the nose after an injury. The nose may be broken.

- If nosebleeds recur often.

Objects in the Ear

Children sometimes put small objects in their ears, or an insect will crawl into the ear. It may be hard to know if an insect is in the ear. Your child may say, "My ear is bumping around."

Home Treatment

For an insect in the ear:

- Don't try to kill it. Pull the ear up and back and point it toward the sun or a bright light. Insects are attracted to light and it may crawl out.

- If the insect doesn't crawl out, fill the ear canal with mineral, olive, or baby oil. The insect may float out.

For other objects in the ear:

- Tilt the head to the side and shake it. Gently pulling the ear up and back may straighten the ear canal and help dislodge the object.

- If the object is soft and can be easily seen, try *carefully* to remove it with tweezers. Do not try this if the person will not hold very still or if the object is in the ear so far that you can't see the tips of the tweezers. Use care not to push the object further in.

- Call a health professional if you cannot remove the insect or object.

Objects in the Eye

A speck of dirt or small object in the eye will often wash out with your tears. If the object is not removed, it may scratch the covering of the eye (cornea). Most corneal scratches are minor and heal on their own in a day or two.

Home Treatment

- Don't rub the eye, it could scratch the cornea. You may have to restrain small children from rubbing.

- Do not try to remove an object that is on the pupil, or that is stuck in the white of the eye. Cover both eyes and call a health professional.

- Wash your hands before touching the eye.

Objects in the Eye – continued

- If the object is at the side of the eye or on the lower lid, moisten a cotton swab or the tip of a twisted piece of tissue and touch the end to the speck. The object should cling to the swab or tissue. Some minor irritation is common after you have removed the foreign body.

- Gently wash the eye with cool water. An eyedropper helps.

- Never use tweezers, toothpicks, or other hard items to remove any object. Eye damage may result.

When to Call Kaiser Permanente

- If the object is on the pupil or is embedded in the eye. Do not pull out an object that is stuck in the eye.

- If you cannot remove the object.

- If pain persists, if it feels like there is still something in the eye, or if vision is blurred after the object is removed. The cornea may be scratched. Keep the eye closed.

- If pain is severe.

Objects in the Nose

Children sometimes put small objects, like beads or popcorn, up their noses. Your first clue may be a foul-smelling green or yellow discharge from just one nostril. The nose may also be tender and swollen.

Home Treatment

- Spray a nasal decongestant (see page 297) in the affected nostril to reduce the swelling.

- Have the child pinch the other nostril closed and try to blow the object out.

- If you can see the object, try to remove it with blunt-nosed tweezers. Hold the child's head still and use care not to push the object in further. If the child resists, do not try tweezers. Some minor bleeding from the nostril is not serious.

- Call a health professional if you are unable to remove the object after several tries.

Poisoning

FOR ANY POISONING: Call 861-3434, 911, or your local poison control number immediately.

Children will swallow just about anything, including poisons. When in doubt, assume the worst. Always believe a child who indicates that some poison has been swallowed, no matter how unappetizing the substance is. You will not harm anyone who has not swallowed poison by following the steps below.

If you suspect food poisoning, see page 51.

Prevention

Develop habits of poison prevention before your child is born, and certainly before she is crawling. About

80 percent of poisonings occur in children age one to four. Infants grow so fast that sometimes they are crawling and walking before you have time to protect them.

- Never leave a poisonous product unattended, even for a moment.

- Lock all drugs away from children. Aspirin is the most common source of childhood poisoning, especially flavored baby aspirin. Lock up drugs between doses.

- Do not keep poisons such as drain opener, dishwasher detergent, oven cleaner, or plant food under your kitchen sink. Keep them completely out of reach of children. Dishwasher detergent is especially dangerous.

- Keep products in their original containers. Never store poisonous products in food containers.

- Use childproof latches on your cupboards.

- Use "Mr. Yuk" stickers and teach your children to recognize them.

- Purchase syrup of ipecac (see page 301) and keep the poison control center number near your phone.

Home Treatment

- Call a poison control center, hospital, or health professional *immediately.* Have the poison container with you so you can tell them what it is. They will tell you whether it is safe to make the person vomit.

- Do *not* have the person vomit if she:

  ○ Is having convulsions.

  ○ Is unconscious.

  ○ Has a burning sensation in the mouth or throat.

  ○ Has swallowed a corrosive agent or petroleum product (dishwasher detergent, lye, bleach, disinfectant, drain opener, floor wax, kerosene, grease remover).

- If suggested by poison control, induce vomiting by:

  ○ Giving syrup of ipecac, if available. See page 301.

  ○ Placing a spoon or finger at the back of the throat.

- When vomiting begins, place the head lower than the chest to prevent vomited material from entering the lungs.

Puncture Wounds

Puncture wounds are caused by sharp, pointed objects that penetrate the skin. Nails, tacks, ice picks, knives, and needles can all cause puncture wounds. Puncture wounds are easily infected because they are difficult to clean and provide a warm, moist place for bacteria to grow.

Home Treatment

- Make sure that nothing, such as the tip of a needle, is left in the wound. Check to see if the object is intact.

- Allow the wound to bleed freely to clean itself out unless there has been a large loss of blood or the blood is squirting out. If bleeding is heavy, see page 219.

Lead Poisoning

Infants and young children exposed to lead are at risk of developing learning disabilities and growth problems.

Lead is present in old paint, water pipes, and other substances. Lead-based paint may be a hazard in older homes, especially if it is flaking and peeling.

To reduce the risk of lead poisoning:

- Keep painted surfaces in good repair, and clean paint flakes and chips from older painted surfaces such as floors and windowsills carefully. The dirt next to a house painted with lead-based paint can become very contaminated.

- Keep young children away from home remodeling and refinishing projects.

- If your home has lead or lead-soldered water pipes, let the water run for a few minutes before using it for cooking or formula.

- If you believe your infant may have been exposed to lead, have your child's blood lead level tested at about age one year.

Call your local health department for more information on preventing lead poisoning.

Puncture Wounds – continued

- Clean the wound thoroughly with soap and water.

- For the next four to five days, soak the wound in warm water several times a day. This will clean the wound from the inside out. If the wound is closed, an infection under the skin may not be detected for several days.

When to Call Kaiser Permanente

- If the wound is in the head, chest, or abdomen, unless it is minor.

- If there is numbness, tingling, loss of feeling, or the person is unable to move a limb below the wound.

- If the object that caused the puncture wound was dirty, such as barbed wire, a rusty nail, or a farm implement, or if a deep wound to the foot occurred through a tennis shoe, you may need a tetanus shot. See page 26.

- If signs of infection develop:

  ○ Increased pain, swelling, redness, or tenderness

  ○ Heat or red streaks extending from the wound

  ○ Discharge of pus

  ○ Fever of 100° with no other cause

Scrapes

Scrapes or abrasions happen so often that they seem unimportant. Good home treatment will reduce scarring and prevent infection.

Home Treatment

- Scrapes are usually very dirty. Remove large pieces of debris with tweezers, then scrub vigorously with soap and water and a wash-cloth. The injured person will probably complain loudly, but cleaning is necessary to prevent infection and scarring. If you have a water sprayer in your kitchen sink, try using that on the scrape with additional scrubbing.
- Apply steady pressure with a clean bandage or cloth to stop bleeding.
- Ice may help reduce swelling and bruising.
- If the scrape is large or in an area rubbed by clothing, apply an anti-biotic ointment and cover it with a non-stick (Telfa) bandage. This type of bandage won't stick and is held in place by adhesive around the edges. Putting the ointment on the bandage first will be less painful.

When to Call Kaiser Permanente

- If your tetanus shots are not up to date. See page 26.
- If the scrape is very large and dirty.
- If you cannot remove dirt and debris embedded under the skin. They may cause tattooing and/or infection if not removed.

- If signs of infection develop:
  - Increased pain, swelling, redness, or tenderness
  - Heat or red streaks extending from the scrape
  - Discharge of pus
  - Fever of 100° or higher with no other cause

Removing Splinters

If you can grasp the end of the splinter with tweezers, gently pull it out. If the splinter is embedded in the skin, clean a needle with alcohol and make a small hole in the skin over the end of the splinter. Lift the splinter with the tip of the needle until it can be grasped with the tweezers and pulled out.

After the splinter has been removed, wash the area with soap and water. Apply a bandage if needed to keep the wound clean; otherwise, leave it open to the air. Watch for signs of infection (see above).

Call a health professional if the splinter is very large or deeply embedded and cannot be easily removed, or if the splinter is in the eye.

Shock

Shock may occur due to sudden illness or injury. When the circulatory system is unable to get enough blood to the vital organs, the body goes into shock. Sometimes, even a mild injury will lead to shock.

The signs of shock include:

- Cool, pale, clammy skin
- Dilated pupils
- Weak, rapid pulse
- Shallow, rapid breathing
- Low blood pressure
- Thirst, nausea, or vomiting
- Confusion or anxiety
- Faintness, weakness, dizziness, or loss of consciousness

Shock is a life-threatening condition. Prompt home treatment can save lives.

Home Treatment

- Have the person lie down and elevate his legs 12 inches or more. If the injury is to the head, neck, or chest, keep the legs flat. If the person vomits, roll him to one side to let fluids drain from the mouth.
- Control any bleeding (see page 219) and splint any fractures (see page 83).
- Keep the person warm, but not hot. Place a blanket underneath him and cover him with a sheet or blanket, depending on the weather. If the person is in a hot place, try to keep him cool.
- Take and record the person's pulse every five minutes.
- Comfort and reassure him to relieve anxiety.

When to Call Kaiser Permanente

- Call for help immediately if signs of shock develop.

Spinal Injuries

Any accident involving the neck or back must be considered a possible spinal injury. Permanent paralysis may be avoided if the injured person is immobilized and transported correctly.

Signs of a spinal injury include:

- Severe pain in neck or back
- Bruises on head, neck, shoulders, or back
- Weakness, tingling, or numbness in the arms or legs
- Loss of bowel or bladder control
- Bleeding or clear fluid discharge from ears or nose
- Unconsciousness

Home Treatment

- If you suspect a spinal injury, do not move the person unless there is an immediate threat to life, such as fire. Don't drag victims from automobile accidents.
- If the person is in immediate danger, keep the head and neck supported

and aligned while you move him to safety.

• If it was a diving accident, don't pull the injured person from the water as you may cause permanent damage. Float the person face up in the water until help arrives. The water will act as a splint and keep the spine immobile.

• If you suspect a spinal injury, call a health professional to transport the injured person.

Unconsciousness

An **unconscious** person is completely unaware of what is going on and is unable to make purposeful movements. Fainting is a form of brief unconsciousness; a coma is a deep, prolonged state of unconsciousness.

Causes of unconsciousness include stroke, epilepsy, heat exhaustion, diabetic coma, insulin shock, head or spinal injury, suffocation, drunkenness, shock, bleeding, and heart attack.

Fainting is a partial loss of consciousness most often due to a momentary drop in blood flow to the brain. When you fall or lie down, blood flow is improved and you regain consciousness. This light-headedness is a mild form of shock, and is usually not serious. If it happens often, there may be a more serious problem. Dizziness and fainting can also be brought on by sudden emotional stress or injury. See page 116.

Home Treatment

• Make sure the unconscious person can breathe. Check for breathing and, if necessary, open the airway and begin rescue breathing. See page 206.

• Keep the person lying down.

• Check the pulse. If there is none, call for help and start cardiopulmonary resuscitation (CPR). See page 206.

• Treat any injuries.

• Do not give the person anything to eat or drink.

• Look for medical identification, such as a bracelet, necklace, or card that identifies a medical problem such as epilepsy, diabetes, or drug allergy.

• If the person has diabetes, he or she may have **insulin shock** (low blood sugar) or be in a **diabetic coma** (too much sugar in the blood).

When to Call Kaiser Permanente

• If someone has completely lost consciousness.

• If unconsciousness follows a head injury. A head injury victim needs to be carefully observed. See page 224.

• If a person with diabetes loses consciousness.

Be true to your teeth or your teeth will be false to you.
Dental Proverb

Chapter 16

Mouth and Dental Problems

Your teeth will last a lifetime if you care for them properly. Regular brushing, flossing, and visits to a dentist will help keep your teeth healthy.

Choose a dentist as carefully as you choose any other doctor. See page 13 for tips on finding a dentist who meets your needs and is concerned about preventive care.

Canker Sores

Canker sores are painful open sores on the inner membranes of the mouth and cheek. Possible causes of canker sores include injury to the inside of the mouth, infection, genetic predisposition, female hormones, and stress. The sores usually heal in 7 to 10 days.

Prevention
- Avoid injury to the inside of your mouth:
  - Chew food slowly and carefully.
  - Use a soft-bristle toothbrush and brush your teeth thoroughly but gently.
- Avoid foods that seem to cause sores.

Home Treatment
- Avoid coffee, spicy and salty foods, and citrus fruits.
- Apply an oral paste, like Orabase, to the canker sore. It will protect the sore, ease pain, and speed healing. Other over-the-counter canker sore medications include Gly-oxide, Amosan, and Cankaid. Ambesol may help relieve pain.

Mouth and Dental Problems

Problem	Possible Causes
White spots, sores, or bleeding in mouth	See Canker Sores, p. 237; see thrush, p. 138. If unexplained sores last longer than 14 days, call a health professional.
Bleeding gums	Gum disease. See Dental Problems, p. 239.
Toothache	See p. 243.
Sores on the lips	See Cold Sores below.
Bad breath	May be a sign of dental problems, indigestion, or upper respiratory infection.
Pain and stiffness in jaw, with headache	See TMJ, p. 243; Tension Headaches, p. 129.

Canker Sores – continued

- Rinse your mouth with a mixture of one tablespoon of hydrogen peroxide in eight ounces of water.

- A thin paste of baking soda and water applied to the sore may bring relief.

When to Call Kaiser Permanente

- If mouth sores developed after starting a medication.

- If a canker sore, or any sore, does not heal in 14 days.

- If a sore is very painful or recurs frequently.

- If white spots that are not canker sores appear in the mouth and are not improving in one to two weeks.

Cold Sores

Cold sores (fever blisters) are small red blisters that appear on the lip and outer edge of the mouth. They often weep a clear fluid and form scabs after a few days. They are sometimes confused with impetigo (see page 140), which usually develops between the nose and upper lip. The fluid that weeps from impetigo is cloudy and honey-colored, not clear.

Cold sores are caused by a herpes virus. Most people will get cold sores at some point. Herpes viruses (chickenpox is another kind) stay in the body after the first infection. Later, something that triggers the virus causes it to become active again. Cold sores may appear after colds, fevers, exposure to the sun, and stressful times. They may also occur during menstruation. Sometimes, they appear for no apparent reason.

Prevention

- Avoid kissing someone who has a cold sore and avoid direct skin contact with genital herpes sores (see page 199). Both types of herpes can affect either the mouth or genitals. Condoms help reduce the risk.

- Use a sunscreen on your lips or wear a hat if exposure to the sun seems to trigger cold sores.

- Reducing stress may help in some cases. Practice relaxation exercises often. See page 252.

Home Treatment

- At the first sign of a cold sore (tingling or prickling at the site where the sore will appear), apply ice to the area. This may help reduce the severity of the sore.

- Apply petroleum jelly (Vaseline) to ease cracking and dryness.

- Apply a paste made of cornstarch and a little water.

- Blistex or Campho-Phenique may ease the pain. Don't share them with others.

- Be patient. Cold sores usually go away in 7 to 10 days.

When to Call Kaiser Permanente

- If sores last longer than two weeks, or occur frequently.

- If you have many or frequent cold sores. A prescription medication may reduce the frequency and severity of outbreaks.

Dental Problems

Dental disease is preventable. You can keep all of your teeth by practicing good home care and having regular professional checkups. Brush and floss regularly. Both tooth decay and gum disease are the result of bacterial plaque.

Plaque and Tooth Decay

Bacteria are always present in the mouth. When they are not removed by brushing and flossing, bacteria stick to the teeth and multiply into larger and larger colonies called plaque. Plaque forms as a sticky, colorless film on your teeth.

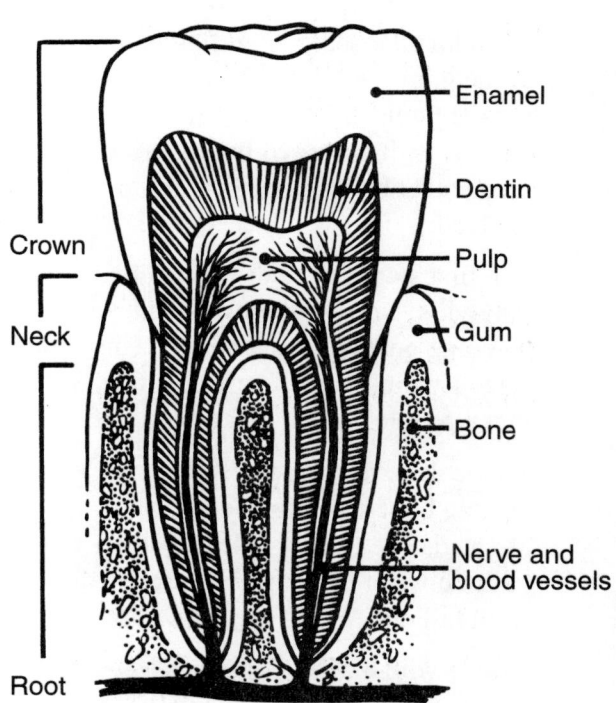

The tooth

Dental Problems – continued

This sticky plaque damages teeth in two ways. First, food particles, especially refined sugars, stick to it. The plaque uses that food to grow more bacteria and to produce acid. Second, the plaque holds the acid against the tooth surface and prevents saliva from mixing with it. Left alone, the acid will eventually eat through the tooth enamel, causing tooth decay.

If you eat only at mealtimes, it takes about 24 hours for bacteria and acid to harm your teeth. This is enough time for you to brush the plaque off and to wash away the acid. If you eat a lot of between-meal snacks, plaque builds up faster and you need to brush more often.

Plaque and Gum (Periodontal) Disease

Periodontal disease, an inflammation of the gums and in the bone supporting the gums, is a major cause of tooth loss. It is caused by bacterial plaque that builds up and sticks to the teeth.

The first stage of the disease, called gingivitis, is marked by swollen, bleeding gums and bad breath. This stage is painless and, unfortunately, many people do not seek treatment.

As the disease progresses, the supporting bones and ligaments are affected. The gum recedes, creating gaps between the teeth. Eventually the teeth fall out.

People with diabetes and those who smoke or chew tobacco are at increased risk of gum disease.

However, everyone is at risk; an estimated 75 to 80 percent of Americans have some form of gum disease.

Occasional bleeding when you brush or floss is an early sign of gum disease. However, with good care, it won't take long to get your gums back to normal. Brush and floss your teeth every day, and follow the prevention guidelines.

Prevention

• Have your teeth checked and cleaned at least twice a year by a dentist or dental hygienist.

• Eat crunchy foods that naturally clean the teeth (apples, carrots, and other raw vegetables), and foods with ample vitamin C, like citrus fruits and broccoli.

Brushing

Brush and floss properly to remove plaque. Brush at least twice a day for three to five minutes each time. Clean every surface of every tooth.

1. Use a toothbrush with soft, rounded-end bristles and a head that allows you to reach all parts of your mouth. Replace your toothbrush every three to four months.

2. Use a fluoride toothpaste and use only a small dab (pea-sized or smaller). Fluoride is a mineral that strengthens tooth enamel and reduces the harmful effects of plaque. Tartar-control toothpastes may help slow the formation of hard plaque buildup (tartar) on the teeth, but daily brushing with any toothpaste and flossing are the best tartar-control methods.

3. Place the brush at a 45° angle where the teeth meet the gums. Press firmly, and gently rock the brush back and forth using small circular movements. Do not scrub if you have a stiff-bristled brush. Vigorous brushing can make the gums recede and scratch your tooth enamel.

4. Brush all surfaces of the teeth: tongue side and cheek side. Pay special attention to the front teeth and behind the back teeth.

5. Brush the chewing surfaces vigorously with short back-and-forth strokes.

6. Brush the tongue. Plaque on the tongue can cause bad breath and is an ideal environment for bacteria to grow.

7. Use disclosing tablets periodically to see if any plaque is left on the teeth. Disclosing tablets are chewable tablets that will color any plaque left on the teeth after brushing. They are available at most drugstores.

Flossing

Brushing properly can remove most dental plaque. Regular flossing is the best way to remove plaque that forms between the teeth and below the gum line. Floss once a day using one of the following methods:

1. The finger-wrap method: Cut off a piece of floss 18 to 20 inches long. Wrap one end around the left middle finger and the other end around the right middle finger, until your hands are about two to three inches apart.

2. The circle method: Use a piece of floss about 12 inches long. Tie the ends together, forming a loop. If the loop is too large, wrap the floss around the middle fingers to make it smaller.

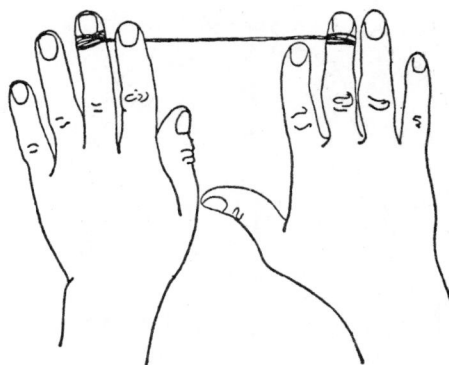

Finger-wrap method

To floss the upper teeth, use the thumb of one hand and forefinger of the other as shown in the illustration.

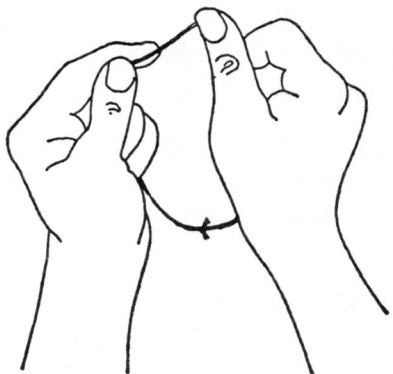

Flossing upper teeth

Flossing – continued

To floss the lower teeth, use both forefingers to guide the floss as in the illustration. The fingers should be about ½ inch apart.

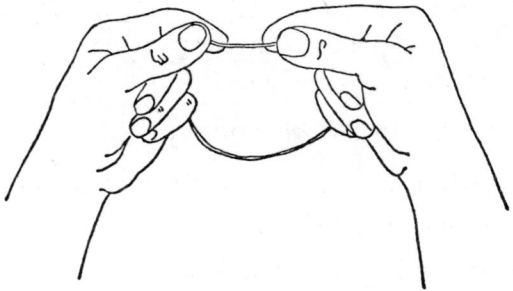

Flossing lower teeth

Curve the floss around each tooth and gently slide it under the gum line. Move the floss firmly up and down several times to scrape off the plaque. Popping the floss in and out without scraping will not remove much plaque.

Flossing tools may be especially helpful for adults who are flossing a child's teeth. Use the same scraping motion to remove plaque.

With practice, flossing will become easy. Any bleeding should subside as gums become healthy.

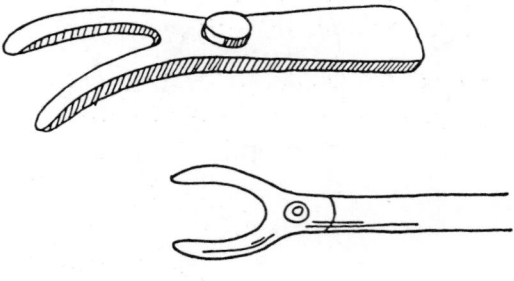

Flossing tools

Dental Care for Children

Children should have their first dental visit by age two to three. Visits every six months for checkups and cleaning are usually recommended for children and adults.

- Start caring for your children's teeth early, before permanent teeth have come in. Do not put an infant or small child to bed with a bottle of juice or milk. Prolonged contact with the sugar in these liquids can cause tooth decay. Nursing an infant to sleep is fine, however.

- Start toothbrushing as soon as the teeth come in. Parents should brush their children's teeth for the first four to five years, until children have enough dexterity to take over the job. A good teaching method is to have the child brush in the morning and the parent brush at night until the skill is mastered. Use disclosing tablets to see if the child is removing all the plaque.

- Start flossing as soon as the child has teeth that touch each other. As with brushing, an adult will have to help with flossing until the child is old enough to manage it. Flossing tools can help.

Sealants and Fluoride

Sealants are a plastic coating applied to the chewing surfaces of the back teeth to protect them from developing cavities. Sealants are especially good for the permanent molars when they first emerge in the mouth, usually between age 6 and age 11. Even with sealants, regular brushing and flossing are essential.

Children and adults need fluoride to build and keep strong teeth. Talk with your dentist about the amount of fluoride in your area's drinking water, and discuss fluoride treatments if needed.

When to Call a Dentist

• For regular cleanings and exams. Every six months is the recommended schedule.

• If your gums bleed when you press on them or bleed often when you brush your teeth.

• If teeth are loose or moving apart or if there are changes in the way your teeth fit together when you bite.

• If gums are very red, swollen, or tender, or if pus is present.

• If you have a toothache. Toothaches are caused when the inside of the tooth (dentin) is exposed. The pain may go away temporarily, but the problem will not. Take aspirin, ibuprofen, or acetaminophen for pain relief until you can get an appointment. A cold pack on the jaw may also help.

TMJ Syndrome

The olive-sized joint that connects your jawbone to your skull is called the temporomandibular joint (TMJ). TMJ syndrome is a set of symptoms that relate to damage, wear and tear, or unusual stress to the joint. The symptoms can include:

• Pain in and around the joint

• Noises such as clicking, popping, or snapping in the joint

• Inability to "open wide"

• Muscle pain and spasms where the jaw muscles attach to the bone

• Headache, neck and shoulder pain, ear or eye pain, and difficulty swallowing

The cause of TMJ syndrome is difficult to determine. The most likely causes include:

• Injury, such as a direct hit on the jaw, whiplash, or forceful stretching of the jaw during dental work

• Chronic tooth grinding, clenching, or gum chewing

• Arthritis in the joint

• Chronic muscle tension due to stress, anxiety, depression, or poor posture (usually affects the jaw muscles more than the joint)

• Teeth that do not fit together when you bite (malocclusion)

TMJ Syndrome – continued

Home treatment and nonsurgical treatments will successfully relieve most TMJ symptoms. Your doctor may recommend use of a plastic mouth plate (splint), physical therapy, or prescription pain relievers. Surgery is needed for a very small percentage of TMJ problems.

Prevention

- Regularly practice progressive muscle relaxation, particularly before going to sleep. See page 252.
- Stop chewing gum or tough foods at the first sign of pain or discomfort in your jaw muscles.
- Avoid biting your nails and nibbling on pencils or other objects, which forces your jaw into an awkward position and may cause pain.
- Maintain good posture with your ear, shoulder, and hip in a straight line. See page 57.

Home Treatment

- Continue the prevention tips.
- Avoid chewing gum and hard or chewy foods.
- Avoid opening your mouth too wide.
- Avoid cradling a telephone receiver between your shoulder and jaw.
- Rest your jaw, keeping your teeth apart and your lips closed. (Keep your tongue on the roof of your mouth, not between your teeth.)
- Put an ice pack on the joint for eight minutes, three times a day. Gently open and close your mouth while the ice pack is on. If the jaw muscle is swollen, apply ice six times a day.
- Take aspirin or ibuprofen to reduce swelling and pain.
- If there is no swelling, use moist heat on the jaw muscle three times a day. Gently open and close your mouth while the heat is on. Alternate with the cold pack treatments.
- If you are under severe stress or suffer from anxiety or depression, see Chapter 19.

When to Call Kaiser Permanente

- If the pain is severe.
- If TMJ symptoms occur after an injury to the jaw.
- If your jaw locks in certain positions.
- If any jaw problem or pain continues more than two weeks without improvement.
- If other mild TMJ symptoms do not improve after four weeks of home treatment.

If exercise could be packed into a pill, it would be the single most
widely prescribed, and beneficial, medicine in the nation.
Robert Butler, M.D.

Chapter 17

Fitness and Relaxation

Staying fit and relaxed is not only good for your health, it is good for you. If you want to enjoy life more, the tips in this chapter can help.

The Benefits of Exercise

No amount of exercise can guarantee a long life. However, even moderate amounts of exercise can improve the likelihood of a healthy life. Along with a positive attitude and a healthy diet, your fitness level plays a major role in how well you feel, what illnesses you avoid, and how much you enjoy life.

Consider the benefits of fitness presented here. Find one or more reasons to commit to your own fitness program.

Your Personal Fitness Plan

No one can prescribe the perfect fitness plan for you. You have to figure it out based on what you enjoy doing and what you will continue to do. The next few pages can be a big help.

Benefits of Exercise

- Relieves tension and stress
- Provides enjoyment and fun
- Stimulates the mind
- Helps maintain stable weight
- Controls appetite
- Boosts self-image
- Improves muscle tone and strength
- Improves flexibility
- Lowers blood pressure
- Relieves insomnia
- Increases "good" (HDL) cholesterol
- Prevents diabetes

Consistency is the most important, the most basic, and the most often neglected part of fitness. Consistency in regular exercise or moderate activity delivers all of the fitness benefits.

Personal Fitness Plan – cont.

A good fitness plan has three parts: aerobic fitness, muscle strengthening, and flexibility. Read the section on each part. Then, see "Setting Your Fitness Goals" on page 249.

Aerobic Fitness

Aerobic conditioning strengthens your heart and lungs. Good aerobic exercises include brisk walking, running, stair climbing, biking, swimming, aerobic dance, or anything else that raises your heart rate and keeps it up for a while.

How Hard Should I Exercise?

Nice and easy does it. Exercise does not have to be intense to be of value. In fact, if you exercise too hard, you get less benefit than if you go at a moderate pace.

Above all, listen to your body. If the exercise feels too hard, slow down. You will reduce your risk of injury and enjoy the exercise much more.

Try the talk/sing test to determine your ideal exercise pace:

- If you can't talk and exercise at the same time, you are going too fast.

- If you can talk while you exercise, you are doing fine.

- If you can sing while you exercise, it would be safe to exercise a little faster.

Your exercise is most effective when you are able to talk, but not to sing.

Target Heart Rate

Another way to see how hard you are exercising is to check your heart rate. You gain the most aerobic benefits when your exercise heart rate is 60 percent to 80 percent of your maximum heart rate. After exercising for about 10 minutes, stop and take your pulse for 10 seconds. Compare the number to the chart below. Adjust the intensity of your exercise so that your heart rate stays between the two numbers.

Target Heart Rate	
Age	10-second heart rate
20	20 - 27
25	20 - 26
30	19 - 25
35	19 - 25
40	18 - 24
45	18 - 23
50	17 - 23
55	17 - 23
60	16 - 22
65	16 - 21
70	15 - 20

Target heart rate is 60 percent to 80 percent of maximum heart rate (maximum heart rate = 220 minus your age).

How Often and How Long Should I Exercise?

Most studies show that exercising 20 minutes three times a week is enough to improve fitness. However, sometimes it's easier to make exercise a habit if you do it every day.

With exercise, harder is not better, but longer is. Although you can get good fitness benefits from as little as 10 minutes of exercise per day, extending your exercise time will increase your rewards. This is true for up to one hour of exercise per day. Beyond that, there may be diminishing health returns and increasing risk of injuries.

Warm Up and Cool Down

For the first five minutes of your exercise routine, start out slowly and easily so your muscles have a chance to warm up.

End your exercise with a little cool-down. Gradually slow your pace, then do a few light stretches to improve flexibility. See page 248.

Drink some extra water before and after exercising.

Muscle Strengthening

Strengthening your muscles improves your work and athletic performance and prevents fatigue. Muscle-strengthening exercises will also improve your posture and help you feel more energetic.

Resistance training, with free weights, weight-training equipment, or inexpensive rubber tubing, can quickly increase your muscle strength.

Other simple, safe, and effective strengthening exercises include bent-knee curl-ups, chin-ups, push-ups, side leg-lifts, and other calisthenics to improve abdominal, neck, arm, shoulder, and leg strength.

Flexibility

Stretching can increase your range of motion and reduce stiffness and pain. Stretching is particularly important during the cool-down phase when your muscles are warm. See the stretches on page 248 and Resource 40 on page 309.

- Stretching should be slow and gradual. Don't bounce. Maintain a continuous tension on the muscle.

- Relax and hold each stretch for a count of 10.

- Exhale as you stretch, inhale as you relax. If it hurts, you have gone too far or you are doing something incorrectly.

Try to stretch a little every day. Try a stretch break instead of a coffee break.

Overcome Barriers to Exercise

There are six barriers to exercise that are all easy to overcome.

1. No time? Try shorter periods of activity spread throughout the day, such as three 10-minute walks.

2. Too tired? It's often lack of exercise that makes you tired. Exercise gives you energy. Try it.

3. Embarrassed? People often are, especially at first. Be proud that you're taking care of your body.

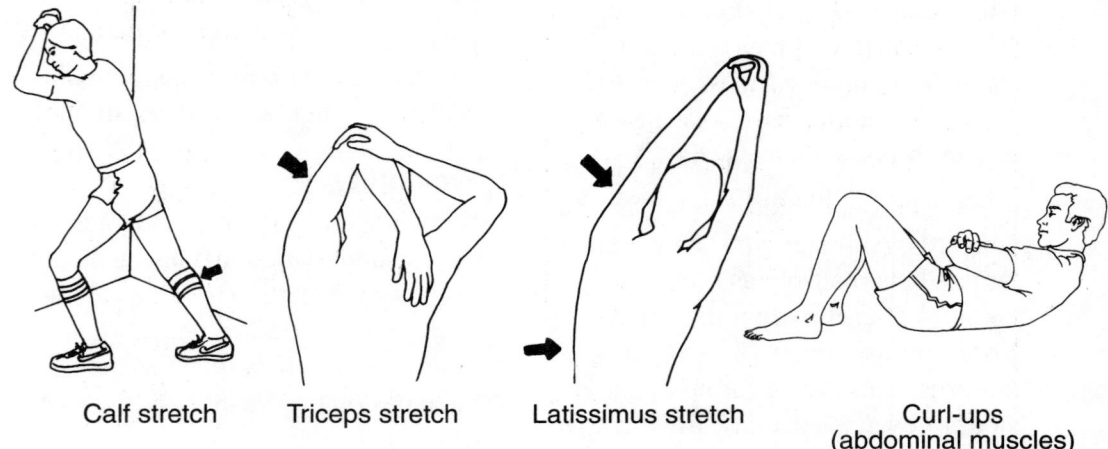

Calf stretch   Triceps stretch   Latissimus stretch   Curl-ups
(abdominal muscles)

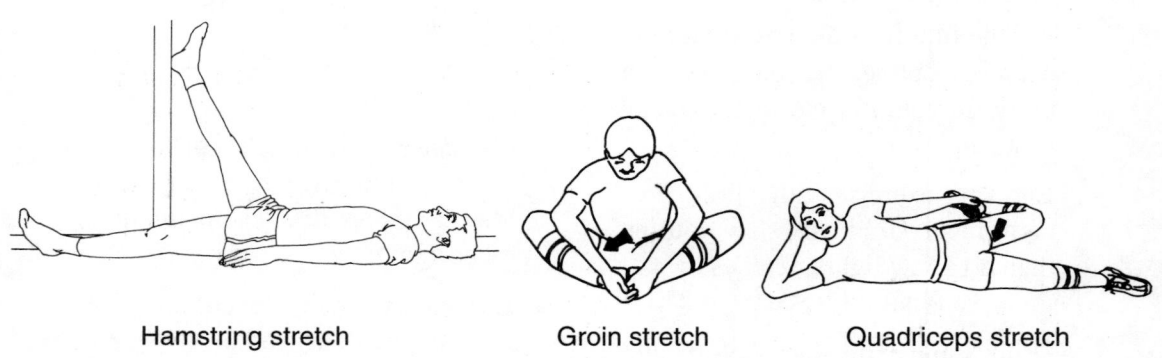

Hamstring stretch   Groin stretch   Quadriceps stretch

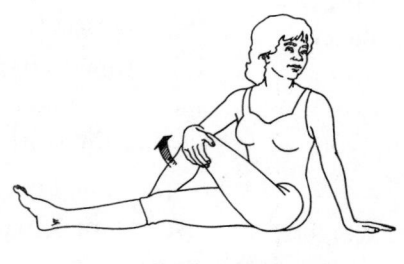

Hip flexor stretch

Stretching exercises

Exercise Caution

For most people, moderate exercise is not a health hazard. To be safe, start slowly and gradually increase the intensity of your exercise. However, if you can answer yes to any of the following questions, talk with your doctor before beginning an exercise program.

- Have you been told that you have heart trouble?

- Do you have undiagnosed chest pains?

- Do you have high blood pressure?

- Do you often feel faint or dizzy?

- Do you have arthritis or other bone or joint problems that might be aggravated by improper exercise?

- Do you have diabetes? You may want to talk with your doctor about how increased exercise affects your insulin needs.

Men over age 40 who have been inactive (sedentary) *or* who have two or more risk factors for heart disease* *and* who plan to start a *vigorous* exercise program (running or fast bicycling or swimming) may wish to talk with their doctors about the possible risk of vigorous exercise.

*Cholesterol over 200, blood pressure over 140/90, smoking, diabetes, or family history of heart disease before age 45.

Overcome Barriers – cont.

4. No partner? Yes, it's fun to exercise with others. If your regular partner quits, find another one.

5. Bad weather? Too hot, too cold, too wet, too windy—it never seems right for exercise. Lots of people exercise come rain or shine. Try a variety of indoor and outdoor activities.

6. Too costly? You had to let the fitness club membership expire. You can't afford a mountain bike. You panic at the price of running shoes. It all costs money. But can you afford not to exercise? Try a low-cost option, such as walking instead of driving.

Setting Your Fitness Goals

Are you as strong, flexible, and physically fit as you would like to be? If you are, good for you. We hope this chapter has helped you reaffirm the exercises you are already doing. However, if you want to make some improvements, here's one piece of advice: try to improve a little bit at a time.

The only way to walk a mile is to take one step at a time. The only way to improve your fitness level is to take it one step at a time.

- Pick one aspect of fitness (aerobic, strength, flexibility) you want to improve first.

- Pick an activity that you enjoy. You're more likely to keep doing something you look forward to.

Setting Fitness Goals - cont.

• Set a one-month goal that you think you can reach. For example, plan to walk for 10 minutes at lunch three days a week, or stretch for five minutes each morning.

• Start today. Keep a record of what you do.

• When you reach your first goal, reward yourself! Then set a new one.

Consistency brings success. Each success may be a small one, but small successes can quickly add up to physical fitness that will make a big difference in your life.

Stress and Distress

Stress is the physical, mental, and emotional reactions you experience as the result of changes and demands in your life.

Stress is part and parcel of common life events, both large and small. It comes with all of life's daily hassles, traffic jams, long lines, petty arguments, and other relatively small irritations. Stress also comes with crises and life-changing events, such as illness, marriage problems or divorce, losing a job, getting a new job, or children leaving home.

All these events may force you to adjust, whether you are ready to or not. Unless you can regularly release the tension that comes with stress, it can greatly increase your risks for physical and mental illness.

Because many major life events are beyond your control, take charge of those aspects of your life that you can

manage. One major change doesn't mean that all areas of your life must change. Continue to participate in the same activities you did before the event happened.

Not all stress is bad. Positive stress (eustress) is a motivator, challenging you to act in creative and resourceful ways. When changes and demands overwhelm you, negative stress (distress) sets in. This chapter has specific techniques you can use to cope with stress in your life and to help you feel your best.

What Stress Does to the Body

The immediate physical reactions to stress are universal:

• Heart rate increases to move blood to the muscles and brain.

• Blood pressure increases.

• Breathing rate increases.

• Digestion slows.

• Perspiration increases.

• Pupils dilate.

• You feel a rush of strength.

At the first sign of alarm, chemicals released by the pituitary and adrenal glands and the nerve endings automatically trigger these physical reactions. Your body is tense, alert, and ready for action. For primitive humans, these reactions were an advantage in the face of sudden danger, preparing them for better survival by either "fight or flight." Today, our bodies still react the same way but it is not as acceptable to either fight or run away (although we often wish we could).

After the natural "alarm" reaction to a real or perceived threat, our bodies stay on alert until we feel the danger has passed. When the stressor is gone, the brain signals an "all clear" sign to the pituitary and adrenal glands. They stop producing the chemicals that caused the physical reaction, and the body returns to normal.

Problems with stress occur when the brain fails to give the "all clear" signal. If the alarm state lasts too long, you begin to suffer from the consequences of constant stress. Unrelieved stress can lead to many health problems.

Recognizing Stress

It's sometimes difficult to recognize or admit that stress is affecting your health. If you can learn to watch for its effects and take corrective action quickly, you will be able to cope with your stress.

The signs of stress are classic. You may get a headache, stiff neck, nagging backache, rapid breathing, sweaty palms, or an upset stomach. You may become irritable and intolerant of even minor disturbances. You may lose your temper more often and yell at your family for no good reason. Your pulse rate may increase and you may feel jumpy or exhausted all the time. You may find it hard to concentrate.

When these symptoms appear, recognize them as signs of stress and think of a way to deal with them. Just knowing why you're crabby may be the first step in coping with the problem. It is your attitude toward stress, not the stress itself, that affects your health the most.

Managing Stress

Some people seek to relieve stress by smoking, drinking, overeating, or taking pills. There is a better way. Avoid the dangerous side effects of tobacco, alcohol, and drugs by learning to control your stress level. You can do this by using your body to soothe your mind and using your mind to soothe your body.

Stress and tension affect our emotions and feelings. By expressing those feelings to others, we are able to better understand and cope with them ourselves. People who develop a source of understanding with their spouse or a good friend have an invaluable assistant in coping with stress in their lives.

Crying can also release tensions. It's part of our emotional healing process. Expressing yourself through writing, crafts, or art may also be a good tension reliever.

Exercise is a natural response to stress; it is the normal reaction to the fight-or-flight urge. Walking briskly will take advantage of the rapid pulse and tensed muscles caused by stress and will release the pent-up energy. After a long walk, the stress level is lower and more manageable.

The rest of this chapter is devoted to skills and techniques other than exercise that will help you increase your resistance to stress and better cope with those stressors you choose to accept.

Relaxation Skills

Regardless of whatever else you do to manage stress, you can benefit from the regular use of relaxation skills. Their effect is the exact opposite to the fight-or-flight response. When learning these skills, it's critical to remove yourself from all outside distractions.

It may take some practice to become comfortable with these techniques. Once you've trained your body and mind to relax (two to three weeks), you'll be able to produce the same relaxed feelings on the spur of the moment.

Of the many methods of relaxation and meditation, the following three are among the simplest and most effective. They should be done twice a day for about 20 minutes. Pick a time and place where you won't be disturbed or distracted.

Roll Breathing

The object of roll breathing is to develop full use of your lungs and get in touch with the rhythm of your breathing. It can be practiced in any position, but it is best to learn it lying on your back, with your knees bent.

1. Place your left hand on your abdomen and your right hand on your chest. Notice how your hands move as you breathe in and out.

2. Practice filling your lower lungs by breathing so that your left hand goes up when you inhale while your right hand remains still. Always inhale through your nose and exhale through your mouth.

3. When you have filled and emptied your lower lungs 8 to 10 times with ease, add the second step to your breathing: inhale first into your lower lungs as before, but then continue inhaling into your upper chest. As you do so, your right hand will rise and your left hand will fall a little as your abdomen falls.

4. As you exhale slowly through your mouth, make a quiet, whooshing sound as first your left hand and then your right hand falls. As you exhale, feel the tension leaving your body as you become more and more relaxed.

5. Practice breathing in and out in this manner for three to five minutes. Notice that the movement of your abdomen and chest is like rolling waves rising and falling in a rhythmic motion. Roll breathing should be practiced daily for several weeks until it can be done almost anywhere, providing you with an instant relaxation tool any time you need one.

CAUTION: Some people get dizzy the first few times they try roll breathing. If you begin to hyperventilate or become lightheaded, slow your breathing. Get up slowly.

Progressive Muscle Relaxation

The body responds to tense thoughts or situations with muscle tension, which can cause pain or discomfort. Deep muscle relaxation reduces the muscle tension as well as general mental anxiety. You can use a pre-recorded tape to help you go through all the muscle groups or you can do it by just tensing and relaxing each muscle group. Deep muscle relaxation is effective in combatting stress-related health problems and often helps people get to sleep.

Muscle Groups and Procedure

Pick a place where you can stretch out comfortably, such as a carpeted floor.

Tense each muscle group for 4 to 10 seconds (hard but not to the point of cramping), then give yourself 10 to 20 seconds to release them and relax. At various points, review the various muscle groups and relax each one a little more each time.

How to Tense Muscle Groups:

1. Hands by clenching them.

2. Wrists and forearms by extending them and bending the hands back at the wrist.

3. Biceps and upper arms by clenching your hands into fists, bending your arms at the elbows, and flexing your biceps.

4. Shoulders by shrugging them. (Review the arms and shoulders area.)

5. Forehead by wrinkling it into a deep frown.

6. Around the eyes and bridge of the nose by closing the eyes as tightly as possible. (Remove contact lenses before beginning the exercise.)

7. Cheeks and jaws by grinning from ear to ear.

8. Around the mouth by pressing the lips together tightly. (Review the face area.)

9. Back of the neck by pressing the head back hard.

10. Front of the neck by touching the chin to the chest. (Review the neck and head area.)

11. Chest by taking a deep breath and holding it, then exhaling.

12. Back by arching the back up and away from the support surface.

13. Stomach by sucking it into a tight knot. (Review the chest and stomach area.)

14. Hips and buttocks by pressing the buttocks together tightly.

15. Thighs by clenching them hard.

16. Lower legs by pointing the toes toward the face, as if trying to bring the toes up to touch the head.

17. Lower legs by pointing the toes away and curling the toes downward at the same time. (Review the area from the waist down.)

18. When you are finished, arouse yourself thoroughly by counting backwards from five to one.

Relaxation Response

The relaxation response is the exact opposite of a stress response. It slows heart rate and breathing, lowers blood pressure, and helps relieve muscle tension.

Technique (adapted from Herbert Benson, MD):

1. Sit quietly in a comfortable position with eyes closed.

2. Begin progressive muscle relaxation. See page 252.

Relaxation Skills – continued

3. Become aware of your breathing. With each exhale, say the word "one" (or any other word or phrase) silently or aloud. Concentrate on breathing from your abdomen and not your chest. Instead of focusingon a repeated word, you may choose to fix your gaze on a stationary object. Any mental stimulus will help you to shift your mind away from external thoughts.

4. Continue this for 10 to 20 minutes. As distracting thoughts enter your mind, don't dwell on them, just allow them to drift away.

5. Sit quietly for several minutes, until you are ready to open your eyes.

6. Notice the difference in your breathing and your pulse rate.

Don't worry whether you are successful in becoming deeply relaxed. The key to this exercise is to remain passive, to let distracting thoughts slip away like waves on the beach.

Practice for 10 to 20 minutes once or twice a day, but not within two hours after a meal. When you have set up a routine, the relaxation response should come with little effort.

For a more complete description of the relaxation response, see Resource 78 on page 311.

Never eat more than you can lift.
Miss Piggy

Chapter 18

Nutrition

This chapter gives some guidelines for good eating and some hints on how to help your children establish healthy eating habits. Children learn best by example, so teach them by practicing good eating habits along with them. For more information about healthy eating, see Resource 68 on page 310.

Seven Simple Guidelines for Eating Well

(Dietary Guidelines for Americans, USDA, 1990)

1. Eat a variety of foods. Include a daily selection of:

- Whole-grain and enriched breads, cereals, and grain products

- Vegetables

- Fruits

- Milk, cheese, and yogurt

- Meats, poultry, fish, eggs, dried beans and peas, tofu

2. Maintain a healthy weight. See page 266.

3. Choose a diet low in fat, saturated fat, and cholesterol. Fats have twice as many calories per gram as any other food. A high-fat diet increases your risk of heart disease and some cancers. See page 259.

4. Eat plenty of vegetables, fruits, and grain products. Complex carbohydrates (grains, vegetables, and starches) and fruits pack the most nutrients per calorie. See page 256.

5. Use sugars only in moderation. Sugars have little, if any, vitamins, minerals, or fiber. See page 259.

6. Use salt and sodium only in moderation. For some people, sodium increases blood pressure. See page 265.

7. If you drink alcohol, do so only in moderation. Alcohol is high in calories and has no nutrients. For men,

Eating Well – continued

this means not more than two drinks per day; for women, not more than one. A drink is equal to 12 ounces of beer, five ounces of wine, or 1½ ounces of distilled alcohol (vodka, gin, etc.).

Eating Well: A Basic Plan

Eat a variety of foods from the Food Guide Pyramid every day. Eat more from the breads and cereals and fruits and vegetables groups than from the other groups. Most people who follow this plan will get all the vitamins, minerals, and other nutrients their bodies need and will have little trouble controlling their weight.

Breads, Cereals, and Starches

Contrary to popular belief, bread, potatoes, rice, and pasta are not fattening! These starchy foods are actually good for you.

Starches are carbohydrates, which have less than half the calories per gram as fat. Unprocessed starches (whole grains, vegetables) also contain large amounts of vitamins, minerals, fiber, and water.

Starchy foods are fattening only when you add fat to them. Try nonfat yogurt or salsa on baked potatoes. Use fresh vegetable and tomato sauces on pasta.

Fruits and Vegetables

Fresh fruits and vegetables are good for you. They provide vitamins, minerals, and fiber and are naturally low in fat. Many fruits and vegetables, contain a lot of vitamins A (beta carotene), and C, especially oranges and other citrus fruits, broccoli, sweet potatoes, winter squash, carrots, spinach, and other leafy greens. As a result, a diet that includes lots of fruits and vegetables helps protect you against heart disease and cancer.

Fruits and vegetables are most nutritious when eaten fresh and raw or lightly cooked. When you cook vegetables, steam or microwave them to retain more vitamins.

Fruits and Vegetables Against Cancer

Fruits and vegetables are important for good basic nutrition. They contain lots of fiber, especially when eaten raw. A diet high in fiber may protect you against colon cancer. Many vegetables and fruits contain the two antioxidant vitamins A (as beta carotene) and C, which may protect against some cancers. Beta carotene is found in carrots, apricots, winter squash, sweet potatoes, cantaloupe, and broccoli. Vitamin C is found in citrus fruits such as oranges, and in cantaloupe, strawberries, peppers, broccoli, and tomatoes.

Vegetables in the cabbage family, including broccoli and cauliflower, appear to protect against several types of cancer.

The National Cancer Institute recommends that you eat at least five servings per day of fruits and vegetables to lower your risk of cancer.

Guide to Eating Well

Grains (breads, cereals, rice, pasta) form the foundation of a healthy diet. Serving sizes: 1 slice of bread, 1 oz. of cereal, ½ bagel, ½ cup of pasta or rice.

Eat plenty of fruits and vegetables. Serving sizes: ¾ cup fruit or vegetable juice; ½ cup raw, canned, or cooked fruits or vegetables, medium apple or banana, 1 cup raw leafy vegetables.

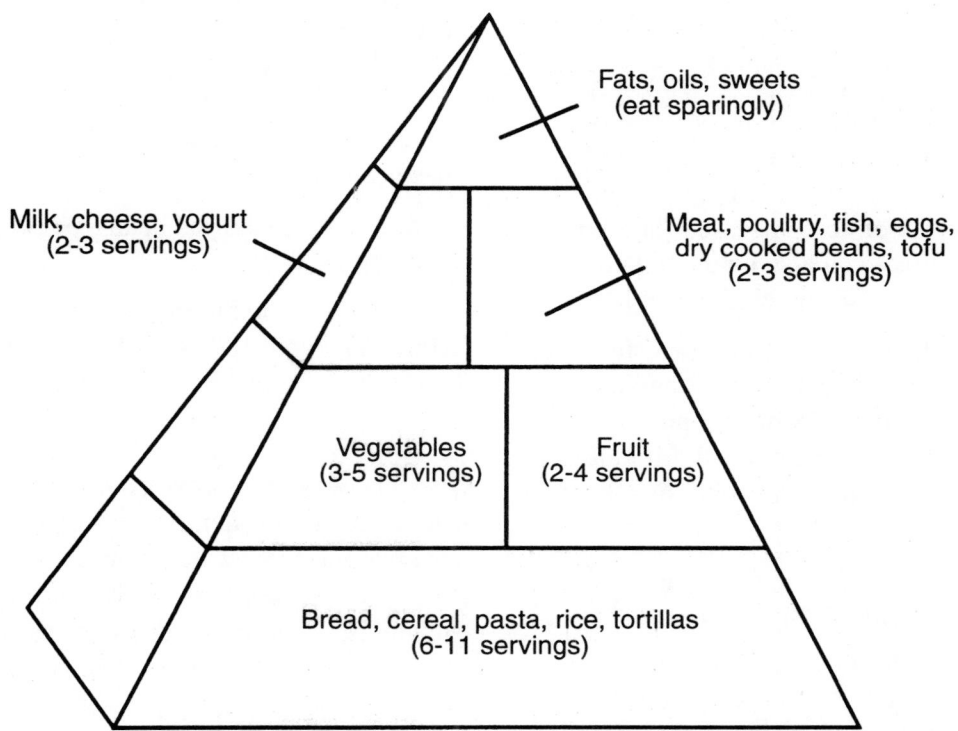

The Food Guide Pyramid (USDA)

Eat more fish, poultry, and dry cooked beans to reduce fat. Serving sizes: 2 – 3 oz. cooked lean meat, poultry, or fish, ½ cup cooked dried beans, 1 egg, 2 tbsp. peanut butter.

Choose nonfat or low-fat dairy products. Serving sizes: 1 cup milk or yogurt, 1½ – 2 oz. low-fat cheese, ½ cup cottage cheese.

Eat foods from the top of the pyramid only in moderation. Examples: cooking oil, butter or margarine, high-fat salty snacks, alcohol, candy.

Eating Well – continued

Fiber

Fiber has no vitamins or minerals, yet it is important to good health. There are two types of fiber.

Insoluble fiber in whole-grain products provides bulk for your diet. Together with fluids, fiber stimulates the colon to keep waste moving out of the bowels. Without fiber, waste moves too slowly, increasing your risk for constipation, colon and bowel cancer, and diverticulosis.

Soluble fiber found in fruit, beans, peas and other legumes, and oats helps lower cholesterol, reducing your risk of heart disease. The fiber in legumes can also help regulate blood glucose and cholesterol levels.

Do you need more fiber? If your bowel movements are soft and easy to pass, you probably get plenty of fiber. If they are hard and difficult to pass, more fiber and water may help.

Small Changes Can Make a Big Difference

You don't have to change your whole diet at once. Pick one easy change at first and stick with it. Add others once you've had success with the first change.

- Buy only whole-grain bread.
- Buy only skim or 1% milk.
- Use less oil for cooking.
- Eat fish at least twice a week.
- Eat a raw vegetable at lunch.
- Drink an extra glass of water when you wake each morning.

See page 42 for more information on constipation.

To increase fiber in your diet:

- Eat at least five servings of fruits and vegetables a day. Eat fruits with edible skins and seeds: kiwis, figs, blueberries, apples, and raspberries. Eat more of the stems of broccoli and asparagus.

- Switch to whole-grain and whole-wheat breads, pasta, tortillas, and cereals. The first ingredient listed should be whole-wheat flour. If it just says wheat flour, it means white flour, from which much of the fiber has been removed.

- Eat more cooked dried beans, peas, and lentils.

- Popcorn is a good high-fiber snack. However, avoid added oil, butter, and salt.

Water

One easy way to improve your diet is to drink more water. Active people need two quarts of water a day. People who exercise regularly need even more water. If you drink other fluids, you can get by with less, but plain water is best.

Caffeine

There is no convincing evidence that a moderate amount of caffeine (two to three cups of coffee or cola per day) will do you any harm if you are healthy.

Caffeine is mildly addictive. Cutting back too quickly may cause a headache. Gradual reductions will prevent this.

Sugar

What's wrong with sugar? It comes from a vegetable (sugar beets or sugar cane), is relatively cheap, tastes good, is fat free, and is even a carbohydrate. Can sugar be all that bad?

From a health point of view, the biggest problem with sugar is that it is stripped of all vitamins, minerals, and fiber. What is left are crystals of pure calories.

In moderation, sugar does little harm. However, if too many of your calories come from sugar, you will either gain weight or not get enough of the other nutrients you need. Sugar also contributes to cavities.

- Be aware of hidden sugars in flavored yogurt, canned, and other processed foods. Check the label for words that end in "-ose," like dextrose, fructose, sucrose, lactose, and maltose, which are forms of sugar. Corn syrup is another common form of sugar.

- Limit foods that list sugar among the first few ingredients.

- Look for breakfast cereals that have six grams or less of added sugar per serving.

- You can reduce the sugar in homemade baked goods by up to one-half without affecting the texture.

- Eat a sweet piece of fruit instead of a sugary dessert.

- All sugars are basically alike. Honey and brown or raw sugar have no advantage over other sugars.

Artificial Sweeteners

Although artificial sweeteners do help you avoid sugar, weight-loss success depends more on reducing calories from fat. Avoid using artificially sweetened foods to justify eating more high-fat food.

Aspartame (NutraSweet) and saccharin are not considered to cause any health problems, but the effects of long-term use are not yet known. Use them in moderation.

Fats in Foods

Fat, butter, lard, cream, oil, margarine, mayonnaise, and grease in foods account for 37 percent of the calories in the average American diet. Fat has more than twice as many calories per gram as carbohydrates or protein.

How much fat is too much? The USDA Dietary Guidelines recommend that less than 30 percent of total calories come from fat. Changing from a diet that contains 37 percent fat to one that contains 30 percent fat may slow the development of heart disease, reduce cancer risk, and improve your overall diet. But is it enough?

Many scientists suggest a 30-percent fat diet is still too high for a healthy heart. A 20-percent fat diet will slow heart disease even more. There is some evidence that a 10-percent fat diet, along with other lifestyle changes, can even reverse the buildup of arteriosclerosis in the arteries. However, a 10-percent fat diet is challenging to maintain.

> ### The 80-20 Rule
>
> If you are generally healthy, you don't need to worry about perfection in a healthy diet. If you make healthy eating choices 80 percent of the time, occasional high-fat or high-calorie foods won't be a problem the other 20 percent of the time.

Eating Well – continued

Based on your heart disease risks, you may wish to set a goal for how much fat to include in your diet. A nutritionist can help you with a menu plan to meet your goal.

15 Simple Ways to Reduce Fat

When eating meat:

1. Eat more poultry and fish. Choose lean cuts of meat, such as tenderloin, top and bottom round, or lean veal.

2. Remove all visible fat before cooking. Poultry skin may be removed either before or after cooking.

3. Broil or bake instead of frying.

4. Reduce serving sizes to two or three ounces and don't take seconds.

5. Replace some meat with cooked dry beans and grains.

When using dairy products:

6. Use skim or 1% milk.

7. Choose low-fat, part skim milk cheeses like gruyere, Farmer's, Jarlsberg Swiss, mozzarella, or ricotta. Look for low-fat or nonfat Cheddar and Monterey Jack cheeses.

8. Substitute low-fat or nonfat cottage cheese and yogurt for cream and sour cream, or use fat-free sour cream and cream cheese.

In cooking:

9. Steam vegetables, saute with one teaspoon of oil or less, or cook with wine or defatted broth.

10. Use non-stick pans or add oil to a preheated pan. Less oil goes further this way.

11. Flavor vegetables with herbs and spices instead of butter and sauces, or try Butter Buds or Molly McButter.

12. Experiment using less oil than is called for in recipes. You may need to increase other liquids. Use applesauce to replace some or all of the fat in baked goods.

In general:

13. Avoid crackers, chips, cookies, and margarines made with hydrogenated oil, palm oil, coconut oil, or cocoa butter.

14. Eat plenty of carbohydrates to fill you up (fruits, vegetables, grains, bread, pasta, etc.).

15. Let salads go naked, modestly dressed with lemon juice, or use fat-free dressings and mayonnaise.

Cholesterol

Cholesterol is a waxy substance that is produced by the human body and is also found in animal products. Some cholesterol is needed for cells to function. Unfortunately, excess cholesterol builds up inside the arteries. Cholesterol deposits (arteriosclerosis) are the major cause of heart attacks and strokes.

The amount of cholesterol in your blood is a good predictor of your risk for heart disease and stroke, along with how much you smoke, how high your blood pressure is, your family medical history, and whether you have diabetes. The higher your cholesterol level, the higher the risk. However, not all cholesterol is bad.

Calculating Percent Fat

Each gram of fat has 9 calories. To calculate the percent of a food's total calories that come from fat, multiply the grams of fat times 9 and then divide by the total number of calories. Multiply your result by 100 to get the percent.

For example, an 8-ounce serving of 2% milk has 5 grams of fat and 130 total calories:

$$\frac{5 \text{ grams fat x 9 calories/gram}}{130 \text{ calories}} =$$

$$= 34.6\% \text{ calories from fat}$$

The new food labels contain information about the percentage of your daily fat allotment in a serving of food.

For example, a food that has 6 grams of fat per serving provides 10 percent of the daily fat allotment in a 2,000 calorie diet.

Balance higher-fat foods with lower-fat vegetables, fruits, and grains.

Good Cholesterol

Fat travels through your bloodstream attached to protein in a combination called a lipoprotein. Two lipoproteins are the main carriers of cholesterol: low-density lipoprotein (LDL) and high-density lipoprotein (HDL).

LDL acts like a fat delivery truck. It picks up cholesterol from the liver and delivers it to the cells. When more cholesterol is ready for delivery than the cells can take, LDL cholesterol drops off the extra cholesterol on the artery walls. A lot of LDL cholesterol in your blood increases your risk of heart disease and stroke.

HDL works like a garbage truck. It removes excess cholesterol from the bloodstream and takes it to the liver. A lot of HDL cholesterol decreases your risk of heart disease and stroke.

Cholesterol Screening

Cholesterol screening is important in assessing your risk for heart disease. Heart disease risk should be assessed at least once between age 20-40, 40-60, and 60-75 years. Ideally, all adults should have cholesterol screening at least twice during their lives. Those who are at increased risk for heart disease (for example, people who smoke, have high blood pressure, have diabetes, are overweight, or have high cholesterol levels) should be reassessed more often as directed by their health care provider.

Cholesterol – continued

Total Cholesterol Scores

Total cholesterol levels are categorized as follows by the National Cholesterol Education Program:

- Under 200 mg/dL: Desirable
- 200 - 239 mg/dL: Borderline high-risk
- 240 or higher: High-risk

However, overall heart disease risk depends on the combination of many factors, not just cholesterol levels. Although cholesterol levels often get the most attention, quitting cigarette smoking, increasing physical activity, and controlling your blood pressure may be even more important for some people than lowering cholesterol.

If your total cholesterol is high, measuring the other types of cholesterol (HDL and LDL) may be useful, especially before considering the use of medications to lower cholesterol. For most people, a low-fat diet is all that is necessary to lower cholesterol. Besides helping to lower cholesterol, a low-fat diet may help control diabetes, blood pressure, and may lower the risk of certain types of cancer.

Because of the potential side effects and risks, medication to lower cholesterol should only be considered in people at the highest risk for heart disease. If you are age 40 to 65, at very high risk for heart disease, and you find that a low-fat diet isn't enough to lower your cholesterol, then adding cholesterol-lowering medication may be helpful.

How to Reduce Your Cholesterol

- Eat less total fat. Because a high-fat diet increases cholesterol, just cutting back on cholesterol is not enough. You must cut back on total fats as well. See page 260.

- Buy a cooking oil that is liquid at room temperature (such as canola, corn, soybean, sunflower, or cotton-seed oil) and use less of it.

- Eat two to three servings of fish per week. Most fish contain omega-3 fatty acids that help lower blood cholesterol and triglycerides. In general, fish with darker flesh, such as mackerel, lake trout, herring, salmon, and halibut, have more omega-3 oils. The safety and value of fish-oil supplements is not yet known.

- Exercise more. Exercise increases your protective HDL cholesterol level.

- Quit smoking. Quitting can increase your HDL levels and reduce your risk of heart disease.

- Lose extra pounds. Losing even 5 to 10 pounds can increase HDL levels and lower your total cholesterol.

- Eat more soluble fiber, which lowers overall cholesterol. See page 258.

- Attend a low-fat eating workshop, consult a registered dietitian, or read Resource 67 on page 310 to learn ways to lower your fat intake to 30 percent, 20 percent, or less of total calories, based on your goal.

Protein

Protein is important for maintaining healthy muscles, tendons, bones, skin, hair, blood, and internal organs. Most adult Americans get all the protein they need.

Protein deficiencies are rare. If you eat animal products (milk, cheese, eggs, fish, meat), your diet will contain plenty of protein. Even if you do not eat any animal products (vegans), if your diet includes a wide variety of vegetables, legumes, fruits, and breads and cereals, you will get all the protein you need.

Reversing Heart Disease

A low-fat diet and lifestyle changes may actually reverse the process of heart disease and help reopen arteries that are clogged by arteriosclerosis.

Participants in the Lifestyle Heart Trial followed a vegetarian diet containing less than 10 percent of calories from fat and no caffeine. They also stopped smoking, got 30 minutes of exercise at least six days a week, and practiced a relaxation technique (deep breathing, stretching, progressive muscle relaxation, etc.) for one hour each day. After a year, over 80 percent of the participants had lost weight, reduced their cholesterol, and most importantly, reduced the amount of blockage in their coronary arteries.

For more information, see Resource 44 on page 309.

Vitamins

Vitamins are exciting! These tiny, unseen elements of food have no calories, yet are essential to good health.

Vitamins A, D, E, and K are fat-soluble and can be stored in the liver or fat tissue for a relatively long time. The other nine are water-soluble and can be retained by the body for only short periods. They include:

- Thiamine
- Riboflavin
- Niacin
- Pantothenic acid
- Biotin
- Folate (folic acid)
- Vitamin B_6
- Vitamin B_{12}
- Vitamin C

For most people, a diet that contains a variety of foods from the Food Guide Pyramid provides all the vitamins needed for good health.

If you eat less than 1500 calories per day, consider a low-dose vitamin/mineral supplement.

Minerals

Minerals help regulate the body's water balance, hormones, enzymes, vitamins, and fluids. The various minerals must be maintained in delicate balance to ensure proper functioning of the systems they serve. Eating a variety of foods is the best way to get all the minerals you need.

Minerals – continued

To date, 60 minerals have been discovered in the body, and 22 are essential to health. We know the most about calcium, sodium, and iron.

Calcium

Calcium is the primary mineral needed for strong bones. Calcium is especially important to growing children and women, especially in the peak bone-building years between the teens and early 30s. Plenty of calcium in the diet helps build and maintain strong, healthy bones and helps women prevent osteoporosis, which can occur after menopause. See page 79.

Children age 1 to 10 need 800 mg of calcium per day. Teens and adults need 800 to 1200 mg per day. A cup of skim milk has about 313 mg of calcium. Nonfat and low-fat yogurt has 442 mg per cup. Other good sources of dietary calcium include broccoli, greens, kidney beans, and low-fat cheese.

While dietary calcium is preferred, low-dose calcium supplements can also help keep bones strong. One 500-mg TUMS (calcium carbonate) tablet provides about 200 mg of calcium. A few TUMS tablets per day can help adults meet their calcium needs, but should not replace natural forms of calcium such as milk and other dairy products, tofu, soy milk, broccoli, greens, or calcium-fortified orange juice.

Lactose Intolerance

People whose bodies produce too little of the enzyme lactase have trouble digesting the lactose sugar in milk. Symptoms of lactose intolerance include gas, bloating, cramps, and diarrhea after drinking milk or eating dairy products.

Tips for dealing with lactose intolerance include:

- Eat small amounts of dairy products at any one time.

- Drink milk only with snacks or meals.

- Try cheese, which usually does not cause symptoms. Most of the lactose is removed during processing.

- Yogurts made with active cultures provide their own enzymes and cause fewer tolerance problems.

- Pretreated milk, enzyme treatments, and enzyme tablets (LactAid, Dairy-Ease) are available in most stores.

- If you cannot tolerate milk in any form, include other calcium-rich foods in your diet. See left.

- Severe lactose intolerance may increase your need for calcium supplements. Ask your doctor.

Sodium

Most people get far more sodium than they need. Our bodies need only 500 mg of sodium per day. Anything over 2500 mg of sodium per day is probably too much.

For some people, excess sodium causes high blood pressure. If you are not sodium-sensitive, salt may not be a problem for you. See page 37.

Salt is the most familiar source of sodium. About 40 percent of salt is pure sodium. Sodium is also hidden in foods that don't taste salty, such as cheddar cheese and processed foods. Sodium is also a major ingredient of monosodium glutamate (MSG), disodium phosphate, and baking powder.

If you want to cut back on the sodium in your diet:

• Beware of ready-mixed sauces and seasonings, frozen dinners, canned soups, and salad dressings, which are usually packed with sodium. Products labelled "low sodium" contain less than 140 mg of sodium per serving.

• Eat lots of fresh or frozen fruits and vegetables. These foods have very little sodium.

• Don't put the salt shaker on the table or get a shaker that lets very little salt come out. Or, use Lite Salt or salt substitute sparingly.

• Always measure the salt in recipes and use half of what is called for.

Iron

Small amounts of iron are needed to make hemoglobin, which carries oxygen in the blood. Adults need about 10 to 15 mg of iron per day. People who have increased blood loss from ulcers or heavy menstrual periods, or who regularly take aspirin, blood thinners (anticoagulants), or arthritis medications may need more iron. An inexpensive blood test can determine if you need additional iron.

For more iron in your blood:

• Vitamin C helps you absorb more iron from food. Drink a glass of orange or other citrus juice and eat a bowl of iron-enriched cereal. High-iron cereals have at least 25 percent of the USRDA or Daily Value of iron.

• Increase absorption of vegetable iron by eating meat, poultry, or fish along with the vegetables. The iron in animal tissue improves the absorption of the iron in vegetables.

Iron Supplements

People who eat less than 1500 calories per day may wish to consider a multivitamin/mineral supplement that contains iron. A low-dose ferrous-form iron supplement containing no more than 20 mg is safe for most people. However, too much iron can cause a number of serious medical problems or mask the development of medical problems. Do not take more than 20 mg without consulting your doctor. Take the supplement with orange or other citrus juice. Keep iron supplements away from children.

Vitamin/Mineral Supplement Buyer's Guide

Although research is showing that vitamins from food intake may prevent some diseases, it remains unproven whether supplements do the same. However, if you choose to take vitamin and mineral supplements, the following guidelines may be helpful:

- Choose a balanced, multiple-vitamin/mineral supplement rather than a specific vitamin or mineral, unless it has been prescribed by a doctor. Too much of any one vitamin or mineral might be toxic and can interfere with the body's ability to use other vitamins and minerals.

- Choose a supplement that provides about 100 percent of the RDA (Recommended Dietary Allowances) for vitamins and minerals.

- Avoid taking much more than 100 percent of the RDA for any vitamin or mineral. This is particularly important for the fat-soluble vitamins A, D, E, and K and minerals. Because they are stored in the body, large doses can build up to toxic levels.

- Don't use a supplement to make up for a poor diet.

- High-priced brand-name vitamins or those sold door-to-door are no better than store or generic brands.

- Check expiration dates.

Minerals – continued

Iron Deficiency Anemia

Chronic blood loss of any kind depletes the body's store of iron. Symptoms of iron deficiency anemia include paleness and fatigue. A blood test is needed to confirm the diagnosis because anemia can be caused by many other things.

A Healthy Weight

People come in all shapes and sizes. Genetics, exercise, and the food you eat all play a role in determining your body's shape and size.

Focus on Health, Not Weight

Eating well, enjoying physical activity, and accepting your body size are the keys to good health. Although excess body fat does increase your risks of heart disease, diabetes, and stroke, it is more important to focus on healthy habits rather than trying to achieve a certain body size or shape.

When you eat healthy, lower-fat foods and add more regular physical activity to your life, you may lose some weight, but more importantly, you will have some health habits that you can maintain for life.

Exercise Makes It Easier

Regular exercise makes you feel stronger, more energetic, and in better overall health. As a bonus, regular exercise makes maintaining a healthy weight a little easier.

Small exercise steps, done every day or every other day, can make a big difference. Pick an exercise you enjoy enough to stick with for a long time. Even a five-minute walk every day is a good start. Add more exercise when you can.

Exercise Keeps You Strong

Exercise helps build your lean muscle mass when you are losing weight. One of the biggest problems with "diets" is that if you don't exercise while you diet, you will lose both fat and lean muscle mass. Dieting in general has not been shown to be healthful, and dieting without exercise can be detrimental. Dieters often suffer from weakness and low energy. If you are trying to lose weight, include a regular exercise program.

Creative Salt Substitute

Mix together and put in a shaker:

½ teaspoon cayenne pepper

½ teaspoon garlic powder

1 teaspoon each:

> Basil
>
> Black pepper
>
> Mace
>
> Marjoram
>
> Onion powder
>
> Parsley
>
> Sage
>
> Savory
>
> Thyme

Never Go Hungry

You may think that skipping a meal is a good way to lose weight. It is not. Going hungry, even for a few hours, can cause your metabolic rate to drop and make you more likely to overeat later. Take time to savor your food and relax during meals.

Focus on Fat, Not Calories

Eat a variety of nutritious, low-fat foods. Focus on eating more fruits and vegetables and on eating less fat, rather than counting calories. See the ways to reduce fat on page 260.

Get Help From Your Friends

The food customs and habits of friends and family affect what you eat. Ask friends and family to:

• Encourage you to respect yourself regardless of what you weigh.

• Celebrate events with a variety of nutritious foods and/or activities that everyone can enjoy.

• Serve low-fat options with meals, and make water and low-fat snacks available.

• Offer small servings, and don't insist on second helpings.

• Join you in a walk, swim, or other enjoyable activity.

Help Yourself to Good Thoughts

Develop a positive attitude about yourself. Think of yourself as healthy, and take pride in making positive nutrition and exercise choices. Focus on living a healthy life regardless of your weight.

Nutrition for Children

- Focus your whole family's diet on whole grains, fruits, vegetables, low-fat dairy products, and lean meats. Offer a wide variety of choices, but don't force a child to eat an unwanted food. Respect your child's ability to decide how much food to eat.

- Limit the amount of sugar in infants' and toddlers' diets. Your children can learn to enjoy healthy sweets, such as fruits.

- Avoid using food as a reward or punishment.

Child-Sized Environment

Imagine yourself eating at a giant's table. That's how a child can feel eating at an adult-sized table in an adult-sized chair.

- Provide a booster seat and child-sized utensils. However, fingers are fine until a child can hold utensils easily.

- Give children smaller plates and smaller servings (one tablespoon per year of age is a good serving size guide). Let the child ask for seconds.

Healthy Snacks

Young children have small stomachs and high energy needs, so they need frequent snacks to supplement meals. Plan between-meal snacks as part of the day's total food intake. They should provide good nutrition, not just empty calories.

- Fruits and fruit juices are good snacks. Other good choices are raw

---

Food Allergies

Less than one percent of adults have true food allergies. Most adverse reactions to foods are due to food intolerances, reactions to food additives, or food poisoning. Most true food allergies are to legumes, nuts, shellfish, eggs, wheat, and milk. An allergic reaction to a food can result in anaphylactic shock. See page 91.

Consider breast-feeding your child for at least the first six months if either parent has a history of any allergy, including hay fever. Children who are breast-fed develop fewer food allergies than those who are not. By gradually introducing simple solid foods into your child's diet, any allergy will be more easily found. Children often outgrow food allergies by age six. If your child was allergic to a food when younger, try reintroducing it as he gets older (unless the reaction was severe).

---

vegetable sticks with fat-free dressing, cereal, yogurt, cheese, or soup.

- When you serve cookies and other desserts, choose those that are low in fat and contain nutrients. Fig bars or oatmeal raisin cookies are good choices.

- Serve meals and snacks on a regular schedule. Do not serve snacks so close to a meal that they interfere with the child's appetite.

- For more information on feeding children, see Resources 27 and 28 on page 308.

Diabetes

The starches, sugars, fats, and protein in the food you eat are converted to glucose, a sugar that your body uses for fuel. Insulin is a hormone produced by the pancreas to control the amount of glucose in the blood. Without insulin, the body cannot use or store glucose, so it stays in the blood.

Type I, or insulin-dependent diabetes mellitus (IDDM), occurs when the pancreas fails to make enough insulin. It usually occurs in childhood or adolescence, but can develop at any age. People with type I diabetes must inject insulin every day.

Type II, or non-insulin-dependent diabetes mellitus (NIDDM), occurs when body cells become resistant to insulin. This reduces the amount of glucose that can be used by the cells at any one time. Type II diabetes is more common among adults, especially those who are overweight and over age 40.

Many people with type II diabetes are able to control their blood sugar through weight control, regular exercise, and a sensible diet. Some may need insulin injections or oral medications to lower blood sugar.

The following are risk factors for type II diabetes:

- Age 40 or over
- Overweight
- Family history of diabetes
- African-American, Hispanic, or Native American

The symptoms of diabetes are vague, and by themselves, seldom lead to a doctor visit. They include:

- Increased thirst
- Frequent urination
- Increased appetite
- Unexplained weight loss
- Fatigue
- Skin infections
- Slow-healing wounds
- Recurrent vaginitis
- Difficulty with erections
- Blurred vision
- Tingling or numbness in hands or feet

A blood test is needed to accurately diagnose diabetes. Blood glucose tests are inexpensive and very low risk. Ask your doctor if you should eat or fast before the test.

Prevention

At this time, there is no known way to prevent type I diabetes.

In most cases, the risk of type II diabetes can be reduced by regular, daily exercise (see Chapter 17) and by maintaining a healthy body weight.

Home Treatment

- Believe that you can control diabetes. Diabetes requires making significant, long-term lifestyle changes, and can be overwhelming at first. Focus on making one change at a time, and soon you will have good control over your life and your diabetes.

Diabetes – continued

- Take good care of your feet. Diabetes impairs nerve function and blood flow to the feet, increasing your risk of infection. Take care to avoid cuts and sores, and promptly treat any injuries to your feet.

- Get regular eye exams. Changes in the eye caused by diabetes often have no symptoms until they are quite advanced. Early treatment may slow their progress and save your sight.

- Eat a healthful diet. A proper diet helps keep your blood sugar in control and helps you maintain a healthy weight. Pay special attention to eating low-fat foods and to the other eating recommendations in this chapter.

- Get regular aerobic exercise to help regulate your blood sugar, reduce your risk of heart disease, and control your weight. Work closely with your doctor to determine how your activity level affects your blood glucose levels and medication needs.

- Track your diabetes for 30 days. Write down:

  ○ The time and content of each meal.

  ○ The kind and amount of exercise you get.

  ○ How tired or energetic you feel.

  ○ If you have a home glucose monitor, check your blood sugar level at least once a day at different times each day.

This will provide you with a lifelong tool for controlling your diabetes. Once you understand how your body reacts to different foods and exercise, you can correct glucose imbalances before they get out of control.

- Manage your medications. If drugs are prescribed to control your blood sugar, take them as directed. Too little medication will make your blood sugar higher than normal; too much will make it lower than normal. As you improve your diet and exercise, your need for medication may diminish. Check with your doctor.

- Each Kaiser Permanente Health Education Department has resources on diabetes, and nutritionists available to provide diet counseling to help you learn how to manage diabetes.

When to Call Kaiser Permanente

- If a person with diabetes loses consciousness.

- If signs of high blood sugar develop in a person who has diabetes:

  ○ Frequent urination

  ○ Intense thirst

  ○ Dim vision

  ○ Rapid breathing

  ○ Fruity-smelling breath

- If signs of low blood sugar persist after the person has eaten something containing sugar:

  - Fatigue, weakness, nausea

  - Hunger

  - Double or blurred vision

  - Pounding heart

  - Confusion, irritability, appearance of drunkenness

- For a blood glucose test, if you suspect diabetes but have not been diagnosed.

He who laughs, lasts.
Mary Pettibone Poole

Chapter 19

Mental Self-Care and Mental Wellness

Mental health problems are pretty much the same as other health problems. Some can be prevented; some will go away on their own with a little care and home treatment; and some need professional attention.

This chapter is organized in two sections. The first section, Mental Self-Care, covers some common mental and emotional health problems and describes what you can do at home and when you should seek professional help.

The second section, Mental Wellness, describes how you can enlist your mind and emotions to help you to better health.

Mental Self-Care

Medical science is discovering that mental health problems often have a physical cause. Psychological problems are no longer thought of as character weaknesses or flaws.

We now know that mental health problems can begin when psychological or emotional stress (such as the loss of a loved one) triggers chemical imbalances in the brain. While some people can withstand more stress than others, nobody is immune to mental illness.

Because the cause of mental health problems is both physical and psychological, both self-care and professional care are often needed. The goal is to reduce stress and to restore the normal chemical balance in the brain.

Seeking Professional Help

This chapter does not cover all mental health problems. If you have mental or emotional symptoms that are concerning and are not addressed here,

Mental Self-Care – continued

contact your health professional. In general, it is a good idea to seek professional help when:

- A symptom becomes severe or disruptive.

- A disruptive symptom becomes a continuous or permanent pattern of behavior and does not respond to self-care efforts.

- Symptoms become numerous and affect all areas of a person's life and do not respond to self-care or communication efforts.

- The person is thinking of suicide.

There is a wide range of professional and lay resources to choose from for mental health problems.

Family doctor: Mental health problems may have physical causes. Your doctor can review your medical history and medications for clues, provide some counseling, prescribe medications, or refer you to other resources.

Psychiatrists and psychologists: Doctors who specialize in mental disorders and counsel patients. Psychiatrists also prescribe medications and order medical treatments.

Social workers and counselors: These professionals have special training to help people deal with mental health problems. They help patients identify, understand, and work through disturbing thoughts and emotions.

Pastors: People often turn to their clergy for counseling and advice in times of emotional distress. Many

---

Therapist Selection Tips

Here are some ways to improve your likelihood of finding the therapy that's right for you.

- Call a Kaiser Permanente Mental Health office.

- Use mental health professionals to help you identify the real problem and develop a self-management plan to resolve it.

- Emphasize the importance of self-care in the treatment plan.

- Ask about group therapy options.

- Cultivate special friends, join support groups, or look for peer counseling opportunities. Understanding and acceptance can help you resolve the problem.

- Check out 12-step programs such as Alcoholics Anonymous, Overeaters Anonymous, and other groups that can help you deal with addiction problems. Such programs are usually free, effective, and available in most communities.

---

pastors have formal training in counseling, and many do not.

Support groups: Focusing on virtually every mental health issue.

Health education classes: Stress reduction, anger management, and a variety of other classes are available at many Kaiser Permanente facilities.

Alcohol and Drug Problems

The overuse or abuse of alcohol or other drugs is called substance abuse. It is common, costly, and associated with many medical problems.

Alcohol Problems

A person has an **alcohol problem** if the use of alcohol interferes with health or daily living. A person develops **alcoholism** if he or she becomes physically or psychologically dependent on alcohol.

Long-term heavy drinking causes liver, nerve, heart and brain damage, high blood pressure, stomach problems, sexual problems, and cancer. Alcohol abuse can also lead to violence, accidents, social isolation, and difficulties at work and home.

Symptoms of an alcohol problem include personality changes, blackouts, drinking more and more for the same "high," and denial of the problem. The person may also have family or work problems, or get in trouble with the law due to their drinking. A person with alcoholism may gulp or sneak drinks, drink alone or early in the morning, and suffer from the shakes.

Alcohol abuse patterns vary. Some people get drunk every day. Some drink large amounts of alcohol at specific times, such as weekends. Others may be sober for long periods and then go on a drinking binge that lasts for weeks or months.

Someone who is physically dependent on alcohol may suffer serious withdrawal symptoms (such as trembling, delusions, hallucinations, and sweating) if he or she stops drinking suddenly ("cold turkey"). Once alcohol dependency develops, it becomes very difficult to abstain without outside help. Medical detoxification in an inpatient program may be needed.

Signs of Drug Use

- Chronic red eyes, sore throat, dry cough, and fatigue (in the absence of allergies).

- Major changes in sleeping or eating habits.

- Moodiness, hostility, or abusive behavior.

- Work or school problems, absenteeism.

- Loss of interest in favorite activities.

- Social withdrawal or changes in friends.

- Stealing, lying, and poor family relationships.

Drug Problems

Drug abuse includes both the use of marijuana, cocaine, heroin, or other "street drugs," and the abuse of legal prescription drugs. Some people turn to drugs as a way to get a "high" or to deal with stress and emotional problems.

Alcohol, Drug Problems – cont.

Tranquilizers, sedatives, painkillers, and amphetamines are misused most often, sometimes unintentionally. Women are at particular risk; over two-thirds of all tranquilizers are prescribed for women.

Drug dependence or addiction occurs when you develop a physical or psychological "need" for a drug. You may not be aware that you have become dependent on a drug until you try to stop taking it suddenly. Withdrawing from the drug can cause uncomfortable symptoms. The usual treatment is to gradually reduce the dose of the drug until it can be stopped completely.

Screening Test

Many people will deny that they have a problem with alcohol or other drugs. The questions in the "Are You a Problem User?" chart on page 277 may help you, or others, recognize a problem.

Answering yes to two or more questions raises the possibility of an alcohol or drug problem and the need for more help.

Prevention

- Look for signs of mental stress. Try to understand and resolve sources of depression, anxiety, or loneliness. Don't use alcohol or drugs to deal with these problems.

- If you drink, do so in moderation: less than two drinks a day for men and one drink a day for women. One drink is 12 ounces of beer, 5 ounces of wine, or 1½ ounces of hard liquor.

- Provide nonalcoholic beverages at parties and meals.

- Ask your pharmacist or doctor if any of your current medications could potentially lead to overuse problems. Be especially cautious of painkillers, tranquilizers, sedatives, and sleeping pills. Follow the instructions carefully, and do not exceed the recommended dose.

- Do not regularly use medications to sleep, lose weight, or relax without careful supervision by your doctor. Seek non-drug solutions.

- Do not suddenly stop taking any medication without your doctor's supervision. Serious symptoms can result if some medications are abruptly withdrawn.

- Avoid alcohol when you are taking medications. Alcohol can react with many drugs and cause serious complications.

Home Treatment

- Recognize early signs that alcohol or drug use is becoming a problem. See page 277.

- Attend an Alcoholics Anonymous meeting (a self-help group devoted to helping members get sober and stay sober).

- If you are concerned about another person's alcohol or drug use:

  ○ Build up his self-esteem. Reaffirm his value as a person. Help him see himself succeeding in life without alcohol or drugs. Let him know you will support his efforts to change.

- Never ignore the problem. Discuss it as a medical problem.

- Ask if he would accept help. Don't give up after the first no. Keep asking. If he agrees, act that very day to arrange for help. Call a health professional or Alcoholics Anonymous for an immediate appointment.

- Attend a few meetings of Al-Anon, a support group for family members and friends of alcoholics. Read some 12-step program information.

When to Call Kaiser Permanente

- If you answer yes to two or more questions on the "Are You a Problem User?" chart below.

- If you recognize an alcohol or drug problem and are ready to accept help.

Are You a Problem User?

Answer the questions honestly for yourself. Answer "yes" if the statement is true for you for alcohol or drugs (including prescribed, recreational, or illegal substances that can be described as mood-altering).

1. Have you ever decided to stop using alcohol or drugs for a week or so but could stop for only a couple days?

2. Do you resent the advice of others who try to get you to stop or cut down your use of alcohol or drugs?

3. Have you tried to control your use of alcohol or drugs by changing from one type of drink or drug to another?

4. Do you envy people who can use alcohol/drugs without getting into trouble?

5. Has your use of alcohol or drugs impaired your family relationships, your work, your driving safety, or any other aspect of your life?

6. During the past year, have you missed days of work because of your use of alcohol or drugs?

7. Do you tell yourself you can stop using alcohol or drugs any time you want?

8. Do you sometimes go on binges with alcohol or drugs?

9. Do you ever have blackouts related to use of alcohol or drugs?

10. Have you ever felt that your life would be better if you did not use alcohol or drugs?

If you answer "yes" to two or more questions, you may have a problem with alcohol or drugs. If so, talk with a health professional.

Anger and Hostility

Anger signals your body to prepare for a fight. Hostility is being ready for a fight all the time.

When you get angry, adrenaline and other hormones are released into the blood stream. Blood pressure goes up. Continual hostility keeps the blood pressure high and may increase your risk for heart attack and other illnesses. Being hostile also isolates you from other people.

Home Treatment

- Notice when you first get angry. Don't ignore anger until it erupts.

- Identify the cause of the anger.

- Express anger in a healthy way:

  ○ Talk about it with a friend.

  ○ Draw or paint to release the anger.

  ○ Go for a short walk or jog.

  ○ Try screaming or yelling in a private place.

  ○ Write in a daily journal.

  ○ Count to 10. Give yourself a little time for your adrenaline level to go down.

- Use "I" statements, not "you" statements, to discuss your anger. Say "I feel angry when my needs are not being met," instead of "You make me mad when you are so inconsiderate."

- Forgive and forget. Forgiving helps lower blood pressure and ease muscle tension so you can feel more relaxed.

- Books on anger can help. See Resources 10 to 12 on page 307.

- See page 286 for additional information on anger and violent behavior.

When to Call Kaiser Permanente

- If anger has led or could lead to violence or harm to you or someone else.

- If anger or hostility interferes with your work, family, or friends.

Anxiety

Feeling worried, anxious, and nervous is a normal part of everyday life. Everyone frets or feels anxious from time to time. However, it is not normal when anxiety becomes overwhelming and interferes with daily life.

Anxiety symptoms can be divided into two categories: physical and emotional.

Physical Symptoms

- Trembling, twitching, or shaking

- Muscle tension, aches, or soreness

- Restlessness

- Fatigue

- Insomnia

- Breathlessness or rapid heartbeat

- Sweating or cold, clammy hands

Emotional Symptoms

- Feeling keyed up and on edge

- Excessive worrying

- Fearing that something bad is going to happen

- Poor concentration

- Excessive startle response

- Irritability or agitation

- Constant sadness

Anxiety from a specific situation or fear can cause some or all of these symptoms for a short time. When the situation passes, the symptoms subside.

Many people, including children and adolescents, develop anxiety disorders in which many of these symptoms occur when there is no identifiable cause.

Phobias and panic disorder are two common anxiety-related disorders. **Phobias** are irrational, involuntary fears of common places, objects, or situations. **Panic disorder** is characterized by distinct periods of intense fear and anxiety that occur when there is no clear cause or danger. Physical symptoms that may occur during a panic attack include hyperventilation, shaking, pounding of the heart, and feeling faint. Self-care, often combined with professional treatment, can be effective in managing these disorders.

Home Treatment

The following home treatment tips relieve simple anxiety and help in combination with medical care.

- Recognize and accept anxiety about specific fears or situations. Then say to yourself, "Okay, I see the problem. Now I'll start to deal with it."

- Be kind to your body:
  - Vigorous exercise relieves tension as does massage.
  - Practice relaxation techniques. See page 252.
  - Get enough rest. If you have trouble sleeping, see Sleep Problems on page 284.
  - Avoid alcohol, caffeine, chocolate, and nicotine. They increase your anxiety level.

- Engage your mind:
  - Do something you enjoy, such as going to a funny movie or taking a hike.
  - Plan your day. Having too much or too little to do can make you anxious.

- Keep a record of your symptoms and talk about them with a friend. Confiding with others sometimes relieves stress.

- Get involved with helping others. Being alone makes things seem worse than they are.

- Learn more about anxiety. See Resources 13 and 14 on page 307.

When to Call Kaiser Permanente

- If anxiety interferes with your daily activities.

- If anxiety is creating significant discomfort, and home treatment does not help.

Anxiety – continued

- If symptoms are severe and one week of home treatment has not helped.

- If you have sudden, severe attacks of fear or anxiety with intense physical symptoms (shaking, sweating) when there is no apparent reason to be afraid.

- If intense, irrational fears of common places, objects, or situations interfere with your daily life.

- If you suffer from nightmares or flashbacks to traumatic events.

- If you are unable to feel certain about things (e.g., whether you unplugged the iron) no matter how many times you check, or if repetitive, compulsive behaviors interfere with your daily activities.

Depression

Most people experience some form of depression at some point in their lives. Depression can range from a minor problem to a major life-threatening illness. Depression is treatable. For many people, treatment can mean a whole new life.

Medical science is getting closer to understanding depression. Most major depressions involve an imbalance of chemical messengers (neurotransmitters) in the brain. Many things can trigger these imbalances:

- Loss of a loved one or something that is highly valued

- Chronic stress or a stressful event

Sadness or Depression?

If you have experienced four or more of the following symptoms nearly every day for more than two weeks, you may be suffering from depression:

- Feelings of sadness, anxiety, or hopelessness

- Lack of interest or pleasure in usual activities or pastimes

- Increase or decrease in appetite or unexplained gain or loss of weight

- Frequent backaches, headaches, stomach problems, or other aches that don't respond to treatment

- Insomnia or excessive sleepiness

- Low energy, fatigue, tiredness

- Feeling restless or irritable

- Feeling worthless or guilty

- Inability to concentrate, remember, or make decisions

- Frequent thoughts of suicide or death

Home treatment (see page 281) may be all that is needed for mild depression. However, if suicide is a risk or if home treatment doesn't help lift your mood within two weeks, contact a health professional. With counseling and medication, combined with continued home treatment, you can successfully deal with most cases of depression.

- Major illness

- Reaction to medications

- Alcoholism, drug abuse, dementia, and other mental health problems

- Reduced daylight during the winter seems to cause a form of depression called seasonal affective disorder in some people. See right.

Some people are genetically susceptible to chemical imbalances in the brain. For these and others at high risk of depression, it is fortunate that effective treatments are available.

Everyone gets sad. Gauging how deep and pervasive your sad feelings are can help you decide what to do. See "Sadness or Depression?" on page 280 to help determine if you are suffering from depression.

Feeling sad doesn't always mean you are heading for a major depression. Bad news or disappointment can make you feel sad, perhaps for several days without relief. This is normal and healthy as long as those sad feelings don't continue indefinitely. Grief can also cause a normal sadness. See page 282.

Home Treatment

No matter how depressed you are, you can recover. Self-care may be enough to pull you out of a mild depression. For more serious depression, self-care can add to the benefits of professional treatment.

- At the first sign of depression, ask a friend for some extra attention. You can lose objectivity about yourself when you feel blue.

Seasonal Affective Disorder (Winter Depression)

There is increasing evidence (not yet conclusive) that a lack of sunlight during winter months can cause depression in some people. Symptoms include melancholy moods, changes in sleeping habits, cravings for sweets and starchy foods, and chronic fatigue. If you notice such a pattern developing during the winter, consider the following:

- When the sun does shine, go outside and soak it up. Protect your skin—it is the eye's exposure to sunlight that makes the difference.

- Go south for a sunny vacation, if you can.

- Some people may benefit from light therapy: sitting in front of bright, full-spectrum fluorescent lights for one to five hours a day. Depression often improves by the end of the first week of daily treatments.

Because it is a new approach to winter depression, the National Institutes of Health recommend that light therapy be supervised by a health professional.

- Consider what might be causing or adding to your depression:

  ○ Are medications causing it? Review your prescription and over-the-counter medications with a pharmacist or doctor.

Depression – continued

○ If it's wintertime or you haven't been out in the sun for a while, read the information about seasonal affective disorder on page 281.

• Keep on going. It is easier to *do* yourself into *feeling* better than to *feel* yourself into *doing* better.

Grief

Grief is a natural healing process that allows a person to adjust to a significant change or loss. Grief may be expressed physically or emotionally, and may have some of the same symptoms as depression. The following tips may help ease the grieving process.

• Take time to grieve. Actively review mementos, play nostalgic music, and read old letters. Take as much time as you need.

• Let yourself cry. If you can let go and sob, do it.

• Talk about your grief with a friend. If your friend tells you to "snap out of it," find a more sympathetic listener. Your clergy may also help you understand and deal with your loss.

• Friends may feel awkward about mentioning your loss. Let them know it is alright to talk about it.

• Get regular exercise. If nothing else, go for long walks. They help to clear the mind.

• Look for a laugh. Laughter, like exercise, can help restore balance to your system.

• Boost your self-esteem. Read the Mental Wellness section of this chapter.

• Tell yourself that this mood will pass. Then, look for signs that it is ending.

• Surround yourself with happy, upbeat people.

• Books can help. See Resource 33 on page 309.

When to Call Kaiser Permanente

Health professionals can do a great deal to help you through depression. The most common form of treatment combines counseling (psychotherapy) with medication. Inpatient treatment is sometimes needed in severe cases or if the risk of suicide is high. Because many things can contribute to depression, combining self-care and professional treatment is often most helpful.

• If you are feeling suicidal.

• If you suspect you are very depressed. See "Sadness or Depression?" on page 280.

• If you suspect you are depressed and two weeks of home treatment has not helped.

Eating Disorders

In a society where "thin is in," many of us have tried skipping meals or going on diets to lose weight. People with eating disorders have taken this to an extreme; their eating patterns have become abnormal.

Anorexia nervosa is a disorder of severe self-imposed dieting. It affects teenage girls most often. Symptoms include a refusal to eat, extreme weight loss, a distorted body image (thinking she's fat when she is actually very thin), a preoccupation with food, low self-esteem, and excessive physical exercise.

Bulimia nervosa is an eating disorder characterized by binge eating and purging (forced vomiting or the abuse of laxatives and diuretics). The binges are usually triggered by emotional upset, not hunger. Other symptoms include dry skin and brittle hair, swollen glands under the jaw from vomiting, depression and mood swings, a distorted body image, and secrecy to keep others from discovering their abnormal eating behaviors.

Unlike anorexia, whose victims look starved, most people who have bulimia maintain a normal weight and look healthy. Generally, people with anorexia deny they have a problem; people with bulimia know that they do, but keep it a secret.

Compulsive overeating is characterized by binging on food. Thousands of calories will be consumed at a time, quickly and without pleasure. Because there is no purging, the compulsive overeater becomes obese.

Eating disorders appear to be caused by emotional and psychological factors. They also tend to run in families, and there may be a genetic link.

Eating disorders require professional treatment. If untreated, they can lead to major health problems or even death. Treatment may include nutritional therapy, individual psychotherapy, and family therapy. A hospital stay may be required in extreme cases. Your Kaiser Permanente Health Education Department can give you more information and referrals to self-help groups for eating disorders.

Prevention

- Teach and model healthy eating and exercise habits at home and at school.

- Help young people develop confidence and self-esteem. Accept them for who they are.

- Be careful about encouraging a young person to lose weight. Communicate that you love and care for her, regardless of how much she weighs.

- Don't put unrealistic expectations on your child. Striving to live up to them may lead to an eating disorder.

- Be alert to the stress in your child's life. Be available to talk over any problems.

When to Call Kaiser Permanente

If you recognize any of these warning signs:

- Using body weight as a primary measure of self-worth.

Eating Disorders – continued

- Unrealistic body image.

- Significant unexplained weight loss or gain.

- Constant dieting on highly restricted diets. Unrealistic fears of gaining weight.

- Obsessive exercise routines, especially leading to injury.

- Withdrawal from family and friends.

Sleep Problems

The term insomnia can mean:

- Trouble getting to sleep (taking more than 45 minutes to fall asleep).

- Frequent wakenings with inability to fall back to sleep.

- Early morning awakening.

However, none of these are problems unless they make you feel chronically tired. If you are less sleepy at night or wake up early, but still feel rested and alert, there is little need to worry.

Short-term insomnia, lasting from a few nights to a few weeks, is usually caused by worry over a stressful situation. Long-term insomnia, which can last months or even years, is most often caused by general anxiety, medications, chronic pain, depression, apnea (breathing problems that disrupt sleep), or other physical disorders.

Prevention

- Get regular exercise but avoid strenuous exercise within two hours before bedtime.

- Avoid alcohol and smoking before bedtime. Drink caffeine in moderation and not after noon.

- Avoid drinking more than a glass of fluid before bedtime.

Home Treatment

- Don't take sleeping pills. They can cause daytime confusion, memory loss, and dizziness. Continued use of sleeping pills actually increases sleeplessness in many people. Instead, get regular exercise and drink a glass of warm milk before bedtime.

- Try the following six-step formula for two weeks:

  1. Use your bed for sleeping. Don't eat, watch TV, or even read in it.

  2. Sleep only at bedtime. Don't take naps. (However, naps are fine if you don't have sleep problems.)

  3. Forget "bedtime." Go to bed only when you feel sleepy.

  4. Get out of bed and leave the room anytime you lie awake for more than 15 minutes.

  5. Repeat steps 3 and 4 until it is time to get up.

  6. Get up at the same time each day, no matter how sleepy you are.

- Review all of your prescription and over-the-counter medications with a pharmacist to rule out drug-related sleep problems.

- Read about anxiety on page 278.

When to Call Kaiser Permanente

- If you suspect medications are causing sleep problems.

- If a month of self-care doesn't solve the problem.

Suicide

If you are very depressed or feel overwhelmed, you may sometimes think of taking your own life. Occasional thoughts of suicide are not a problem. However, if thoughts of suicide continue, or if you have made suicide plans, it becomes a very serious matter.

People who are considering suicide are often undecided about choosing life or death. With compassionate help, they may choose to live.

Prevention

When you are depressed, or when someone you know is depressed, be alert to the warning signs:

- Verbal warning. Up to 80 percent of people who commit suicide mention their intentions to someone.

- Preoccupation with death. The suicidal person may talk, read, draw, and write about death.

- Previous suicide attempt. Failed attempts are often followed by a successful attempt.

- Giving away prized possessions.

- Depression and social isolation. See page 280.

Home Treatment

- Use your common sense and a direct approach to determine if the risk is high. Ask yourself or the person who you feel is at risk:

  ○ Do you feel there is no other way?

  ○ Do you have a suicide plan?

  ○ How and when do you plan to do it?

- Arrange for a trusted person to stay with you or with the suicidal person until the crisis has passed.

- Encourage the person to seek professional help.

- Don't argue with the person ("It's not as bad as that"). Also, don't challenge the person ("You're not the type").

- Don't ignore warning signs, thinking that you or another person will snap out of it.

- Talk with the person as matter-of-factly as possible. Show understanding and compassion.

When to Call Kaiser Permanente

- For urgent, life-threatening situations, call 861-3434, 911, or other emergency services.

- Call your doctor, Kaiser Permanente Mental Health office, or your local Suicide Prevention hotline (look in the Yellow Pages):

  ○ If you are considering suicide.

  ○ If you suspect someone has made suicide plans.

Violent Behavior

Anger and arguments are normal parts of healthy relationships. However, anger that leads to violence such as hitting, hurting, or threatening, is not normal or healthy. Physical, verbal, or sexual abuse is not an acceptable part of any relationship.

Violent behavior often begins with relatively minor incidents or threats, but over time can become more serious, involving physical harm. Violent behavior seems to be mostly learned, so it is especially important to help your children learn that violence is not a healthy solution to conflict.

Prevention

- Seek nonviolent ways to resolve conflicts. Arguing is fine, even healthy, so long as it does not turn violent. See page 278 for more on controlling anger.

- Avoid physical discipline so that your children will learn that violence is not a solution. If you have concerns about parenting, consider taking a course on parenting skills. Also see page 154.

To prevent violence with firearms and other weapons:

- Make sure that no one in the home will have access to firearms or weapons unless they know how to use them safely.

- Lock up firearms unloaded. Lock ammunition in a separate place.

- Do not keep loaded firearms in a home where there are children or where there is someone who has a drug or alcohol problem, who is prone to violent behavior, or who has threatened suicide.

If a family member or someone else has threatened to harm you or your child:

- Confide in someone: a trusted friend, clergy, or health professional. In Colorado, mental health professionals and doctors are required by law to report physical assault to the local law enforcement authorities.

- Identify local resources that can help in a crisis. Your local YMCA, police department, or hospital has information on shelters and safe homes.

- Be alert to warning signs, such as threats or drunkenness, so that you can avoid a dangerous situation. If you can't predict when violence will occur, have an "exit plan" for use in an emergency.

When to Call Kaiser Permanente

- If you or someone in your family is physically abused or the victim of violence. Physical abuse is a crime, no matter who does it.

- If you have any concerns about violent behavior in yourself, a family member, or friend.

Check the Yellow Pages for hotlines and other resources for victims of abuse. Your Kaiser Permanente Mental Health offices also have resources available.

Mental Wellness

Mental wellness means thinking and feeling positive about yourself. You may have heard of psychosomatic illness, when a person "thinks" himself into being sick. Evidence now supports the idea of psychosomatic wellness. For sickness and for health, what you think has some influence on your health and well-being.

The Mind-Body Connection

Medical science is making remarkable discoveries about how expectations, emotions, and thoughts affect our health. This science is called psycho-neuroimmunology, or PNI. It studies how the brain communicates with the rest of the body by sending chemical messengers into the blood.

Researchers have found that one function of the brain is to produce substances that can improve your health. Your brain can create natural painkillers called endorphins, gamma-globulin for fortifying your immune system, and interferon for combatting infections, viruses, and even cancer.

Your brain can combine these and other substances into a vast number of tailor-made prescriptions for what ails you. The substances that your brain produces depend in part on your thoughts and feelings.

Your immune system's ability to heal the body is linked to your state of mind and your state of mental wellness. Your level of optimism and your expectations of what could happen can affect what goes on inside your whole body.

Positive Thinking

People with positive attitudes generally enjoy life more. Aside from that, are they any healthier? The answer is often yes.

Optimism is a resource for healing. Optimists are more likely to overcome pain and adversity in their efforts to improve their medical treatment outcomes. For example, optimistic coronary bypass patients generally recover more quickly and have fewer postoperative complications than people who are less hopeful.

Conversely, pessimism seems to aggravate ill health. One long-term study showed that people who were pessimistic in college have significantly higher rates of illness through age 60.

We seem to develop a tendency toward either optimism or pessimism at an early age. However, even if your outlook on life tends to be gloomy, you can enjoy psychosomatic wellness by using your brain to support your immune system.

Boosting Your Immune System

Your immune system responds to your thoughts, emotions, and actions. In addition to staying fit, eating right, and managing stress, the following three strategies will help your immune system function better:

1. Create positive expectations for health and healing.

2. Open yourself to humor, friendship, and love.

3. Appeal to the Spirit.

Mental Wellness – continued

1. Create positive expectations for health and healing.

Mental and emotional expectations can influence medical outcomes. The effectiveness of any medical treatment depends in part on how useful you *expect* it to be.

The placebo effect is proof that expectations affect health. A placebo is a drug or treatment that provides no medical benefit except for the patient's belief that it will help. On the average, 35 percent of patients who receive placebos report satisfactory relief from their medical problem, even though they received no actual medication.

Changing your expectations from negative to positive may give your immune system a boost. Here's how:

- Stop all negative self-talk. Make statements that promote your recovery.

- Write your illness a letter. Tell it that you don't need it anymore and that your immune system is now ready to finish it off.

- Send yourself a steady stream of affirmations. An affirmation is a phrase or sentence that sends strong, positive statements to you about yourself, such as "I am a capable person," or "My joints are strong and flexible."

- Visualize health and healing. Add mental pictures that support your positive affirmations.

- Become a cheerleader for your immune system. Talk to it and encourage it to keep up the fight.

2. Open yourself to humor, friendship, and love.

Positive emotions strengthen the immune system. Fortunately, almost anything that makes you feel good about yourself helps you stay healthy.

- Laugh. Life with a little humor mixed in is richer and healthier. Laughter increases creativity, reduces pain, and speeds healing. Keep an emergency laughter kit of funny videotapes, jokes, cartoons, and photographs. Put it with your first-aid supplies and keep it well stocked.

- Seek out friends. Friendships are vital to good health. Close social ties help you recover more quickly from illness and reduce your risk of developing diseases ranging from arthritis to depression.

- Volunteer. People who volunteer live longer and enjoy life more than those who do not. By helping others, we help ourselves.

- Plant a plant and pet a pet. Plants and pets can be highly therapeutic. When you stroke an animal, blood pressure goes down and your heart rate slows. Animals and plants help us feel needed.

3. Appeal to the Spirit.

If you believe in a higher power, ask for support in your pursuit of healing and health. Faith, prayer, and spiritual beliefs can play an important role in recovering from an illness.

Your sense of spiritual wellness can help you overcome personal trials and things you cannot change. If it suits you, use spiritual images in visualizations, affirmations, and expectations about your health and your life.

Hardiness

Some people seem to have more protection from disease than others. Their immune systems appear to be more efficient. Researchers studying these hardy people have identified three personality factors that stand out.

1. Hardy people have a strong commitment to self, work, family, and other values.

2. Hardy people have a sense of control over their lives.

3. Hardy people generally see change in their lives as a challenge rather than a threat.

Developing a Hardy Personality

Can you develop more commitment, control, and acceptance of life's challenges? Apparently so, particularly if you start at an early age. You can help your children become hardy by encouraging them in the following ways:

• Help them develop a sense of commitment by providing strong parental encouragement and acceptance. The more accepted a child feels, the more he will be able to commit himself to others.

• Help them develop a sense of control by continually providing a variety of tasks that are neither too difficult nor too simple. Experience with both success and failure followed by success helps to build a sense of control.

• Encourage children to see changes as opportunities for enrichment rather than losses. Accentuate the positive and teach them that some losses are a part of life.

Adults can also develop hardiness. Training to develop more commitment, control, and challenge has proven to be effective.

Remaining Guiltless

There is no value in feeling guilty about health problems. While there is a lot we can do to reduce our risk of health problems and improve our chances of recovery, some illnesses develop and persist no matter what we do. Try to avoid feeling guilty, especially in applying the mental self-care suggestions in this chapter. If what you do helps, terrific. However, if your illness persists despite your best efforts, don't blame yourself. Some things just are. Do the best you can.

Chapter 20

Your Home Health Center

More health care happens in your home than anywhere else. Having the right tools, medicines, supplies, and information on hand will improve its quality.

Store all your self-care resources in one central location, such as a large drawer in the bedroom or family room. Use the charts on tools and supplies, and the list of resources in this chapter as checklists for keeping your home health center well stocked.

Note: If small children are around, keep your supplies out of reach or protected by childproof safety latches.

Self-Care Tools

Self-care tools are the basic equipment of your home health center.

Cold Pack

A cold pack is a plastic envelope filled with gel that remains flexible at very cold temperatures. Buy two cold packs and keep them in the freezer. Use them for bumps, bruises, back sprains, turned ankles, sore joints, or any other health problem that calls for ice. A cold pack is more convenient than ice and may become the self-care tool you use the most.

You can make your own cold pack:

• Half fill a one-gallon heavy duty plastic freezer bag with one pint rubbing alcohol and 3 pints water.

• Seal the bag and then seal it in a second bag. Mark it "Cold pack: Do not eat," and place it in the freezer.

A bag of frozen vegetables will also work as a cold pack.

Self-Care Tools – continued

Humidifier and Vaporizer

Humidifiers and vaporizers add moisture to the air, making it less drying to your mouth, throat, and nose. A humidifier produces a cool mist and a vaporizer puts out hot steam.

A humidifier has several advantages: it can't burn you; it makes tinier particles of water that get into your respiratory system better; it can't hurt the furniture; and the cool mist is more comfortable than hot steam.

However, humidifiers are noisy, produce particles that may be irritating, and they need to be cleaned and disinfected after each use. This is especially important for people who have mold allergies.

A vaporizer's hot steam does not contain any irritating particles, and may feel good when you have a cold, but the hot water can burn anyone who overturns it or gets too close.

Humidity in the air can help to soothe a scratchy throat, ease a dry, hacking cough, and make it easier for someone with a stuffy nose to breathe. Added humidity will make your home more comfortable, especially in the winter when dry air is a problem.

Medicine Spoon

Medicine spoons are transparent tubes with marks for typical dosage amounts. A medicine spoon makes it easy to give the right dose of liquid medicine. While the spoons are convenient for anyone, they are a particular blessing for young children. The tube shape and large lip get most

---

Self-Care Tools

For every household:

- Blood pressure cuff*
- Cold pack*
- Dental mirror
- Eyedropper
- Heating pad
- Humidifier or vaporizer
- Medicine spoon*
- Nail clippers
- Penlight*
- Scissors
- Stethoscope*
- Thermometer*
- Tweezers

For children under six, add:

- Bulb aspirator/syringe
- Rectal thermometer*
- Otoscope*

*Described in text

---

of the medication inside the child without spilling. Buy one at your local pharmacy.

Otoscope

An otoscope is a flashlight with a special attachment for looking into the ear. With practice, using an otoscope can help you decide if an ear infection is present. Inexpensive consumer model otoscopes are available but do not illuminate the ear canal and eardrum as well as the one your doctor uses. They can also be used as high-intensity penlights. One product is the Earscope, which can be ordered for around $26.95 from Notoco, P.O. Box 300, Ferndale, CA 95536, (707) 786-4400.

Penlight

A penlight has a small intense light that can be easily directed. It is useful for giving a physical exam and is easier to handle than a flashlight.

Stethoscope and Blood Pressure Cuff

If you have high blood pressure, it's a good idea to have both a stethoscope and a blood pressure cuff (sphygmomanometer) to monitor your blood pressure regularly.

For a stethoscope, purchase a flat diaphragm model rather than a bell-shaped one. The flat surface makes it easier for you to hear.

Blood pressure cuffs come in many models. If you have difficulty reading

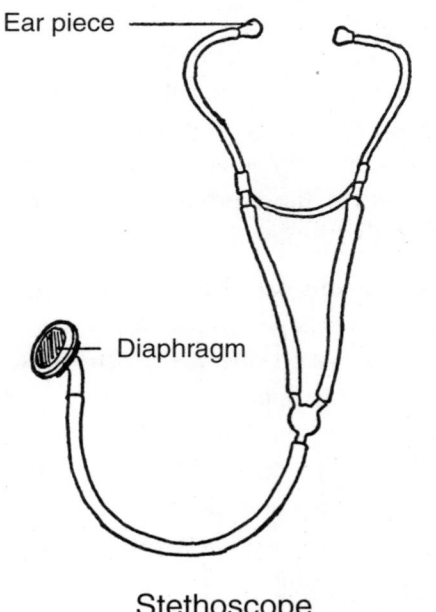

Ear piece

Diaphragm

Stethoscope

the gauge on a regular cuff, look for one attached to an upright mercury column, or an electronic digital model. Ask your pharmacist or Kaiser Permanente Health Education Department staff to recommend a blood pressure kit and show you how to use it.

Thermometer

Buy a thermometer with easy-to-read markings. Digital electronic thermometers are accurate and easy to read. Temperature strips are very convenient and safe, but are not as accurate as mercury or electronic thermometers and should only be used to measure axillary (armpit) temperature. Thermometers that measure the temperature in the ear are fast, easy to use, and can be quite accurate, but are expensive.

Rectal thermometers with enlarged bulbs are helpful for children under six or anyone who cannot hold an oral thermometer in his mouth. See page 32 for instructions on taking a temperature.

Self-Care Supplies

See the Self-Care Supplies chart (next page) for a list of supplies that are useful to keep on hand in your home health center. These products are inexpensive, easy to use, and generally available at any drugstore or pharmacy.

Over-the-Counter (OTC) Medications and Products

An over-the-counter (OTC) medication is any drug that you can buy without a doctor's prescription. However, don't assume that all OTC drugs are safe for you. These drugs

OTC Medications – continued

can interact with other medications and can sometimes create serious health problems.

Carefully read the label of any over-the-counter drug you use, especially if you also take prescription medications for other health problems. Ask your pharmacist for help in finding the one best suited to your needs.

Some common OTCs include:
- Antacids
- Antidiarrheals
- Cold and allergy remedies
- Laxatives
- Pain relievers, such as aspirin, ibuprofen, naproxen, and acetaminophen

These drugs can be very helpful when used properly, but can also create serious problems if used incorrectly. The following tips will help you use these common OTC drugs wisely and safely. In some cases, you may find that you don't need to take them at all. The chart on page 295 lists common health problems and suggestions for OTC products to treat them.

These medications are available at discounted prices to members at Kaiser Permanente Pharmacies.

Antacids

Antacids are taken to relieve heartburn or indigestion caused by excess stomach acid. While they are safe if used occasionally, antacids may cause problems if taken regularly. There are several kinds of antacids. Get to know what ingredients are in each type so that you can avoid any adverse effects.

Self-Care Supplies

Keep these on hand:
- Adhesive strips ("Band-aids") in assorted sizes
- Adhesive tape (one inch wide)
- Butterfly bandages
- Sterile gauze pads (two inches square)
- Elastic ("Ace") bandage (three inches wide)
- Roll of gauze bandage (two inches wide)
- Cotton balls
- Safety pins
- Dental disclosing tablets and dental floss

- Sodium bicarbonate antacids (Alka-Seltzer, Bromo Seltzer) contain baking soda. If you have high blood pressure, or if you are on a salt-restricted diet, avoid these antacids because of their high sodium content. If used too frequently, they may interfere with kidney or heart function.

- Calcium carbonate antacids (TUMS, Alka-2) are sometimes used as calcium supplements (see page 264). However, these products may cause constipation.

- Aluminum-based antacids (Amphojel) are less potent and work slower than other products. They may also cause constipation. Some may cause calcium depletion and should not be taken by postmenopausal women. Check with your doctor before using aluminum antacids if you have kidney problems.

OTC Products for Home Use

Problem	OTC Product (example)	Comments
Allergies	Antihistamine (Chlor-Trimeton, Benadryl)	Useful for allergies and itching. See page 297.
Colds	Decongestant	See page 297 for precautions.
Constipation	Laxative or bulking agent (Metamucil)	Avoid long-term or regular use of laxatives. See page 299.
Cough, non-productive	Suppressant (Robitussin-DM)	Ease a dry, hacking cough. See page 298.
Cough, productive	Expectorant (Robitussin)	Thin and help clear the mucus. See page 298 for precautions.
Diaper rash	Protectant (A&D Ointment, Desitin)	Protects skin from urine and stool. See page 161.
Diarrhea	Antidiarrheal (Kaopectate)	Avoid long-term use. See page 296.
Dry skin	Lubricating cream (Vaseline Intensive Care)	Few side effects, inexpensive. Also see page 136.
Heartburn	Antacid (TUMS, Maalox)	Avoid long-term use. See page 46.
Itching	Hydrocortisone cream (Cortaid)	Antihistamines are also helpful. See page 297.
Pain, fever, inflammation	Aspirin, naproxen, or ibuprofen	Help relieve swelling and pain. May cause stomach upset. See page 299.
Pain, fever	Acetaminophen (Tylenol)	Less stomach irritation. Safe for children. See page 300.
Poisoning	Syrup of ipecac	To start vomiting if poisoning occurs. See page 301.
Scrapes, skin infections	Antibiotic ointment (Bacitracin, Polysporin)	May cause local allergic reaction. Keep creams cool and dry. Discard if out of date.

Antacids – continued

- Magnesium compounds (Phillip's Milk of Magnesia) may cause diarrhea.
- Aluminum-magnesium antacids (Maalox, Di-Gel, Mylanta, Riopan) are less likely to cause constipation or diarrhea than aluminum-only or magnesium-only antacids.

Antacid Precautions

- Try to eliminate the cause of frequent heartburn instead of taking antacids regularly. See Heartburn on page 46.

- Consult your doctor or pharmacist before taking an antacid if you take other medications. Antacids may interfere with the absorption and action of some drugs, such as antibiotics, digitalis, and anticoagulants. Also consult your doctor if you have ulcers or kidney problems.

Antidiarrheals

There are two types of antidiarrheal drugs: those that thicken the stool and those that slow intestinal spasms.

The **thickening** mixtures (Kaopectate) contain clay or fruit pectin and absorb the bacteria and toxins in the intestine. Although they are safe in that they do not go into the system, these antidiarrheals also absorb bacteria needed for digestion. Long-term use is not advised.

Antispasmodic antidiarrheal products slow the spasms of the intestine. Loperamide (Imodium A-D) is an example of this type of preparation. Donnagel and Parepectolin contain both thickening and antispasmodic ingredients.

Antidiarrheal Precautions

- Because diarrhea often helps rid your body of an infection, try to avoid using antidiarrheal medications for the first six hours. After that, use them only if the diarrhea continues to cause cramping and pain.

- Do not use an antidiarrheal if there is a fever.

- Be sure to take a large enough dose. Take antidiarrheal preparations until the stool thickens, then stop immediately to avoid constipation.

- Replace depleted body fluids. Dehydration can develop when a person, especially an infant, child, or older adult, has diarrhea. See page 44 for a rehydration drink you can make at home to prevent dehydration.

Cold and Allergy Remedies

In general, if you take drugs for your cold, you'll get better in about a week. If you take nothing, you'll get better in about seven days. Rest and liquids are probably the best treatment for a cold (see page 99). Antibiotics will not help. However, medications help relieve some cold symptoms.

Do not give cold medicines to children under six months of age without a doctor's supervision. Over-the-counter cold medicines have not been shown to be effective for preschool children.

Allergy symptoms, especially runny nose, often respond to antihistamines.

Antihistamines

Antihistamines dry mucous membranes, and are commonly used to treat allergy symptoms and itching. They are also found in many cold medications, often together with a decongestant. However, the value of antihistamines in treating cold symptoms is under debate.

If your runny nose is due to allergies, an antihistamine will help. For cold symptoms, home treatment and perhaps a decongestant (see below) will probably be more helpful. It is usually best to take only single-ingredient allergy or cold preparations.

Chlor-Trimeton (chlorpheniramine) and Benadryl (diphenhydramine) are single-ingredient antihistamine products.

Dristan, Coricidin, and Triaminic are products containing both a decongestant and an antihistamine.

Antihistamine Precautions

- Do not give antihistamines to infants under age four months. For children between four months and one year, ask your doctor first.

- Drink extra fluids when taking cold or allergy medications.

- Antihistamines can cause problems for people with certain health problems, such as glaucoma, epilepsy, and enlarged prostate. They may also interact with some drugs, such as certain antidepressants, sedatives, and tranquilizers. Read the package carefully and ask your pharmacist or doctor to help you choose one that will not cause problems.

- The drowsiness that antihistamines often cause usually diminishes with continued use. If it continues, or if the medication isn't helping your allergies after one week, call your doctor for advice.

- Nonsedating antihistamines are available by prescription. These drugs carry some additional risk.

Decongestants

Decongestants make breathing easier by shrinking swollen mucous membranes in the nose and allowing air to pass through the nose. They also help relieve runny nose and postnasal drip, which can cause a sore throat.

Decongestants can be taken orally or used as nose drops or sprays. Oral decongestants (pills) are probably more effective and provide longer relief. Sudafed (pseudoephedrine) is an oral decongestant.

Sprays and drops provide rapid but temporary relief. Neo-synephrine (phenylephrine) is an effective nasal spray. Sprays and drops are less likely to interact with other drugs than oral decongestants.

Decongestant Precautions

- Do not give oral decongestants to infants under age 6 months.

- *Do not* use medicated nasal sprays or drops for more than three days or more than three times a day. Continued use will cause a "rebound effect": the mucous membranes swell up more than before using the spray.

Cold and Allergy – continued

- Decongestants can cause problems for people with certain health problems, such as heart disease, high blood pressure, glaucoma, diabetes, and overactive thyroid. They may also interact with some drugs, such as certain antidepressants and high blood pressure medications. Read the package carefully and ask your pharmacist or doctor to help you choose one.

Cough Preparations

Coughing is your body's way of getting foreign substances, phlegm, and mucus out of your respiratory tract. Often coughs are useful and you don't want to eliminate them. Sometimes, though, coughs are severe enough to impair breathing or prevent rest.

Water and other liquids, such as fruit juices, are probably the best cough syrups. They help soothe the throat, and also moisten and thin mucus so that it can be coughed up more easily.

You can make a simple and soothing cough syrup at home by mixing one part lemon juice with two parts honey. Use as often as needed. This can be given to children over one year old. Also see page 101.

There are two kinds of cough medicines. **Expectorants** help thin the mucus, making it easier to "bring up." Robitussin is an expectorant cough syrup. Look for products containing guaifenesin.

Saline Nose Drops

The easiest nasal drop for a stuffy nose is homemade saline solution. Saline nose drops will not cause a rebound effect. They keep nasal tissues moist so they can filter the air.

Mix ½ teaspoon salt in 1 cup of body temperature water (too much salt will dry nasal membranes).

Place the solution in a clean bottle with a dropper (available at drugstores). Use as necessary. Discard and make a fresh solution every three days.

To insert drops, lie on your back with your head hanging over the side of the bed. This helps the drops get farther back. Try to prevent the dropper from touching your nose.

Over-the-counter saline sprays (NaSal, Ocean) are particularly convenient, inexpensive, and sterile.

Suppressants control or suppress a nagging cough. They subdue the cough reflex and work best for the dry, hacking cough that keeps you awake. Look for suppressant medications containing dextromethorphan, such as Robitussin-DM.

Don't suppress a productive cough too much (unless it is keeping you from getting enough rest).

Cough Preparation Precautions

- Cough preparations can cause problems for people with certain health problems, such as asthma, heart disease, high blood pressure, and prostate enlargement. They may also interact with some drugs, such as sedatives and certain antidepressants. Read the package carefully and ask your pharmacist or doctor to help you choose one.

- Use with caution if you have chronic respiratory problems; cough suppressants can stifle breathing. Use care when giving cough suppressants to the very old or frail.

- Read the label so you know what ingredients you are taking. Some cough preparations contain a large percentage of alcohol; others contain codeine. There are many choices. Ask your pharmacist to advise you.

Laxatives

There are two types of products to ease the passage and elimination of bowel movements.

Laxatives (Correctol, Ex-Lax, Senokot, Dulcolax) speed up the passage of stool by stimulating the intestines.

Bulk-forming agents such as bran or Metamucil are not laxatives, but ease constipation by increasing the volume of stool and making it easier to pass.

There are many other ways to treat constipation, such as drinking more water. See page 42.

Laxative Precautions

- Take any laxative or bulking agent with plenty of water or other liquids.

- Do not take laxatives regularly. Overuse of laxatives decreases tone and sensation in the large intestine, causing dependence on the laxative. (Regular use of bulking agents is safe and increases their effectiveness.)

- Regular use of some laxatives (Correctol, Ex-Lax, Feen-A-Mint) may interfere with your body's absorption of vitamin D and calcium, which may weaken your bones.

Pain Relievers

Aspirin is widely used for relieving pain and reducing fever in adults. It also relieves minor itching and reduces swelling and inflammation. Most tablets contain 325 mg. Although it seems familiar and safe, aspirin is a very powerful drug.

Aspirin Precautions

- More childhood poisonings are caused by aspirin than by any other drug. Keep all aspirin, especially baby aspirin, out of children's reach.

- Aspirin can irritate the stomach lining, causing bleeding or ulcers. If aspirin upsets your stomach, try a coated brand, such as Ecotrin. Talk with your doctor or pharmacist to determine what will work best for you.

Pain Relievers – continued

- Aspirin use increases the risk of Reye's Syndrome in children. Do not give aspirin to children and teens under age 20 years unless recommended by a doctor.

- Some people are allergic to aspirin. (They may also be allergic to ibuprofen.)

- Do not take aspirin:
  - If suffering from gout
  - If taking blood thinners (anticoagulants)
  - For a hangover. Aspirin used with alcohol increases the risk of stomach irritation.

- High doses may result in aspirin poisoning (salicylism). Symptoms of aspirin poisoning include:
  - Ringing in the ears
  - Visual disturbances
  - Nausea
  - Dizziness
  - Rapid, deep breathing

Stop taking aspirin and call a health professional if any of these symptoms occur.

Other Uses of Aspirin

In addition to relieving pain and inflammation, aspirin is effective against many other ailments. Because of the danger of side effects and the interactions aspirin may have with other treatment, **these uses of aspirin should not be tried without a doctor's supervision.**

Heart Attacks and Strokes

Aspirin in low but regular doses helps prevent heart attacks and strokes. Doses as low as 30 mg per day have helped. Aspirin may also help as a first-aid measure for heart attacks. A half a tablet chewed may be enough to help.

Stomach and Colon Cancer

Some studies have shown that one aspirin per day can reduce the risk of cancers in the digestive system.

Migraines

Regular, low-dose aspirin use may reduce the frequency of migraines.

Ibuprofen (Advil, Nuprin) and **naproxen** (Aleve) are other non-steroidal anti-inflammatory drugs (NSAIDs). Like aspirin, they relieve pain and reduce fever and inflammation. Also like aspirin, they can cause nausea, stomach irritation, and heartburn. Both drugs should be used with caution by people who take blood thinners (anticoagulants).

For liquid forms, follow the dosage instructions on the label. For adults and children over age 12 years, take one to two 200-mg tablets three times a day.

Acetaminophen (Tylenol) reduces fever and relieves pain. It does not have the anti-inflammatory effect of aspirin and ibuprofen, but also does not cause stomach upset and other side effects. For liquid forms, follow the dosage instructions on the label. Take every four hours, as needed:

- 12 pounds or less: consult your doctor.
- 13 – 23 pounds: 60 – 80 mg
- 24 – 35 pounds: 160 mg

- 36 – 47 pounds: 240 mg

- 48 – 59 pounds: 320 mg

- 60 – 71 pounds: 400 mg

- 72 – 95 pounds: 480 mg

- Adults: 500 – 1000 mg (maximum of 4000 mg per day)

Do not exceed dosage limits. Excess use of acetaminophen can contribute to alcohol-induced liver damage. People who drink more than three alcoholic beverages a day should discuss use with their doctors.

Syrup of Ipecac

Syrup of ipecac (ip-uh-kack) is a drug given to cause vomiting when a poison has been swallowed.

In most cases of poisoning, the best treatment is to get the substance out of the victim's stomach as quickly as possible. Syrup of ipecac is excellent for this.

Sometimes, causing the patient to vomit can be harmful. *Do not* use ipecac if the patient has swallowed any of the following:

- Alkalis, such as dishwasher detergents or cleaning solutions.

- Petroleum distillates, such as furniture polish, kerosene, gasoline, oil-based paints, etc. Give water to dilute the poison without inducing vomiting.

With *all* poisonings, call your doctor, emergency department, or poison control center *immediately!*

Dosage for Ipecac

For children over one year, give 1 tablespoon. Follow with at least 12 ounces of water, which is essential to ensure vomiting. Try to keep the person walking around.

Repeat in 20 minutes if the person has not yet vomited. Repeat only once. When he vomits, have him lie on his side with mouth lower than chest so the vomited material will not enter the airway and cause more trouble. If he leans over a toilet, be sure his chest is lower than his stomach.

The vomiting caused by ipecac is *very* violent and it should *not* be used in the following situations:

- If the victim is over five months pregnant.

- If the victim has a history of heart disease.

- If the child is under 12 months old.

- If the person might choke on the vomited material or inhale it into the lungs:

  ○ Persons over age 65

  ○ Persons who have taken Valium or any other drug that may cause unconsciousness

  ○ Person is drunk

  ○ Person is drowsy

Keep ipecac on hand and replace it every five years if you haven't used it. After opening, the product will be effective for one year.

Poisons

Do NOT induce vomiting:

- Dishwasher detergent (e.g., Cascade)
- Gasoline, kerosene
- Drano
- Oven cleaner
- Oil-based paints
- Furniture polish
- Cleaning solutions

Induce vomiting:

- Dishwashing liquid (e.g., Dawn)
- Plant food
- Aspirin and other medications
- Ink
- Fingernail polish remover
- Rat poison

Prescription Medications

There are thousands of different prescription medications, used to treat hundreds of different medical conditions. Your best sources of information about your prescription medications are your doctor and your pharmacist. There are also good books available that contain information on many different prescription drugs. See Resource 2 on page 307.

Guidelines for taking every kind of prescription medication could fill several books. Two common types are covered here: antibiotics and minor tranquilizers/sleeping pills.

Antibiotics

Antibiotics are prescription drugs that kill bacteria. They are only effective against bacteria, and have no effect on viruses. Antibiotics will not cure the common cold, flu, or any other viral illness. Unless you have a bacterial infection, it's best to avoid the possible adverse effects of antibiotics, which may include:

- Side effects, including allergy. Common side effects of antibiotics include nausea, diarrhea, and increased sensitivity to sunlight. Most side effects are mild, but some, especially allergic reactions, can be severe. An allergic reaction can be life-threatening. If you have any unexpected reaction to an antibiotic, tell your health professional before another antibiotic is prescribed.

- Secondary infections. Antibiotics kill all the bacteria in your body that are sensitive to them, including those that help your body. They may destroy the bacterial balance in your body, leading to stomach upset, diarrhea, vaginal infections, or other problems.

- Bacterial resistance. Bacteria build resistance to antibiotics that are used frequently, especially when only part of a dose is taken, leaving the stronger bacteria to survive.

When you and your health professional have decided that an antibiotic is necessary, follow the instructions with the prescription carefully.

- Take the whole dose for as many days as prescribed, unless you have severe unexpected side effects. Antibiotics kill off many bacteria quite

---

Medication Guidelines

Basic guidelines for taking prescription and over-the-counter medications include:

- Use medications only if non-drug approaches are not working.

- Know the benefits and side effects of a medication before taking it.

- Limit the medication to the minimum effective dose.

- Never take a drug prescribed for someone else.

- Follow the prescription instructions exactly or let your doctor know why you didn't.

- Keep medications in their original containers with the caps on tightly and stored according to directions.

- Do not take medications in front of small children. They are great mimics. Don't oversell the "candy" taste of children's medicines or leave children's vitamins accessible to small children.

- Add a consumer's guide to medications to your home health library. See Resource 2 on page 307.

---

quickly, so you may feel better in a few days. If you stop taking it too soon, the weaker bacteria will have been eliminated, but the stronger ones may survive and flourish.

- Be sure you understand any special instructions about taking the medication. These should be printed on the label, but double check with your doctor and pharmacist.

- Store antibiotics in a dry, cool place. They will usually keep their potency for about a year. However, most are prescribed for a specific illness in an amount needed to cure that illness. Liquid antibiotics are always dated. Check carefully to see if they need refrigeration.

- Never give an antibiotic prescribed for one person to someone else.

- Do not take an antibiotic prescribed for another illness without a health professional's approval.

Minor Tranquilizers and Sleeping Pills

Minor tranquilizers like Valium, Librium, Xanax, and Tranxene, and sleeping pills like Dalmane, Restoril, and Halcion are widely prescribed. However, these drugs can cause problems; for example, memory loss, mental impairment, addiction, and injuries from falls due to drug-induced unsteadiness.

Minor tranquilizers can be effective for short periods of time. However, long-term use is of questionable value and introduces the risk of addiction and mental impairment.

> ### Adverse Drug Reactions
>
> Side effects, drug-drug and food-drug interactions, over-medication, and addiction may cause:
>
> - Nausea, indigestion, vomiting
> - Constipation, diarrhea, incontinence, or difficulty urinating
> - Dry mouth
> - Headache, dizziness, ringing in the ears, or blurred vision
> - Confusion, forgetfulness, disorientation, drowsiness, or depression
> - Difficulty sleeping, irritability, or nervousness
> - Difficulty breathing
> - Rashes, bruising, and bleeding problems
>
> Don't assume any symptom is a normal side effect that you have to suffer with. Call your doctor or pharmacist any time you suspect your medicines are making you sick.

Minor Tranquilizers – cont.

Sleeping pills may help for a few days or even a few weeks, but using sleeping pills for more than a month generally causes more sleep problems than it solves. For other approaches, see page 284.

If you have been taking minor tranquilizers or sleeping pills for a while, talk with your doctor about discontinuing the medication or reducing its dosage. Be sure to report any problems you have had with unsteadiness, dizziness, or memory loss.

Medication Problems

Several kinds of adverse medication reactions can occur:

Side effects: Predictable, but unpleasant reactions to a drug. They are not usually serious, but can be inconvenient. In some people, they are severe and dangerous.

Allergies: Some people have severe, sometimes life-threatening reactions (called anaphylaxis) to certain medications. See page 93 for signs of an allergic reaction.

Drug-drug interactions: When two or more prescription or over-the-counter drugs mix in the body and cause an adverse reaction. The symptoms can be severe and may be misdiagnosed as a new illness.

Drug-food interactions: When medications react with food. Some drugs work best when taken with food, but others should be taken on an empty stomach. Some drug-food reactions can cause serious symptoms.

Over-medication: Sometimes the full adult dose of a medication is too much for small people and those over age 60. Too much of a drug is very dangerous.

Addiction: Long-term use of some medications can lead to dependence on them and severe reactions if they are withdrawn suddenly. Narcotics, tranquilizers, and barbiturates should all be used with care to avoid addiction. See page 275.

Home Medical Tests

Many common medical laboratory tests are now available in home kits. When combined with regular visits to your health professional, these home tests can help you to monitor your health and, in some cases, detect problems early.

Home medical tests must be very accurate (over 95 percent) to be approved by the Food and Drug Administration. However, they must be used correctly to give such accurate results. Follow the package directions exactly. If you have questions, ask your pharmacist or check the label for the company's toll-free phone number to call.

Home medical tests are especially helpful if you have a chronic condition that requires frequent monitoring, such as diabetes, asthma, or high blood pressure. Ask your doctor which home medical tests would be appropriate for your use. Some common tests are described below.

Medicine Chest

Look inside your medicine chest and chances are you will find a history of illnesses going back for years. Since you should never give a prescription drug to anyone other than the person for whom it was prescribed, and because most medications lose their potency after a few years, throw out any medication that:

• Was prescribed for a particular illness that is now over.

• Has expired (see date on label).

• Has no label.

Home Urinalysis

Some of the more common medical lab tests on urine can also be done at home. Home urinalysis can help you monitor diabetes. It is also useful if you have frequent urinary tract infections.

Home Blood Glucose Monitoring

If you have diabetes, you may already monitor your blood sugar levels (glucose) using a finger prick and a test strip and/or an electronic monitor.

This test should always be used under a doctor's supervision. Never adjust your insulin dose based on a single abnormal test, unless your doctor has specifically instructed you to do so. Check with your doctor if you have symptoms of abnormal blood sugar levels, even if the test is normal. See page 269.

Home Blood Pressure Monitoring

If you have high blood pressure, it is important that you monitor your blood pressure frequently. Blood pressure testing can be done easily at home with a little instruction.

By checking your blood pressure at home, when you are relaxed, you will be able to track changes due to your home treatment and medications.

• Do not make any changes to your medications based on your home blood pressure readings without consulting your doctor.

Home Medical Tests – cont.

• Check your blood pressure at different times of day to see how rest and activities affect it. For regular readings, check it at the same time of day. Usually, blood pressure is lowest in the morning and rises during the day.

• For the most accurate reading, sit still for five minutes before taking your blood pressure.

• Calibrate (adjust) the blood pressure device yearly.

Home Tests for Blood in Stool

The fecal occult blood test can detect hidden blood in the stool, which may indicate colon cancer or other problems. If the test is positive, your doctor may recommend additional testing such as flexible sigmoidoscopy or colon X-ray to look at the inside of your colon to determine whether a cancer may be present. See page 30.

Home Pregnancy Tests

Home pregnancy tests are reliable and require only a few steps. Follow the package instructions and report all positive results to your doctor. See page 174.

Home Medical Records

Your home health center is a good place to keep your family's medical records, too. A three-ring binder or wire-bound notebook with dividers for each member of the family is helpful. Each person should have a cover sheet listing:

• Diagnosed chronic conditions: arthritis, asthma, diabetes, high blood pressure, etc.

• Any known drug, food, or other allergies.

• Information that would be vital in an emergency: Does the person have a pacemaker, a hearing aid, diabetes, epilepsy, or is he or she deaf or blind?

• Name and phone number of primary doctor.

Other important information that should be put on additional pages:

• An up-to-date list of medications. Include name of drug, purpose, dose, instructions, doctor and date prescribed.

• Immunization records: Childhood immunizations, tetanus, influenza, pneumonia.

• Health screening results: Blood pressure, cholesterol, vision, hearing.

• Records of major illnesses and injuries, such as pneumonia, bronchitis, broken bones, or major infections.

• Records of any major surgical procedures and hospitalizations.

• Records listing major diseases in members of your family: heart disease, stroke, cancer, diabetes.

Your Home Health Library: Self-Care Resources

The most important self-care resource for the home is good information. Many of the resources listed below are available at your local bookstore or public library. If not, ask the bookstore to order the ones you want.

Three Books Every Home Should Have.

1. D. W. Kemper, et al., *Healthwise Handbook* (11th ed.), Healthwise, 1994. Available from Healthwise, Inc., P.O. 1989, Boise, ID 83701, (208) 345-1161.

2. J. W. Long, MD, *The Essential Guide to Prescription Drugs 1992: Everything You Need to Know for Safe Drug Use,* Harper-Collins, 1992.

3. E. Pinkney and C. Pinkney, *Patient's Guide to Medical Tests,* Facts on File.

General Purpose Resources

4. D. Vickery, MD, and J. Fries, MD, *Take Care of Yourself* (5th ed.), Addison Wesley, 1993.

5. D. E. Larson, MD, ed. *Mayo Clinic Family Health Book,* William Morrow, 1990.

Special Concerns Resources

AIDS

6. *AIDS: A Self-Care Manual* (2nd ed.), 1993. Available from AIDS Project, Los Angeles, 1313 N. Vine St., Los Angeles, CA, 90028, (213) 993-1487.

Alcohol Problems

7. *Alcoholics Anonymous: The Story of How Thousands of Men and Women Have Recovered from Alcoholism* (3rd ed.), Alcoholics Anonymous World Services, Inc., 1976.

8. *The Twelve Steps of Alcoholics Anonymous,* interpreted by The Hazelden Foundation, Harper and Row, 1987.

Alzheimer's Disease/Dementia

9. N. L. Mace and P. V. Rabins, MD, *The 36-Hour Day: A Family Guide to Caring for Persons with Alzheimer's Disease, Related Dementing Illnesses, and Memory Loss in Late Life,* The John Hopkins University Press, 1991. Also available from the Alzheimer's Association, (800) 272-3900.

Anger

10. R. Williams, MD, and V. Williams, *Anger Kills: 17 Strategies for Controlling the Hostility That can Harm Your Health,* Random House, 1993.

11. A. Ellis, *Anger,* Carol Publishing Group, 1985.

12. H. Lerner, *The Dance of Anger,* Harper Row, 1989.

Anxiety

13. E. Bourne, *The Anxiety and Phobia Workbook,* New Harbinger, 1990.

14. R. Z. Peurifoy, *Anxiety, Phobias, and Panic: Taking Charge and Conquering Fear,* Life Skills, 1992.

Self-Care Resources – cont.

15. A. Seagrave and F. Covington, *Free From Fears,* Poseidon Press, 1989.

Arthritis

16. K. Lorig and J. Fries, MD, *The Arthritis Helpbook,* Addison-Wesley, 1991.

Also see Resource 32.

Asthma

17. The American Lung Association, *Help Yourself to Better Breathing,* 1991. Available from your local chapter of the American Lung Association.

18. A. Weinstein, MD, *Asthma: The Complete Guide to Self-Management of Asthma for Patients and Their Families,* McGraw-Hill, 1987.

Also see Resource 32.

Back Pain

19. R. McKenzie, *Treat Your Own Back,* Spinal Publications, 1989.

20. R. Cailliet, MD, *Low Back Pain Syndrome,* Davis Co., 1988.

Cancer

21. M. Dollinger, E. H. Rosenbaum, G. Cable, *Everyone's Guide to Cancer Therapy*, Somerville House Books, 1991.

22. D. Spiegel, *Living Beyond Limits: New Hope and Help for Facing Life-Threatening Illness*, Times Books, 1993.

Child Health

23. S. P. Shelov, MD, ed., *Caring for Your Baby and Young Child,* Bantam Books, 1991.

24. Boston Children's Hospital, *The New Child Health Encyclopedia,* Delacort, 1987.

25. A. Eisenberg, et al., *What to Expect the First Year,* Workman Publishing, 1989.

26. R. Pantell, et al., *Taking Care of Your Child,* Addison-Wesley, 1990.

27. E. Satter, *How to Get Your Child to Eat...But Not Too Much,* Bull Publishing, 1991.

28. E. Satter, *Child of Mine: Feeding With Love and Good Sense,* Bull Publishing, 1991.

29. P. Leach, *Your Baby and Child From Birth to Age Five*, Alfred A. Knopf, New York, 1989.

30. D. Dinkmeyer, Sr., G. D. McKay, J. S. Dinkmeyer, *Parenting Young Children*, American Guidance Service, 1989.

31. J. L. Wykoff, PhD, B. C. Unell, *How to Discipline Your Six- to Twelve-Year-Old Without Losing Your Mind*, Doubleday Books, 1991.

Chronic Illnesses

32. K. Lorig, H. Holman, D. Sobel, et al., *Living a Healthy Life with Chronic Conditions: Self-Management of Heart Disease, Arthritis, Stroke, Diabetes, Asthma, Bronchitis, Emphysema, and Others*, Bull Publishing, 1993.

Depression

33. M. Seligman, *Learned Optimism,* Random House, 1991.

Also see Resources under Mental Self-Care.

Diabetes

34. L. Jovanovic-Peterson, MD, C. M. Peterson, MD, and M. B. Stone, *A Touch of Diabetes: A Guide for People Who Have Type II, Non-Insulin Dependent Diabetes,* DCI Publishing, 1991.

Also see Resource 32.

Elder Care

35. M. Mettler, et al., *Healthwise for Life: Medical Self-Care for Healthy Aging,* Healthwise, 1992.

36. D. W. Kemper, et al., *Growing Wiser: The Older Person's Guide to Mental Wellness,* Healthwise, 1986.

Both available from Healthwise, P.O. Box 1989, Boise, ID, 83701, (208) 345-1161.

37. J. Fries, MD, *Aging Well,* Addison Wesley, 1989.

First Aid

38. *American Red Cross First Aid and Safety Handbook,* Little, Brown, and Company, 1992.

Fitness

39. P. Lyons, D. Burgard, *Great Shape: The First Fitness Guide for Large Women,* Bull Publishing, 1990.

40. B. Anderson, *Stretching,* Shelter Publications, 1992.

Grief

41. M. Colgrove, H. Bloomfield, P. McWilliams, *How to Survive the Loss of a Love,* Bantam, 1991.

42. E. Neeld, *Seven Choices,* Crown, 1990.

43. H. S. Schiff, *Living Through Mourning: Finding Comfort and Hope When a Loved One Has Died,* Penguin Books, 1986.

Heart Disease

44. D. Ornish, MD, *Dean Ornish's Program for Reversing Heart Disease,* Ballantine, 1992.

Also see Resource 32.

Incontinence

45. K. L. Burgis, MD, K. L. Pearce, and A. L. Lucco, MD, *Staying Dry: A Practical Guide to Bladder Control,* The Johns Hopkins University Press, 1989.

Insomnia

46. P. Hauri, S. Linde, *No More Sleepless Nights,* John Wiley & Sons, 1990.

Irritable Bowel Syndrome

47. E. F. Shimberg, *Relief From Irritable Bowel Syndrome,* Ballantine, 1988.

Medical Consumerism

48. D. W. Kemper, et al., *It's About Time: Better Health Care in a Minute (or two),* Healthwise, 1993. Available from Healthwise, P.O. Box 1989, Boise, ID 83701, (208) 345-1161.

Self-Care Resources – cont.

49. C. Inlander and E. Weiner, *Take This Book to the Hospital With You,* Pantheon, 1991.

50. D. R. Stutz, MD, and B. Feder, *The Savvy Patient: How to be an Active Participant in Your Medical Care,* Consumers Union, 1990.

51. R. Arnot, MD, *The Best Medicine,* Addison-Wesley, 1992.

52. C. B. Inlander, *Good Operations, Bad Operations: The People's Medical Society's Guide to Surgery,* Penguin Books, 1993.

Medical Tests

53. P. Shtasel, *Medical Tests and Diagnostic Procedures,* Harper/Collins, 1991.

Mental Self-Care

54. D. Burns, MD, *The Feeling Good Handbook,* New American Library/Dutton, 1990.

55. D. Sobel, MD, and R. Ornstein, *The Healing Brain,* Simon and Schuster, 1988.

56. S. Locke, MD, and D. Colligan, *The Healer Within,* New American Library, 1986.

57. D. Goleman, J. Gurin (eds.), *Mind/Body Medicine: How to Use Your Mind for Better Health,* Consumer Reports Books, 1993.

58. G. Emery and J. Campbell, *Rapid Relief From Emotional Distress,* Fawcett, 1987.

59. F. I. Kass, *The Columbia University College of Physicians and Surgeons Complete Guide to Mental and Emotional Health,* Holt Henry & Company, 1992.

60. B. Moyers, *Healing and the Mind,* Doubleday, 1993.

Men's Health

61. *Staying Strong For Men Over 50: A Common Sense Health Guide.* Available from AARP, Stock no. D15296, 601 E Street NW, Washington, DC 20049.

Neck Pain

62. R. McKenzie, *Treat Your Own Neck,* Spinal Publications Ltd. (New Zealand), 1989.

Newsletters

63. *Personal Best,* 420 5th Avenue South, Suite D, Edmonds, WA 98020-3584, (800) 888-7853.

64. *University of California at Berkeley Wellness Letter.* Available from Health Letter Associates, P.O. Box 420148, Palm Coast, FL 32142.

65. *Columbia University Health And Nutrition Newsletter.* Available from P.O. Box 5000, Ridgefield, NJ 07657.

66. *Mental Medicine Update,* The Center for Health Sciences, P.O. Box 381062, Cambridge, MA 02238-1062. Phone (800) 222-4745.

Nutrition

67. *Health Counts.* John Wiley and Sons, Inc., 1991.

68. E. R. Blonz, *The Really Simple, No-Nonsense Nutrition Guide,* Conari Press, 1993.

Pain

69. E. M. Catalan, *The Chronic Pain Workbook: A Step-by-Step Guide for Coping With and Overcoming Your Pain,* New Harbinger Publications, 1987.

70. M. Caudill, *Managing Chronic Pain: A Behavioral Medicine Program Workbook*, Guilford, 1994.

Pregnancy

71. A. Eisenberg, *What to Expect When You're Expecting,* Workman Publishing, 1991.

72. P. Simkin, et al., *Pregnancy, Childbirth, and the Newborn,* Meadowbrook, 1984.

73. C. Marshall, *From Here to Maternity: Your Guide for the Nine-Month Journey Toward Motherhood,* Prima Publishing, 1991.

Self-Help Groups

74. B. White, E. Madara, *The Self-Help Sourcebook: Finding and Forming Mutual Aid Self-Help Groups*, Saint Clares-Riverside Medical Center, 1992.

Smoking

75. T. Ferguson, MD, *The No-Nag, No-Guilt, Do-It-Your-Own-Way Guide to Quitting Smoking,* Putnam, 1988.

76. U.S. Department of Health and Human Services, *Clearing the Air,* NIH Publication No. 92-1647, 1989. Available from the Office on Smoking and Health, (404) 488-5705.

Shyness

77. P. Zimbardo, *Shyness,* Addison-Wesley, 1990.

Stress

78. H. Benson and M. Klipper, *The Relaxation Response,* Avon Books, 1976.

79. M. Davis, et al., *The Relaxation and Stress Reduction Workbook*, New Harbinger, 1994.

Wellness

80. H. Benson and E.M. Stuart, *The Wellness Book,* Carol Publishing Group, 1992.

81. D. W. Kemper, et al., *Pathways: A Success Guide for a Healthy Life,* Healthwise, 1985. Available from Healthwise, P.O. Box 1989, Boise, ID 83701, (208) 345-1161.

82. R. Ornstein and D. Sobel, MD, *Healthy Pleasures,* Addison-Wesley, 1989.

Women's Health

83. The Boston Women's Health Collective, *The New Our Bodies, Ourselves, A Book By and For Women,* 1992.

84. K. Johnson, *Trusting Ourselves: The Complete Guide to Emotional Well-being for Women*, Atlantic Monthly Press, 1991

85. B. D. Shephard, MD, and C. A. Shephard, *The Complete Guide to Women's Health,* Penguin Books, 1990.

86. *The Womanly Art of Breast-feeding,* La Leche League International, New American Library, 1991.

87. K. Huggins, *Nursing Mother's Companion*, Harvard Common Press, 1991.

Also see entries under Pregnancy.

Index

K

Kaiser Permanente System
    advice nurse, 4, 13, 14
    choosing a provider, 4
    emergency services, 5
    health education services, 6
    identification card, 7
    making appointments, 4
    questions, 4
    pharmacy services, 6
Kaopectate, 295
Knee problems, 77
K-Y Jelly, 178, 187

L

Labyrinthitis, 117
Lacerations (cuts), 219
Lactaid, 264
Lactose intolerance, 264
Laryngitis, 103
Laxatives, 299
    caution with appendicitis, 42
    eating disorders and, 283
Lead poisoning, 231
Learned Optimism, 309
Leg pain, 78
    see Sciatica, 57
Lethargy
    dehydration and, 45
    following head injury, 224
    with headache, fever, stiff neck, 102
Lice, 144
Lifting, proper posture, 59
Lightheadedness, 116
Limbs, freeing trapped, 222
Living a Healthy Life with Chronic
    Conditions, 308
Living Beyond Limits, 308
Living Through Mourning, 308
Lockjaw, see Tetanus, 26
Low back pain, 55, 185, 193
Low Back Pain Syndrome, 308
Low-density lipoprotein (LDL) cholesterol,
    261, 262
Lump
    on anus, 47
    in breast, 169, 171
    in groin or scrotum, 191, 192
    in scrotum or on testes, 191
Lungs, see Chest and respiratory problems
Lyme disease, 148

Lymph nodes, swollen, 107, 108
Lytren, 44

M

Maalox, 47, 54
Mammogram, 31, 172
Managing Chronic Pain, 311
Mayo Clinic Family Health Book, 307
Measles
    symptoms of, 166
    vaccine, 27, 28
Medical consumer
    emergency services, 19, 21
    finding the right doctor, 13
    partnership with doctor, 11, 13
    questions about medications, 16
    questions about medical tests, 15
    questions about surgery, 17
    research, 21
    shared decision making, 14
    ways to cut costs, 18
Medical records, home, 306
Medical research, doing your own, 21
Medical tests, also see Home medical tests,
    305
    cholesterol, 261
    clinical breast exam, 31, 172
    during pregnancy, 32
    flexible sigmoidoscopy, 30, 31
    mammograms, 31, 172
    Pap test and pelvic exam, 31, 173
    questions to ask, 15
    reducing costs, 16
    screening, chart, 31
Medical Tests and Diagnostic Procedures,
    310
Medications
    acetaminophen, 300
    adverse effects of, 304
    allergies, 296
    antacids, 294
    antibiotics, 302
    antidiarrheals, 296
    antihistamines, 297
    anti-inflammatories, 300
    aspirin, 299
    cold remedies, 296
    cough preparations, 298
    decongestants, 297
    depression and, 281
    dry eyes and, 118
    erection problems and, 191

T

U